T0221169

AESTHETIC MEDICINE

GROWING YOUR PRACTICE

AESTHETIC MEDICINE

GROWING YOUR PRACTICE

By

MARIE CZENKO KUECHEL, MA

Consultant and Founder,
Czenko Kuechel Consulting, Ltd.,
Chicago, Illinois

Quality Medical Publishing, Inc.
St. Louis, Missouri ▪ 2009

Copyright © 2009 by Quality Medical Publishing, Inc.

All rights reserved. No part of this publication may be reproduced, stored in a retrieval system, or transmitted in any form or by any means, electronic, mechanical, photocopying, recording, or otherwise, without prior permission of the publisher.

Printed in United States of America

This book presents current scientific information and opinion pertinent to medical professionals. It does not provide advice concerning specific diagnosis and treatment of individual cases and is not intended for use by the layperson. Medical knowledge is constantly changing. As new information becomes available, changes in treatment, procedures, equipment, and the use of drugs become necessary. The editors/authors/contributors and the publisher have, as far as it is possible, taken care to ensure that the information given in this text is accurate and up to date. The authors and publisher will not be responsible for any errors or liable for actions taken as a result of information or opinions expressed in this book.

PUBLISHER   Karen Berger

EDITORIAL DIRECTOR   Michelle Berger

DIRECTOR OF EDITING   Suzanne Wakefield

VICE PRESIDENT OF PRODUCTION AND MANUFACTURING   Carolyn Reich

PRODUCTION   Elaine Kitsis, Sandra Hanley

COVER AND SECTION DESIGN   Grip Design, *www.gripdesign.com*

COVER IMAGE   Mark Weiss/Photodisc/Getty Images

TEXT DESIGN   Amanda Behr

Quality Medical Publishing, Inc.
2248 Welsch Industrial Court
St. Louis, Missouri 63146
Telephone: 1-314-878-7808
Website: *http://www.qmp.com*

Library of Congress Cataloging-in-Publication Data

Kuechel, Marie Czenko.
    Aesthetic medicine : growing your practice / by Marie Czenko Kuechel.
        p. ; cm.
    Includes index.
    ISBN 978-1-57626-314-3 (pbk.)
    1. Surgery, Plastic--Practice. I. Title.
    [DNLM: 1. Practice Management, Medical. 2. Surgery, Plastic. 3.
Marketing of Health Services. WO 600 K95a 2009]
    RD118.K84 2009
    617.9'5068--dc22

                                        2009024128

QM/EB/EB

5 4 3 2 1

To those who live, work, and grow
with passion, integrity, and faith

CONTRIBUTORS

Bradley P. Bengtson, MD, FACS
Founding Member, Center for Aesthetics and Plastic Surgery, Grand Rapids, Michigan

Gene Colón, ESQ.
Assistant Vice President, Medical and Medical Relations, Active Cosmetics, L'Oreal, New York, New York

Julius W. Few, MD, FACS
Clinical Associate, Department of Surgery, Division of Plastic Surgery, University of Chicago Pritzker School of Medicine; Director, The Few Institute for Aesthetic Plastic Surgery, Chicago, Illinois

Heather Frayn
School of Journalism, University of Missouri, Columbia, Missouri

Alan H. Gold, MD, FACS
Attending Surgeon, Department of Surgery, Division of Plastic Surgery, North Shore University Hospital, Manhasset, New York

John E. Gross, MD, FACS
Clinical Associate Professor, Department of Surgery, Keck School of Medicine, University of Southern California, Los Angeles, California

Victoria Hulett-Gross
Founder, *www.venusstock.com* (Exclusive—Beauty Stock Photo Company); Art Director and Producer, Los Angeles, California

Jack P. Gunter, MD, FACS
Clinical Professor in Plastic Surgery and Clinical Professor in Otolaryngology, University of Texas Southwestern Medical Center, Dallas, Texas

Steven M. Harris, ESQ.
McDonald Hopkins LLC, Chicago, Illinois

Mark L. Jewell, MD
Assistant Clinical Professor, Department of Plastic Surgery, Oregon Health Science University, Portland, Oregon

Mary Lind Jewell, RPT
Corporate Practice Manager for Mark Jewell MD, PC, Eugene, Oregon

John N. Kuechel, CPA
Partner, Burton Partners LLC, Schaumburg, Illinois

Mary P. Lupo, MD, FAAD
Clinical Professor, Department of Dermatology, Tulane Medical School;
Director, The Lupo Center for Aesthetic and General Dermatology,
New Orleans, Louisiana

Kevin McConkey
Principal, Grip Design, Chicago, Illinois

Daniel C. Mills, MD, FACS
Associate Clinical Professor, Department of Surgery, Division of Plastic
Surgery, Loma Linda University School of Medicine, Loma Linda;
Aesthetic Fellowship Director, Aesthetic Plastic Surgical Institute, Inc.,
Laguna Beach, California

Foad Nahai, MD, FACS
Clinical Professor of Plastic Surgery, Department of Surgery, Emory
University; Paces Plastic Surgery, Atlanta, Georgia

Marian D. O'Hagan, RN, BSN
Clinical Training Specialist, Laser and IPL Specialist, Palomar Medical
Technologies, Burlington, Massachusetts

Steven L. Ringler, MD, FACS
Clinical Professor of Plastic Surgery, Department of Surgery, Michigan
State University, Grand Rapids, Michigan

Renato Saltz, MD, FACS
Former Associate Professor of Plastic Surgery, Department of Surgery,
University of Utah, Salt Lake City; Medical Director, Saltz Plastic Surgery
and Spa Vitória, Salt Lake City and Park City, Utah

Karen A. Zupko
President, Karen Zupko & Associates, Inc., Chicago, Illinois

FOREWORD

Running a successful medical practice requires the physician to use proven business-management techniques effectively. However, such concepts are rarely taught in medical school or during residency. To survive and prosper, doctors must understand and employ a valid business approach in their medical practices. Marie Czenko Kuechel's book, *Aesthetic Medicine: Growing Your Practice,* details virtually every aspect of developing and maintaining a successful aesthetic medical practice.

I have personally witnessed her vast knowledge and experience as an educator and a resource for practice management. She has extensive experience as a guest lecturer at physicians' meetings. She is media savvy and has real-life experience as a journalist, television resource, consumer advocate, and consultant to a variety of medical practices.

Conditions have changed dramatically in the last decade; far more options are available to physicians and the public, partly because of improved technology and an emphasis on "cosmetic medicine," which includes services that were not previously within the province of classic aesthetic surgery practices. Consumers want these services and the refined results they offer. Although noninvasive therapies do not produce the same results as surgical procedures, effective aesthetic practices incorporate these options into their armamentarium to improve results as well as to successfully compete in the marketplace. How these can be integrated into a practice is outlined in these pages.

Building a successful aesthetic practice also requires more than bringing patients into the office; it entails keeping satisfied patients within the practice and maintaining their loyalty to develop a stable, long-term business. There are no shortcuts to achieving these goals.

Aesthetic Medicine: Growing Your Practice outlines sensible, reproducible approaches with an emphasis on service, communication, ethics, honesty, and integrity to guide physicians to meet their own goals and expectations, and what is more important, to meet their patients' desires and expectations. This book offers a broad spectrum of considerations on practice management and how to avoid the pitfalls associated with running a practice. Chapters include information on marketing, positioning, staffing, and growing the practice as well as on safety, communication, and financial concerns.

Trends come and go, but the fundamentals don't go out of style. This book thoroughly addresses the basics while offering many fresh ideas. It is essential to analyze any practice to improve and compete, because if you stay in one place, you will move backward as the rest of the world advances. Marie Czenko Kuechel's book provides methods to improve any practice. It is thought provoking and practical and provides an excellent vantage point from which to review one's trajectory toward a successful aesthetic practice.

Robert Singer, MD, FACS
Clinical Professor of Surgery (Plastic), University of California, San Diego;
Past President of the American Society for Aesthetic Plastic Surgery;
Past Chairman of the Board of Trustees of the American Society of Plastic
Surgeons

PREFACE

Aesthetic medicine has existed for centuries—even before Cleopatra commanded her physicians to find the secret of eternal youth. She is said to have bathed in the milk of asses, but the pursuit of youth and beauty has lived on in other forms. In our science- and technology-driven society, we are continually adding years to the average life expectancy. In addition, through aesthetic procedures we are able to slow the visible signs of aging, alter the appearance, and elevate a person's self-confidence.

The field of aesthetic medicine is burgeoning with new procedures—it has become big business. Much is at stake—today's medical practitioners, from plastic surgeons to dermatologists, have a common concern: to be competitive in providing nonpayor or aesthetic services, they must also be consummate business professionals. Business acumen is critical to their success. Aesthetic medicine extends far beyond surgery to include cosmetic medicine, aesthetic services, and skin care—even dentistry, weight loss, and what some call "antiaging medicine." Today you must offer more than the very best care, services, and expertise; you must know how to run a service business, how to distinguish your practice from the multitude of others in the marketplace, and how to respond quickly and effectively to changes in technology and the economic climate.

Whether you are a sole practitioner or a partner, whether your practice is purely aesthetic or a mix of payor and nonpayor services, whether you are just beginning your career in aesthetic medicine or are a veteran attempting to keep pace with your competition and market opportunities—you must recognize that you are fulfilling the personal desires of other people, a truly rewarding endeavor.

Who are these people? They aren't customers; they don't come in to purchase something tangible, pay and leave, perhaps to return again. Nor are they merely patients seeking medical treatment. They are *clients*—people with whom you must build a relationship. Then, building on that relationship, you must convert that client to become a patient—someone who undergoes medical treatment not out of necessity, but to fulfill personal desire through your expertise, artistry, and skilled care. The ultimate goal is to retain that patient so that you may provide treatment again at a future date.

Research on consumers of aesthetic medicine affirms that the vast majority who undergo a procedure will choose additional services at a later time—men as well as women. A typical progression is for a client or patient to request a noninvasive therapy, such as a skin treatment, then opt for a minimally invasive rejuvenative procedure, and ultimately consider more invasive surgical approaches to maintain a youthful appearance. Aesthetic medicine is the only segment of medicine that reaches beyond basic health care to assist patients to look as young as they feel, to enhance what heredity has bestowed, or to fulfill their desire to create the physical image they have always wished to present to the world.

In my work with physicians, I don't impose or insist—I report and reason. The business of aesthetic medicine has only three absolutes: training, motivation, and integrity. You are trained as a board-certified core specialist, you are motivated to place your patients' goals above your own, and you hold yourself to the highest standards of training and practice.

Aesthetic Medicine: Growing Your Practice is an intersection at which the experiences and the principles of successful business practices and aesthetic medicine meet. I don't claim to have invented, defined, or devised a system of success; I only strive to report what works, to respond to needs, and to assist others to reason through conflict.

This book was written based on the many years and vast range of experiences I've had in consulting with aesthetic physicians. Seasoned doctors and other authorities with diverse backgrounds from all facets of business and with diverse backgrounds have contributed their expertise. Examples and case histories throughout demonstrate key points. These cases are all based on real-life situations faced by my clients as they struggled to master the business principles, variables, and challenges of aesthetic medicine.

Aesthetic Medicine: Growing Your Practice is designed to help you understand all the essential components to the business of medicine and to respond to the dynamic world of aesthetic care. It is organized in an easy-to-follow format that focuses on the variables that define any venture: who, what, where, when, why, and how. The chapters provide a detailed overview defining each aspect of an aesthetic practice, followed by a step-by-step plan of the actions necessary to succeed.

Section I helps readers define who they are as practitioners and what role they will play in aesthetic medicine, whether in establishing a new practice, entering a partnership, or expanding an existing business. Chapters address the supporting players for the enterprise, including administrative staff, the clinical team, and legal and financial advisors, as well as defining the target market and identifying the competition.

Section II considers the importance of developing an image and consistent branding for the practice and selecting a sound, effective practice model. Patient expectations and the risks inherent in running a practice are discussed. Section III explores the realities of finding or building an ideal facility and communicating both inside and outside the practice. Section IV focuses on privacy issues and the timing of opportunities, using the natural cycles of patients' desires to best advantage.

Section V addresses setting and accomplishing personal, professional, client/patient, and practice goals, as well as maintaining safety for everyone associated with the facility. Finally, Section VI weaves together the principles of the earlier sections to help the physician to formulate a sound plan for success, identify personal and practice limitations, and maximize resources and relationships.

Aesthetic Medicine: Growing Your Practice is intended for those who believe as I do that aesthetic medicine has value only when practiced by those with appropriate training and skill, who can take this segment of medicine and make it a business in which unqualified providers simply cannot compete. This book can serve as the basis for you to begin, review, grow, or reshape your practice to evolve into a business that thrives. It is my fervent hope that you will employ the principles and strategies outlined here, and that you will fulfill your commitment to your role in this industry with honesty and serve your patients' desires with integrity. Success will then undoubtedly be yours.

Marie Czenko Kuechel

Acknowledgments

There is much more to people than how they appear. Faces, bodies, and expressions are visible, but so much more lies deep within each person. What is so remarkable is that the appearance can mask what is deep within one's soul.

I've had the privilege of knowing master physicians who not only refine patients' outward aspect to match their inner spirits, but who also recognize that patients must first engage in self-discovery before undertaking a potentially life-changing procedure. These are truly aesthetic physicians. They include my professional clients, friends, and individuals so near to me they are like family.

When I wrote my first book, my sons, Nicholas and Andrew, were happy toddlers. Today they are amazing young men who accept that there are times when they must share me, and others when they can enjoy meeting the aesthetic masters. One such master is Robert Singer, MD, whom I asked to write the foreword for this book. He is a man whose success is built on his integrity, his skill, and his passion; he has taught me many lessons, including his ethical philosophy, which is quoted within the pages of this book and which I hope you too will embrace. Nicholas, 11, and Andrew, 9, conclude the book with their own message. May their view of the adult world of work give you pause to embrace those you love.

To my family I owe the deepest gratitude. Nicholas and Andrew, thank you for your patience, discipline, and love. As you grow, you continue to amaze me with your curiosity, determination, candor, and ambition. John, thank you for encouraging me to be my own woman while still making me feel like a girl who is loved, and for listening, caring, and understanding. Mom and Dad, I will always be grateful for the foundation you gave me, and now, with Mom and Pop, for taking care of things on the home front when I am away.

My grandmother Ana was a woman not defined by means, but by grace. She represented true beauty in a conflicted world. Nearly 25 years after her death, she remains my strength, my guardian, my conscience.

Lulu, thank you for reminding me that play, obedience, and instinct are essential; trust has to be earned.

There are many individuals who helped me to shape the messages conveyed in these pages. To the contributors to this book, I know how precious time is, and I am grateful to you all for sharing your experience, vision, and wisdom. The list of my friends, advisors, and supporters could become a book of its own if I tried to name everyone whose shared knowledge and experience to make this book possible. It has been my privilege to count the masters as well as their family members as my friends and contributors; my life has been enriched by the special moments and laughter we've shared together through the years. My thanks, respect, and love to Mark and Mary Jewell; Hillary Jewell; Robert Singer and Judith Harris Singer; Simon and Rhoda Fredricks; Renato and Flavia Saltz; Julius and Jennifer Few; Foad and Shahnaz Nahai; Hani and Amal Zeini; John and Victoria Gross; Dan and Jan Mills; Alan and Cindi Gold; Gus and Carmen Colon; Jim and Lisa Matas; Bob and Linda Stanton; Gene Colón; Jack Gunter; Steven Harris; Mary Lupo; Marian O'Hagan; Steven Ringler; Karen Zupko; John O'Leary; Brad Bengtson; Heather Frayn; Suzy Couturier; Kevin McConkey; Kelly Kaminski; Jamie Hammer; Joan Kron; Michael Rogers; Annabel Newell; Todd Rosenberg; Valerie McNair; and Mark Bennett.

Special thanks are due to Renato Saltz for connecting me to a capable, involved, and innovative publisher, Karen Berger, President and CEO of Quality Medical Publishing. To Michelle Berger, Suzanne Wakefield, Andrew Berger, Amanda Behr, and the entire QMP team, thank you for the privilege of being an author among the leaders and innovators in your library.

Nothing grows without passion. I wish you the desire and the passion to define your success, to sow your own garden, and to always embrace those you love.

CONTENTS

SECTION IV   WHEN

SECTION V   WHY

SECTION VI   HOW

AESTHETIC MEDICINE

GROWING YOUR PRACTICE

SECTION I

Who

Only as an aesthetic phenomenon is the world justified.
— FRIEDRICH NIETZSCHE

I don't believe that the world is only an aesthetic phenomenon. But to those who sincerely appreciate an aesthetic world, beauty is an extraordinary thing.

CHAPTER 1

Who Are You?

Who are the providers of aesthetic medicine?
This is not a matter defined by turf; it is a
matter defined by training.

THE PROVIDER AND PRACTICE

You are a medical professional with a degree from an accredited medical school. You have completed your residency and possibly elected a fellowship in accredited programs that include training in aesthetic medicine and surgery, namely, plastic surgery, otolaryngology, dermatology, ophthalmology, and perhaps dentistry, and you have received board certification related to your specialty. If you do not see yourself in this description, be cautioned: today's prospective client/patient is better informed and places more emphasis on credentials than you might realize. Who you are as a medical professional, by definition and by recognized credentials, is essential to your success.

Unfortunately, it is not always easy for the public to determine a medical professional's qualifications. There are other specialists providing aesthetic services; some are nonphysicians, whereas others are qualified providers who are crossing into territory beyond their scope of training. Establishing your specialty and services should be the simplest portion of your plan for a nonpayor practice: provide what your patients want; supply where there is a demand. But it's not that easy.

Your patients may sometimes be motivated to request the latest treatment of the moment, a procedure that may not even be appropriate for them. However, if the service you provide is not of genuine value, you'll lose credibility. What your patients want may not be within your scope of training. If you choose to build a practice by providing services outside the scope of your specialty, be prepared for a tough climb. A dentist should not augment lips and a plastic surgeon should not offer dental veneers; a dermatologist should not perform breast surgery, and a facial plastic surgeon or ophthalmic plastic surgeon should not perform body contouring.

If you practice without value or perform procedures outside the scope of your specialty, you build your practice on pillars of sand. Without a strong foundation, your patients, public, peers, and even staff will eventually question your credibility. Aesthetic medicine is a service and a business; it is based on your reputation and credibility. Your credibility is not measured by the visible outcome alone, but by the clinical outcome, the service experience, and the value paid to accomplish your patient's—your customer's—goals. Before you can endeavor to practice successfully, you must first define your practice, legitimately and conventionally, and with coyote wisdom.

RELATIVE WISDOM: Coyote Wisdom*

When I was 12, my father put a .22 rifle in my hands at our family's lake house and taught me to hit a target—a can propped on a stump facing the woods. Not common practice for a suburban girl and her Fortune 500 dad, but I had good aim.

Thirty years later, I have coyotes in my yard. I have experience with a .22. I have good aim. But I know how to handle this: I research the problem. I call a specialist licensed by the state to deal with wildlife hazards. I ask his experience and credentials, ask for his references and plan of action. I ask for a cost estimate, how long he thinks this will take, how it will disrupt our lives, and what risks are associated with all of the options he has presented. Then I hire him to accomplish my goal: remove a threatening brood of wild animals to prevent them from harming the pets and children who populate my yard with snowball fights, tire swing conversations, and nighttime games of flashlight tag.

Comparing aesthetic medicine to hunting coyotes may seem a stretch, but it is relevant. Knowing how to use a scalpel, a cannula, or a needle, watching someone demonstrate techniques, and then practicing for a short time on an animal model may make you capable of performing certain procedures, but it certainly does not mean you should overreach—and ultimately fail by being overly ambitious.

Coyote Wisdom is the title of a book by Lewis Mehl-Medrona, MD, that explores the mind-body connection to healing patients through storytelling.

You will not succeed in the business of aesthetic medicine based on the services you provide alone. Your patients and peers will measure your success by the following parameters:

- *Outcomes:* The physical results you achieve, and how those results and the means to produce them meet your patients' goals and respect their limits.

- *Experience:* The connections to your practice, including every detail and every person in your practice that interrelate to create an experience. Success is affected by each encounter or variable, by each experience as a whole, and by the collective experiences resulting from your services.

- *Value:* The product of your practice or its value consists of your investment and sacrifice in time, money, patience, humility, and stress.

When you define, refine, or change your practice, invest in a new skill or technology, hire a new employee, or redecorate your reception area, you must consider how your actions will affect outcomes, experiences, and value.

YOUR ROLE

The vast majority of physicians practicing aesthetic medicine are in private practice. As a private practitioner, you are the proprietor making both clinical and business decisions or delegating them. Ultimately the responsibility is solely yours. You may time-share offices, facilities, equipment, or even staff, but the business entity is wholly owned by you. There are many other roles you may fulfill from both a medical and business perspective. They are not all mutually exclusive and include:

- *Partner:* You and another physician of the same, complementary, or different specialties may share the ownership of the business entity—your practice.

- *Fellow:* Before you establish your practice or during the course of your practice you may train and work under the supervision of another physician. You should accept only accredited fellowships. In this capacity, you will learn new skills, techniques, and practice lessons from your mentor; you will also observe and absorb experiences that will help you shape how you do or do not wish to practice.

- *Employee:* You may work for another physician, practice group, or even a corporate entity, hospital, or university. You may have only clinical duties, or defined management or administrative duties as well. Like any employee, you are part of a team and part of a hierarchy with an opportunity to grow.

- *Contractor:* In this situation, you are a fee-for-service contractor, or you have a contract wherein you collect fees and pay a percentage to the business entity to which you are contracted. Contract positions are most often short-term opportunities that can evolve into more serious business relationships, or not.

- *Professor:* You teach your specialty and accordingly practice your specialty.

- *Supervisor:* You oversee a group of physicians or providers or oversee a facility.

- *Director:* You lend your expertise to shape the policy and operations of a practice, program, or business entity.

- *Network participant:* You are part of a group of physicians with some common ground, such as belonging to the same hospital group. Network participants are also commonly those who are preferred providers to specific insurance companies and who agree to prenegotiated rates or to see a specific number of patients. In the practice of aesthetic medicine you may perform reimbursable procedures that include appearance enhancement. You must know what is permissible and appropriate to submit for reimbursement and what is not, and practice accordingly.

🌿 IN PRACTICE: The Business of Medicine

Some things are not taught in medical school; namely, how to run a business (or practice). This fact was emphasized to me during a recent conversation with a training program director as we discussed the unmet needs of residents. He said, "The one thing every doctor must learn for himself or herself is how to run a business. As an academician I don't run a private practice; I can't teach that. In fellowships, residents don't get close enough to the decision-making process to learn from it. The only chance to learn about the business of medicine is hands on, and as doctors, we just don't make good businessmen."

I disagreed. "You are a physician. Each day you must make decisions for your patients. The path to your own decision-making process and to measuring the potential impact of solutions is no different." As applied to your practice, it includes the ability to:

1. *Examine:* Look at the "signs and symptoms" around you to make a diagnosis. Collect all relevant facts and define your goals.

2. *Diagnose:* Determine what decision needs to be made and the motivation for making it. Identify all the options and the factors that influence those options.

3. *Prescribe:* Make the best recommendation for this situation, and outline the course necessary to achieve the goal.

4. *Follow through and follow up:* Monitor the situation after your decision is made and throughout the course of the action. Collect feedback, and revise the plan as necessary.

6. *Measure outcomes:* Sound evidence is indisputable—in life, in medicine, and in decision-making. Measure your outcomes from all relevant points; is your decision a "best practice," or can you find ways to improve it? What have you learned that you can apply in the future?

Who you are as a physician is vital to your practice. How you practice as a physician and a business person is vital to your success. But as the following chapters will demonstrate, no one can do it alone.

CHAPTER 2

Who Is on Your Team?

The speed of the boss is the speed of the team.

— LEE IACOCCA

You are a physician, and your practice is your business, but you cannot do it all alone—you need a team. Business organizations have as many hierarchies as there are business models. More important than whether your practice is a top-down or spoke-and-hub model are the people and functions that compose your team. You will have your core day-to-day operational team, your staff, clinical support, and a full team of professionals essential to keep the business not just running, but competitive. The critical functions of your practice or the decisions related to those functions may be fulfilled or managed by you, or by a partner, employer, employee, contractor, advisor, or service provider. The functions essential to a successful aesthetic practice are not exclusive or individual roles; they consist of contributions from various people and sources to build a team.

SOURCES TO BUILD A TEAM
Service Providers

The physician, physician assistant, nurse practitioner, registered nurse, licensed practical nurse, aesthetician, medical technician, medical assistant, laser technician, makeup artist, and massage therapist are all potential players on your team. These individuals have diverse abilities and skills and play distinct roles. The service providers in your practice may be employers, employees, consultants, or contractors. Regardless of their titles or roles, it is essential that these providers act within their ethical and reasonable scope of practice and represent your practice wholly—not themselves. You must not allow any service provider in the practice to act with complete autonomy. In theory and in mind, the practice then becomes his or hers, not yours.

Clinical Support

The same individuals who provide service to your patients (with the exception of a makeup artist and massage therapist) may also provide clinical support to the physician or any other member of the service team. Because of this intricate interrelation among roles, it is vital that scope of service and clinical support functions be clearly defined in job descriptions, appropriately scheduled, and well communicated among team members.

Patient Management

The term *patient coordinator* has been coined to describe the role of the individual responsible for patient management. In some practices this function is performed by the nurse or another clinical support person who manages patients. *Scheduler, booker,* and *consultant* are titles that have been used to identify those who engage and complete the transaction for treatment. (Unless you are selling cars or wedding photography, stay away from these titles.) Titles are less important than are the dedication and skills of those who fulfill the patient management function. This person is a vital contributor to your team, responsible for the entire patient experience and all the documentation and communication related to that experience. This position should not be entrusted to a commissioned, contracted, or consulting individual; patient management must be a vested function in your practice.

Administration

Office manager and *receptionist* are common titles for those who fulfill the administrative functions of the practice. Most often these are employees, but there are also office management consulting firms that can be contracted to run the business of your practice. The most important role of administration is to be timely, systematic, and well organized: this includes management of vital information, including licenses, certifications, and patient records. Administrative positions may be very focused, or diverse to include operations, financial responsibilities, property and facility management, and human resource management. I don't believe in hiring someone whose only function is to serve as a receptionist: every person in the office must be capable of, trained for, and responsible for answering the phone and greeting people in the manner you have defined for your practice.

Operations

Operations include all the things necessary to make the office run smoothly, from medical, IT, and telecommunications equipment and supplies to cleaning and utilities. A consultant may initially define and secure your equipment or service needs and make certain recommendations tailored to *your* needs, not to a predetermined set of guidelines issued by some unknown authority. An administrator on the staff generally coordinates or maintains the practice's operational needs, although clinical needs will require input and involvement from members of the clinical team.

Accreditation review and facility licensure is a vital role of the operational team; its management must be assigned to a designated in-house team member. A number of consultants can guide you through this process, although it is manageable in-house with the great detail and guidance provided by accrediting organizations such as the American Association for the Accreditation of Ambulatory Surgical Facilities (AAAASF) and the Accreditation Association for Ambulatory Health Care (AAAHC), or the Joint Commission on Accreditation of Healthcare Organizations (JCAHO), or in some practices accreditation by Medicare and state licensure.

Property and Facility

You will require a trusted team to locate, design, build, and furnish a complete facility that will represent you, welcome and serve your patients, and be adaptable over time.

Your property and facility will require daily maintenance. Day to day, the condition and function of your property and facility must be addressed in terms of cleanliness, security, safety, and appearance. You may have cleaning, floral, and landscape contractors. Members of your administrative or operations team may take on these and additional roles, such as changing light bulbs and performing regular safety checks. The time of year may require added services, such as snow and ice removal, or may require someone to prompt the landlord to remove the messy nest of birds above the front door. The property and facility require daily attention—observation and action.

Accounting/Banking/Finance and Investment

Accounts payable and receivables, insurance and adjustments (if you are accepting insurance or Medicare); payroll, benefits, taxes, and interest income and expenses; leases, equipment, and supplies; service and retail fees, sales taxes—the list of different financial transactions that relate to your business is a long one, but if well planned, categorized, and recorded, these functions should be straightforward. Today's software and practice management systems are comprehensive and effective, permitting you to maintain an internal function for processing collected income (service fees) and paying the bills. Outsourcing your bookkeeping and payroll to a service is an option (payroll services often provide human resource functions as well). Taxes, loans, and finance matters are best left to a qualified CPA who acts both as an advisor and a team member who knows when to delegate to the banker or the broker for mortgages or investments.

Legal

It is essential to have a lawyer on your team (not on retainer, but on the team) so that you can turn to this professional on a moment's notice to handle legal matters or direct you to a trusted, specialized colleague. All leases, loans, employment contracts, and other contracts should be reviewed by this expert. You will need expert advice on estate planning, as well as intellectual property, mergers and acquisitions, litigation, or defense. It is vital to have a legal advisor you trust and who understands all aspects of your business.

Human Resources

The human resources function to the practice is more than hiring, payroll, benefits, and policy. Within your team there must be a leader, someone you trust to make decisions, keep confidences, and reinforce the messages and policies you want to convey. That person must be an integral part of the team, not a consultant. In fact, that person may be you. You may choose to outsource the payroll, benefits, and other human resources functions; you should also outsource drug testing or competency tests.

Insurance

You will need malpractice, liability, property and casualty, key-man or disability, and disruption insurance. You may choose to carry health insurance and/or life insurance for yourself and your staff. Insurance needs are many and can be costly, but to forego an insurance advisor and essential forms of insurance could be disastrous.

Information Technology

Computer hardware, software, networks, and backup systems, imaging equipment and programs, telephones and security all fall under information technology. It's best to have expert support to define and design these systems and help you determine when it is appropriate to update your systems. It's important to have emergency services in the event things don't work as expected. Internally, you should have someone who keeps track of upgrades, updates, backups, and data management.

Marketing and Communication

Defining your brand, planning an event, running an ad, building your website, or defining and implementing protocols for patient contact all require an in-house team member to plan, organize, and execute needed marketing communications and to delegate specific tasks to trusted outside resources. Marketing need not be handled by a department or a single person; it may be based on the project, the need, or the intended audience or goal. Two areas should be entrusted to an outside resource: the design and the message. You are not an amateur; therefore don't let your image and brand look or sound amateurish.

Media Relations/Publicity

Whether you want to or are invited to engage the media, you will require an expert who knows how to manage content, messages, and situations. Protecting your image and time and making certain that the best possible information is communicated are essential to any public relations endeavor. Moreover, anyone entrusted with your public relations must accept and abide by the clear difference between quality media coverage and advertising.

Amenities

The flowers, beverages, massages, or soft terry exam robes that your practice may offer are amenities. Most of these will be provided by outside sources, but internally you need quality control and a point person to make certain that the amenities are available as needed, and that these are suited to your patients' and your service needs. Whether you send out the laundry or launder it on-site, whether you buy flowers from a florist or at the market, someone needs to be responsible for maintaining the flow of these activities.

Retail

If you choose to supply your patients with skin care, garments, prescriptions, vitamin drinks, skin care devices, or cosmetics, you are in the business of retail. Your team will require someone to prescribe, present, or educate patients about the retail products. Someone must monitor inventory, supply and demand, decide the right products to carry, and account for them accordingly. Don't forget some things require sales tax. Your team also includes the suppliers of retail goods. The salesperson who simply fulfills orders but never asks, answers, engages, or arrives is not interested in you or your patients' needs. Find another resource.

The team you will need is multifaceted, multitalented, and broad reaching. They are instrumental in launching your practice and in your practice's evolution, progress, and responsiveness to changing times and conditions. You may encounter the need for some degree of all of these functions in your daily practice without requiring a multitude of team members. You and your internal team—your staff—will multitask to carry out the daily functions essential to the practice and will engage and provide services to your patients on a daily basis.

YOUR PERSONAL TEAM

Whether they are part of your formal or informal team, spouses, partners, family, and friends can be cheerleaders, advisors, participants, or simply silent supporters. Whatever the role they choose or are asked to play, you must set the guidelines for encouraging—or declining—participation. You must decide the level of involvement you will allow from those close to you, and this must be accepted and respected by those you love and those you employ. The participation and influence of family and friends may evolve, just as your practice does. But two constants must remain: your practice is a business, first and last. Your spouse, family, and friends are personal, always.

HIPAA CONSIDERATIONS

Privacy became a common topic in medical practices when the Health Insurance Portability and Accountability Act (HIPAA) became law. Privacy has been and remains a vital element of any aesthetic practice. Not only are you and your staff required to abide by HIPAA standards, you must also ensure that any service provider to your practice, who has access to patient information or may be on the premises when patients are present, signs an associate's privacy agreement. Legal resources, practice management resources, and your own professional society may have sample documents you can use to protect your practice.

STAFF

Staff are an extension of you; they are the first and last contacts individuals have with you and your practice. They are essential to your practice and must be positively unforgettable.

Staff Roles

Once you establish the parameters of the services you will provide, staff members are the essential and most visible members of your practice team—often more visible to prospective and current patients than you are. Only you can determine your staffing needs based on the pace and productivity of the practice. Only you can define your staffing image based on your expectations, market, and brand. Aside from you, the provider, there are generally three key roles that staff fulfill:

1. Practice administration

2. Patient administration

3. Service provider, service extender, or support provider

Staff may be employees, or contractors; they are essential to your daily operation and part of your day-to-day team. Each person must be loyal to you and to the practice. All team members must thoroughly understand your specialty, as they should in any medical practice or business. In addition, they must be willing to continuously learn and remain current on all of the changes and advances in your specialty, even on services you do not provide. In an aesthetic practice, the three roles of practice—administration, patient coordination, and service provider—require individuals who understand the unique nature of providing nonpayor services and are willing to meet the expectations of patients seeking cosmetic treatments. They must be discreet, warm, compassionate people who also know when and where to draw the line, because they will regularly become involved in the most intimate details of your patients' lives, bodies, and choices.

Personality and Presence

Your staff, particularly those with direct contact with clients and patients, must be chosen based not only on their skill set, but on their personality and presence as well. An individual with the wrong personality or image for the position does not easily change, but with the right foundation, skills can be honed or acquired. Personality is the most critical variable. Staff represent your practice as much as you do; in fact, in almost every case, they are the first in-person impression an individual receives of your practice. The people who work for you are your messengers, gatekeepers, spokespersons, and advocates. They do not need to be a physical model of aesthetic perfection or a mirror of your finest work. They do need to be articulate, kind, patient individuals who understand and reflect that appearances are important personal issues for patients.

A patient visiting your office must enter an environment staffed by individuals who are focused on overall health and self-improvement, who foster confidence and help to allay anxiety, and who are current on the latest treatments and products.

▼ IN PRACTICE: The Shoemaker and the Diva

There is an old adage: *Beware the shoemaker who has holes in his soles.* There is a new adage: *Divas need not apply.*

A competent, qualified young woman was interviewing with the doctor for a key patient service position as a laser and skin care provider. She had all the right stuff, but she also had horrible excoriated acne. The doctor wanted to hire her; he felt she simply needed to have her condition properly treated. I advised against it. He hired her, and in her first days with the practice, he offered her treatment suggestions and options. Not offended, she politely declined. Her acne didn't bother her one bit; she had learned to live with the chronic condition that, according to her, no one could treat. As her first days progressed, her overall appearance went downhill rapidly. In fact, some days it was downright roll-out-of-bed horrible. Other staff members were dismayed. Patients were a bit puzzled; a few even commented on this new nurse's condition and appearance. Within a few days the doctor realized that the image of his staff was as important as qualifications. He let her go.

Lesson learned: Make certain that the first impression your office, staff, and you present is appropriate to patients with the desire for self-improvement. Would you let someone with holes in his shoes fix your shoes? Would you want someone who looks like a diva—overdone, undone, or simply done— to be a part of your cosmetic enhancement decisions? Do not let a first impression leave your patient thinking more about an unpolished or over-the-top office or staff or untreated acne more than his or her motivations to seek out your service.

Staff Cycles

Throughout the course of your practice your staff will cycle, whether by your actions or by their own choosing. The phases you and your practice encounter will affect not only you and the individual staff member, but also your staff as a whole:

- *Recruitment:* Finding the right people to work in your practice.

- *Training:* Instruction on specific job-related tasks, and the nuances of how you expect service to be delivered.

- *Retention:* Keeping your staff, happy, growing, and productive.

- *Compensation:* All the things that are provided to your staff in exchange for services, including salary, bonuses, or commissions, insurance, and even perks such as treatments.

- *Evaluation:* The process of reviewing staff contributions, goals, and growth is the most often overlooked basic component of a staff cycle in any small business.

- *Challenges and growth:* Whether self-initiated by a team member or initiated by you, challenge and growth are essential for some and frightening for others. You must not only challenge each individual to grow, but also apply the same scrutiny to the practice and the team as a whole.

- *Termination:* There will be times when you must terminate an employee, whether for performance issues, economic pressures, or other reasons. It is essential to have an initial probationary period, careful employment agreements that strictly define that employment is at will, and maintain employee performance records to minimize the stress of termination. *At will* means that you may terminate an employee or your employee may elect to resign at one's will, at any time. State employment laws vary, so it is important to have a lawyer review your employment policies and procedures to protect you and your practice from wrongful-termination litigation.

- *Contractors, service providers, and per diem workers:* Although they may not be part of your close inner employment circle, if these personnel are critical to your day-to-day operations, make certain that these nonemployees are viewed in the same cycle as your entire staff.

Although you may not take on the responsibility to manage all the details of your staff, if this is your practice and your business you must empower a capable individual to manage the staff cycle.

Recruitment

Who you will hire is a result of how you go about recruiting individuals to work in your practice. However, more important than the means is the end result.

- Traditional means of recruitment include job postings in the community, in specialty or industry publications, and through online networks. Hiring sites and services such as *Monster.com* and *Careerbuilder.com* are broad reaching but can be very focused in defining and presenting your needs. Most of these are affordable, but they are not always effective in recruitment for a very specialized field such as aesthetic medicine.

- Recruiters and services may look through their bank of candidates or use networking to find candidates and will do pre-screening to send you the right candidates, but these services can be very expensive, costing as much as 30% of the candidate's first-year wages.

- Networking on your own through colleagues, industry resources, and all the individuals who contribute to or are on your team is an inexpensive and focused approach: they know the brand and the image you are building, and they know something about your limits and expectations.

Screening candidates for employment is not a matter for snap decisions, but a painstaking process. Interviews are essential to hiring the right person and should be conducted not once, not twice, but at least three times. The interview process should include the following:

- Email correspondence beyond the presentation of resume and credentials

- A telephone dialog for a set period at a set time

- Face-to-face meetings with other team members and with the physician on one or more occasions

Before or during the process of interviewing, you must check the person's employment history, references, gather salary expectations, and present the need for drug testing, a credit report, or other screening, such as a criminal background check, before the individual may be hired. As you get closer to identifying the right candidate for a position, two things are essential: demonstration of skills and shadowing. Invite the candidate to spend a few hours or a day within the practice to get a feel for the pace, position, responsibilities, and office environment.

Recruiting takes a great deal of energy and time and has a serious impact on your practice. For this reason, nurturing and growing your staff as well as managing them are essential to maintaining a strong team.

IN PRACTICE: The Perfect Hire

She was well known in a tight community: a neighbor with a great background, a great family, and the right motivation for working—she wanted to get out and be productive. She was a patient of the practice, so she had empathy and understanding for the reasons an individual would seek aesthetic procedures. She was a sharp business woman; she had skills. She fit the image and the demographic of the practice's patients. She was interviewed and hired. She lasted until the moment someone she knew walked through the door and she said, "Hello, Susie, so great to see you! I didn't know you came here, too. I just saw your neighbor, Helen, here earlier today, and she looks fabulous."

Medical ethics and the confidentiality that any employee of your practice adheres to (in the form of a document signed the day that he or she becomes a part of the practice) is not enough. Your staff must be discreet in everything from client conversations to staff banter around the water cooler. They must practice this discretion both inside and outside the office. It is essential to the privacy of your clients; it is vital to the success of your practice.

Loyalty, Motivation, and Rewards

Recruiting and hiring staff require an immense effort, and a weakness or void in a staff position is taxing for everyone. Loyalty between you and your staff, motivation for your team, and rewards that recognize staff accomplishments are critical to staff contributions and retention and lead to consistency and continuity in your operation.

Loyalty requires mutual trust, mutual benefit, and individual leadership and takes time to evolve. As the owner of the business, the physician is the leader. But not all physicians want to lead the entire staff or are comfortable in this role. Some simply want to treat patients and let others on the staff handle the leadership role. Unfortunately, this simply does not work: you can have leaders on staff and on your team who take responsibility for certain functions, but the overall leadership of your practice, and of all those who work for you, is not only by default but by design your responsibility, in the same way that any clinical outcome in your practice is your responsibility and potential liability.

- Loyalty among clinical staff means that no matter who provides treatment, it is well understood by all that these are the practice's—the physician's—patients. It requires mutual respect among staff so that no one questions or contradicts the physician or other team member in the patient's presence. It requires mutual respect to credit the individual and praise the team who supports the individual.

- Loyalty among administrative staff is demonstrated by acknowledging that every function of the practice has value, because the whole cannot function without the efficient efforts of all the parts.

Different people are motivated by different stimuli. For some it is money; for others it is praise. Some are motivated by advancement; others simply by the fulfillment and satisfaction they receive from accomplishing daily tasks and specific goals; and others in the business of aesthetics are motivated by their role in helping patients achieve personal goals. Inspiring your staff requires three things:

1. Knowing what motivates the individual

2. Knowing what motivates the team

3. Finding consistent and common means to motivate without creating conflict

Money as a reward may be team oriented and based on individual merit. This should be reviewed at least annually. Praise is something that should occur naturally, regularly, and when warranted. Praise is used for a job well done, but it becomes ineffective when it is overused. *Thank you, great job, well done, kudos, fabulous, outstanding*—no matter the words, use them when you mean them.

Advancement is motivating; training is essential. Clinical staff have a duty not only to keep abreast of practical knowledge, but to also keep current on skills and training. Encourage this, reward this, display the certificates, and communicate your staff's level of knowledge and training to your clients and patients. Your credibility is the core of a successful practice; so is the credibility of those who work for you and with you. Administrative staff have a duty to keep abreast of market, operational, and business knowledge. Reward this and communicate the value of advancement to the entire group, because it should inevitably benefit everyone in the practice when administrators can improve the tasks that bind the practice together.

Achieving patient goals is something we only seem to stop and recognize when we exceed what was thought to be possible, when the patient expresses joy and thanks, or when we fail. The truth is, the exceptional accomplishments or occurrences at either end of the spectrum are not what provide your daily bread: it is those usual, daily, common situations that result in good outcomes that must be recognized, because without them, your practice would be limited.

🦋 IN PRACTICE: Lesson Learned

A busy, quality practice had a great structure of rewarding employees and maintaining a team spirit. Fair salaries and individual provider productivity fees were standard. Fair commissions were earned for retail sales. A monthly bonus for the entire team was defined as a percentage of practice revenue goals. Staff members loved working together. They were loyal to one another, and loyal as a team. Then hard times hit. It was nothing more than a downturn related to economic conditions. The physician chose to let one of her providers go to reduce expenses; she selected the provider with the lowest productivity fees and the lowest retail sales. Jackie, who had been with the doctor since she graduated nursing school, was fired.

Several weeks later, I got a call from the physician. "The office is a mess; everyone is miserable. No one is keeping up on ordering supplies. We fell behind on sterilization. The sample cabinet is empty. There is a stack of patient messages no one wants to take. Suddenly I am addressing rep meetings every day. I just did not realize how much Jackie contributed to this office, in addition to treating patients. The staff is grumbling without her, and I need her back." The problem was that Jackie had a loyal following among the patients she treated. She had set up shop down the street in a nonspecialized physician's office, and she was flourishing in that setting, her client list booming.

What I wanted to reply was this: "Before letting her go, did you look at the whole equation, all the things Jackie contributed other than revenue? Did you consider other options, such as cutting everyone back a little instead of letting one person go? Do you expect that I can fix this, when you fired a woman who was loyal to you for 9 years? Did you consider the fallout of your actions before you made a mistake that is costing you more than the economy has?"

My actual reply was this: "Your staff are going to have to take assignments among themselves to pick up the slack. We'll have to set some policy for rep calls so your time is not overtaxed. You can also contact all the patients Jackie has treated, warmly introduce the other providers, and affirm that such services are still readily and happily available in your practice. You can only try to do damage control."

Lesson Number 1: Money is not the only measure of how essential any one team member may be to your equation. Lesson Number 2: Loyalty should be mutual.

THE ART OF PERSONNEL MANAGEMENT

Mary Lind Jewell, RPT

Hire Staff With the Right Stuff

There are challenges facing your practice every day that require a well-trained staff, including increased competition, patients' expectations, control of practice overhead, economic downturns, diminished reimbursement, and government regulation. As CEO of your practice, you need to implement human resource techniques to ensure that you hire capable, genial, hardworking employees. It pays to be a thoughtful leader who attends to the details of staff development. Developing their talents and encouraging to reach their potential represents a true strategic asset for your practice.

Patient satisfaction is in direct correlation to the efforts and the efficiency of your staff—your staff will either make or break your plastic surgery practice. When it comes to patient satisfaction and customer service, you must hire employees who speak your clients' language. Each time you go through the hiring process, you need to assess how this potential employee will relate to your patients. I am often asked, "Is it more important to hire personality, or knowledge and skill?" You can teach your staff skills and develop their knowledge, but personality is who they are and how they will interact with your patients. I believe that attention to detail is not written in training manuals—it's in our DNA.

Customer service is not a department—it's in the attitude of excellent employees. You must hire people who will promote you and who are hardworking, friendly, empathetic, intelligent, stable, team players. Another important component of their personality must be uncompromising honesty. You should feel as though you could place yourself or a family member into their care and know that you could trust them implicitly.

A Smart Hire Is Worth Thou$ands

The *right* people are an inestimable asset to your practice. It costs you time and considerable money each time there is a turnover, so you should be selective. Even highly skilled new employees take time to get up to speed in a new setting, so it is in your best interest to retain excellent staff members. Hire people whose judgment you can respect so you do not have to micromanage.

Before the interview process begins, you should research pay scales and benefits in your vicinity so you are certain you're offering a competitive wage and a generous package of benefits.

It is important to evaluate candidates' motivational hierarchy; doing their utmost to help build the success of your practice should be at the top of their list.

If you pay a little extra, you may actually get more in the long run. A probationary period is prudent. An interview allows the prospective employer a very narrow glimpse of the interviewee, and hiring the wrong person can be a costly mistake. Legal, financial, and professional problems can arise if an inappropriate candidate is selected, not to mention potential damage to office morale. Always check references with a phone call and listen for what is not being shared with you. Of former employers, ask: Is this person a team player, or best at working autonomously? Would you rehire this person?

Training requires a plan with clearly defined expectations that are written in a training manual. The best training comes from a motivated, patient teacher who is geared for the new employee's success. Expect quality customer service, innovation, and teamwork from the very beginning. Your practice will grow more efficient and effective if you cultivate problem-solvers and risk-takers.

If you do not see growth and benefit for the practice within 90 days, it is best to terminate the individual's employment during the probationary period, or at least extend their probation. Termination of employment requires knowing the rules. Employer's rights on termination belong in the policy manual. If you think competent people are expensive, try hiring incompetents.

Effective Leadership Is the Key

You cannot demand commitment, excellence, or creativity from your staff, but you can encourage and evaluate it. Effective leadership is the key element in motivating and retaining the right staff. Evaluate all employees' performance regularly and with fairness. Empower your staff to identify improvements that can help make the team more efficient, improve the quality of care, and increase patient satisfaction. Evaluations recognize work well done and project tomorrow's goals. Immediate feedback is the most effective form of performance appraisal; recognize excellence and innovation as it occurs. Sometimes mistakes are made. Instead of ignoring the problem, shine a light on the situation and ask the entire team to help resolve the issue. Remember that active listening can help to keep problems small. An employer should praise in public and reprimand in private. Create a trusting environment where each employee is willing to take risks to achieve better outcomes. Having a measure of control over one's area of responsibility pays dividends in staff satisfaction. Coaching your team involves being ready to applaud their efforts, whatever the success of the outcome. Creativity breeds happiness for individuals and the team; regularly ask for their input. Have an education allowance to ensure that learning is ongoing.

Continued

THE ART OF PERSONNEL MANAGEMENT—cont'd

To develop a team focused on the business of patient satisfaction, choose intelligent patient advocates who enjoy innovation and have excellent critical thinking skills. Provide a work environment that welcomes challenges and is open to debates to find solutions and opportunities. What happens when leaders, even the smartest, cut themselves off from employee insights? You can lose the power of parallel processing and the diversity of knowledge. Smart leaders who become players keep their team motivated to innovate, which is your practice's lifeblood.

MAKING IT RELATIVE: Cake and Icing

Birthday cake is a tradition: cake, icing, and of course, a name and birthday message decorated on the top. I love to watch how the way we enjoy birthday cakes changes over a lifetime. Small children love to get their fingers in the icing and lick it away. Older children vie for and demand a specifically decorated portion of the cake. Still others don't care what the cake looks like—they just gobble down the icing, the cake, or both. Adults carefully eat the cake and leave the icing. The reason: as you get older you simply know the consequences of something that is too sweet and too much.

Your staff members are skilled and smart, poised and prepared. They are discreet. Yet they have to be more.

The clients coming to you are doing so by choice, and they won't make that choice if the entire experience is not personalized, is not refreshing and satisfying, and does not meet their expectations. This means that the core staff your clients interact with must also be genuinely caring, personable, patient, and flexible—not sugary, disingenuous, or overindulgent.

Aesthetic medical treatment is the cake; it is an important part of your patient's passage through life. If you want someone to buy your cake, your staff had best be genuine—not loaded with icing.

CHAPTER 3

Who Defines Your Market?

People seeking to fulfill personal desires for youth, curves, balance, or beauty—this is the population from which you will draw your patients.

It is essential to know as much as possible about your patients before you recommend a procedure: their motivations, goals, desires, needs, tolerances, limits, expectations, health concerns, and ability to comprehend and comply with the specifics of a course of treatment.

KNOWING YOUR PATIENTS

A vital first step in connecting to your patients is knowing what has motivated them to consult with you. To shape your practice optimally to attract patients/clients and provide services to them, you must consider the similarities and opportunities presented by your current and prospective patients, and what trends are indicated.

Who are the people who want to look better and feel better about the way they look, and how do they find you? In this communication-saturated world, they come to you in many ways:

- Some will be drawn to you as a result of your efforts.
- Some will be referred to you by another physician or health care provider.

- Others will be referred to you by patients you treated previously.

- They may be referred to you by people who know you and are confident about recommending your services.

- Some will come to you by chance.

- Some patients will return to you, and some will not.

It may be difficult to find your potential clients/patients and connect with them individually. Therefore you must have a means to define your market, your patients, and those who through the course of your professional life will change in their demographics and desires.

- Geography defines where they live.

- Demographics defines their income, age, sex, race, education, and interests.

- Economics defines whether they can afford your services.

- Interest defines their potential desires, spending habits, and limits and will help you to make a broad connection with them.

PATIENT VERSUS CLIENT VERSUS CUSTOMER

A patient is someone under your medical care; a client is someone to whom you provide a service; a customer is someone to whom you sell goods. The people you serve may be any one or all these at any given time. Treat them as the valuable assets to your practice that they are.

LOCATION

The first factor that defines your potential population is geography. Although many affluent clients will travel the world to benefit from the services of a particular practitioner of aesthetic medicine, most will come from a relatively close proximity to your practice.

Geographic Market Areas

The geographic market from which you draw your patient/client population has three related areas:

- The immediate community in which your practice is located.

- The community in which your practice is located, and adjacent communities of similar demographics through which your potential patients travel for work, commerce, and school.

- Your overall *demographic market area* (DMA), a term used to define media markets for advertisers. Understanding your DMA means knowing the region that your dominant local print (newspaper and magazine) and electronic (broadcast television and radio) media sources cover.

Knowing how far your patients are willing to travel and the geographic area in which they are concentrated is more important than simply selecting a location for your practice and understanding your physical reach. It can define your limits and offer new opportunities for attracting patients.

IN PRACTICE: Going the Distance

She was young and opened her practice during challenging times. She carefully studied the opportunities and communities where there was a need for her services. Eighteen years later, in this remote and beautiful part of the world, she had a busy practice where patients came to her from a 150-mile radius. Hers was the only practice in her specialty in the area, and then another physician moved into town, and her practice's monopoly was at an end.

Panicked, the physician decided to reinvent her practice and expand her services. She wanted to add a spa and an on-site recovery center for surgical patients. She envisioned concierge services and attention-getting television commercials about the expanded facility. She wasn't going to let anyone invade her turf and draw away even one patient.

After many conversations and meetings, I asked the physician, "Do the people who have traveled to see you want or need all these things you are proposing to offer?" After some thought, she realized that if people wanted

Continued

🦋 IN PRACTICE: Going the Distance—cont'd

treatment by her hands, they had no other choice; her practice was the most convenient option for them. I had the office manager run one simple report: a zip code breakdown of all her patients over the past 36 months. In this nearly 71,000-square-mile area, patients were concentrated in three specific locations.

The resulting move for this physician: she established two satellite offices, where she practices several days each month. The resulting outcome: the new competition in town has not been a significant factor. By choosing to locate in the areas from which her patients had to travel, she not only retained her loyal patients, but also garnered many new ones.

MEDICAL TOURISM

Foad Nahai, MD, FACS

Searching for excellence in health care at home or even by leaving one's country is nothing new. Throughout history those who have had the means have traveled to centers of excellence in search of the best care.

Affordability, the dramatic growth of medical centers and clinics, media coverage, and the loss of certain stigmas have all contributed to unprecedented growth in the number of people who seek medical services outside their own country. To give this phenomenon a name, the support industries that have fostered inbound medical services coined the phrase *medical tourism.*

Over the past two decades we have seen remarkable growth of people from developed countries traveling to other developed and developing countries in search of bargains in health care. The travel and tourism ministries of many developing countries are supportive of this trend. Recent studies show that outbound medical tourism by far outnumbers inbound tourism, in some instances by as much as twentyfold. Although there are no hard data on the number of medical tourists, it is estimated that 4 million medical tourists per year receive health care services outside their home countries.

Medical tourism is a huge business. It is estimated that the industry generates between $20 and $40 billion annually, with predictions that revenues from medical tourism could reach $100 billion within a few years.

Medical tourists inbound to the United States and Western Europe travel to world-famous medical centers and seek out individual surgeons renowned for excellence. Too often, outbound patients are motivated by only one thing: saving money. This phenomenon is not unique to aesthetic plastic surgery; millions of medical tourists travel for bargains in numerous specialties.

Leading specialties include organ transplantation, heart surgery, joint replacement, and dentistry.

Asian countries top the list of medical tourism destinations because of lower medical care costs, a legal environment more favorable to a variety of procedures, government subsidies, and quality medical professionals. All of these factors contribute to competitive or comparatively bargain prices that cannot be matched by health care providers in the West.

As with any growing trend, the multibillion-dollar medical tourism industry has attracted entrepreneurs from other industries, specifically tour operators, tourist boards, hotel groups, hospital groups, and individual medical and paramedical personnel who see the increase in medical tourism as a perfect opportunity to cash in on the boom. Most of these entrepreneurs promote their bargain-priced aesthetic surgery through glossy brochures as if it were a commodity. They emphasize attractive pricing, vacation destinations, and tourist attractions, with the surgical procedure mentioned as an incidental part of the trip and the seriousness of a surgical operation downplayed. Very few, if any, of these medical tourism operators discuss the qualifications of the surgeons involved or the safety records of the clinics or physicians' offices where such procedures will take place. Some patients leave home without even knowing the name of the surgeon or whether they are suitable candidates for the procedures around which they have organized a vacation.

The most troubling aspect of this scenario is how the entrepreneur or travel organizer displaces the medical professional and becomes an intermediary, supplanting what should be a doctor/patient relationship with a contact person who knows little about medicine and more about local hot spots.

There is no question that some patients are operated on by well-qualified surgeons in certified and safe facilities with good results for a fraction of the price they would have paid in their home country. Regrettably, this is not always the case. It is estimated that as many as 20% of the cosmetic tourists returning to the United Kingdom have a complication that requires attention by a specialist or even hospitalization. A recent report[1] in the *Journal of Plastic, Reconstructive, and Aesthetic Surgery* (JPRAS) addressed the financial burden this puts on the United Kingdom's National Health Service. Medical tourists who return with complications are often unable to afford private care to treat these complications, so they turn to the government. In some instances physicians in the home country are reluctant to deal with complications resulting from medical tourism; this may be related to the legal issues involved. In response to problems such as this, certain insurance companies are beginning to offer policies to cover complications incurred by medical tourists.

Continued

MEDICAL TOURISM—cont'd

These medical forays raise safety issues for patients and moral and ethical issues for surgeons. In response to these challenges, the International Society of Aesthetic Plastic Surgery (ISAPS) and the American Society for Aesthetic Plastic Surgery (ASAPS) have developed guidelines not only for would-be medical tourists, but also for surgeon-members who receive and treat them (see *http://www.surgery.org*).

It is the ethical duty of the surgeon involved to insist that he or she be the focus in establishing the physician/patient relationship, not the tour operator. The physician must reveal his or her credentials, training and expertise in the procedure requested; enter into formal consent discussions with the patient, describing the nature of the procedure, alternative procedures, risks, the likely outcome, and potential complications. The surgeon must outline plans for dealing with complications should they occur, either in the host country or on the patient's return home. These discussions should include delineation of responsibility for additional expenses or an unexpected hospitalization incurred as a result of complications. Continued care on return to the home country must also be discussed and arrangements made.

Discussion should also cover the use of medical devices. Not all prostheses and implants are created equal. Inferior-quality implants and prostheses may be available at a fraction of the price in developing countries compared with costs in the West. A frank discussion concerning any prostheses or implants, such as breast implants, should be part of this consultation in establishing the physician/patient relationship.

Finally, there is an underlying issue that is rarely addressed. It is unethical for a physician to engage in fee-splitting or other financial arrangements with a third party or corporate entity for the procurement and referral of patients. For tour operators whose goal is to make as much money as possible from as many sources as possible, the possibility of commissions from physicians for referrals becomes a problem that threatens the integrity of our profession.

Like it or not, medical tourism is here to stay. It will continue to grow, and it will continue to attract those who wish to profit from this multibillion dollar industry. The question that remains to be answered is: What price will the public and the profession pay for this largely unregulated practice?

REFERENCE
1. Cosmetic tourism and the burden on the NHS [editorial]. J Plast Reconstr Aesthetic Surg 61:1423-1424, 2008.

DEMOGRAPHICS

*I hate the way market forces try to separate us out
into the appropriate demographic—basically in order
to sell us things. We need to find stories that we can
enjoy together, not separately.*
— EMMA THOMPSON, ACTOR

Choosing to undergo an aesthetic procedure is a very personal and intimate decision. Your patients are individuals, and you must consider them as such. While locating prospective patients by geography is the most basic segmentation, pinpointing a market of existing or prospective clients/patients includes a study of demographics—income, age, sex, race, education, and interests.

Income

In some regions there is significant income disparity among populations; other regions are fairly homogeneous based on housing and industry. An area with great disparity in income levels will also have great disparity in education, race, and perhaps age.

Aesthetic procedures are not government subsidized or covered by insurance anywhere in North America or Europe. You need to target individuals with the ability to pay for your services, and populations with higher income levels generally encompass people with a personal desire for your services as well as the ability to pay for them. However, do not discount those in lower income brackets; the value of your services may be equally desired by those to whom a small change in appearance can lead to newfound confidence and opportunities in life.

Age

You must decide whether your practice will encompass all ages or target a specific age-defined segment. Age defines a client population's most likely aesthetic needs. Those in a younger segment may be more interested in maintaining their youth, refining their appearance, or reshaping their bodies. Older individuals are more likely to be interested in restorative procedures, from a desire to either stop the clock or to look like a younger version of themselves. A population with a balance between the age groups presents the option of targeting one or the other or embracing both.

Sex

Many make the assumption that those who seek aesthetic surgery or medical treatments are women. In some markets this may hold true, but do not misjudge your male population. Aesthetic medicine, more than surgery, has been demonstrated to be a successful niche among men. Men want to improve their appearance, but some are averse to more involved procedures, such as surgery.

Race

If there is a dominant ethnic or racial makeup in your geographic market, you should determine whether you are capable of attracting these individuals and understanding their aesthetic requirements, and whether you are qualified to handle the special needs of this group. If the potential population is strong enough, you may decide to cater to this segment, creating a unique practice niche.

Education

Knowing your potential patients' level of education is essential to effectively communicate with that population on an appropriate level. If you communicate below that level, you may insult someone or appear unsophisticated. If you communicate above that level, you may be misunderstood or tuned out.

Although most practices target the majority population's educational level, some may choose to cater to a niche group. The greater value of understanding educational levels is not in attracting patients, but in appropriately communicating the expectations, options, risks, and instructions for treatment. Assuming, without verifying, that a patient comprehends these options and risks puts both your patient's well-being and your practice's reputation at risk.

ON TARGET

Procedural statistics and data from recognized professional groups supporting the specialties that include aesthetic medicine, as well as your own practice's procedural statistics and data, are important tools for defining your practice mix and growth efforts. For example, ASAPS reported that in 2008 there was a surprising increase in the number of cheek implant procedures performed, but there was a slight decrease in the cosmetic injectables used in recent years to enhance or augment the cheeks. Does this mean that your patients will start asking for more cheek implants or that cheek implants are a new trend you should begin to offer patients more readily? Research trends carefully—statistics are not absolutes, but they help to define and build a practice, its mix of services, and the audience to which that mix is targeted. Using the right tools helps to build your practice.

YOUR TARGET POPULATION
Interest

Although individuals may be geographically close, have the money to pay for your services, meet the age, sex, and race that you have targeted, and be educated enough to understand what you and your practice provide, they may simply not be interested in your services.

There are two significant indicators for measuring overall interest within a target population: lifestyle interests and retail purchasing habits. Whether you are tapping an existing interest or creating an interest in your services among a target population, a look at their lifestyles and retail purchasing habits will yield key information about how significant the potential interest is among the target group. These factors will also help you determine the appropriate messages and the means to communicate with that population.

LIFESTYLE

If the lifestyle interests of your target population are high on self (fitness, sports, and health) and what is demographically defined as "the good life" (arts, travel, fashion, food, and wine), this group is also likely to be interested in aesthetic procedures and therapies. Quite simply, these are people who have an interest in and the financial ability to pay for self-improvement. Therefore these people represent a high potential for becoming clients.

RETAIL PURCHASING

Retail buying habits are another indicator of interest, and they relate to how you will build your practice and what messages you will convey to the target population. Consider these questions:

- Do your potential patients/clients spend a significant amount on health, beauty, and fashion?

- Will they spend more for something of greater quality or design? Are they label or value conscious?

- Do they focus on needs, or trends?

There are varying degrees of lifestyle and retail purchasing habits among any population. Uncovering these factors is essential to building a successful practice, because you will refer to these factors when defining:

- The best channels of communication for the target population

- Opportunities to connect with this group

- Cycles that influence the target population

Understanding the nuances of your marketplace and existing patient population is important in identifying needs and trends. It is also essential to use your resources effectively to bring potential clients to your door, to continue to serve those already in your practice, and to draw on those within your practice to help you grow by generating referrals. Population studies are not reserved for the people you hope to attract; the data you have in your patient records are invaluable to better identify the group of people you currently treat or recently treated. The more you know about your patients, the better you are able to evolve to meet the changing characteristics, preferences, and needs of your patients.

Social Indicators

There are social indicators that can greatly influence your success and the goals your patients pursue. The community may be high on self or on selflessness, may appreciate and understand the desire for self-improvement, or may label such desires as vain. In some cultures, the desire for aesthetic procedures can be viewed as denying one's ethnicity and therefore may be severely condemned, whereas in other cultures, seeking out a provider of aesthetic procedures to find a true balance and harmony of appearance is desirable, as has been documented in Muslim cultures, where women's public appearance is cloaked with a chador, burka, or veil. Even an individual who has left a gang has separated from a type of community that has its own influences, and this person may want to erase the signs of belonging, including removal of tattoos, piercings, and other identifying alterations to appearance.

Economics will play a role in the patient population. The matter of personal wealth is not as significant as economic desires are; those who want to alter or enhance their appearance will find the means to pay for what they want. For some, aesthetic improvements are desired to increase acceptance and better opportunities for employment and compensation, or may stem from the attraction of those who have greater economic resources.

Additionally, economic status often compels competition for material things and among individuals to be fit, slim, youthful, or beautiful. Other services desired by your patients can also have an influence on your practice, or they may conflict with your opportunities to attract and provide services to a community, culture, or social group.

RELATIVE WISDOM: Exactly What I Want

When you buy a gift, do you select it with the recipient in mind, or do you select the present based on your own tastes?

A brilliant physician with a solid practice understood the concept of evolving and growing to meet one's market. He regularly reviewed the content of his website, ads, and patient communications; he was completely hands-on in his approach. He often looked at revisions or additions and proudly told me, "I have everything exactly the way I want it."

I replied, "It is not what you want—it must be what your patients want and expect."

Relative wisdom: Whether you are changing the paint on the walls, the photos or message on your website, or the location of your office, make certain that it reflects your image, but delivers value for your patients. It is no different than presenting a gift: the gift may reflect your taste, but it must make your recipient happy.

DATA COMPENDIUMS

Data on your region are everywhere and in many cases can be obtained for free. This simply requires an investment of your time to gather data about your patients and your market.

Practice Management and Electronic Medical Record Software

You can learn many things by simply isolating the data you've already collected about your patients. Each month, look at the breakdown of services provided. Each year, look at the age range of patients per service provided. There are innumerable combinations of data you can collect and review. Don't just make it a practice to run data—use it to build the practice.

Media Kits

Although you may not want to advertise your practice, obtaining rate cards and media kits for local print and broadcast media can provide valuable information. Most media kits contain demographic information about a specific geographic market and the demographics of the audience they reach;

some profile audience interests. Consider the quality, content, and purpose of the publication according to their target audience and how they have selected their market. An unsolicited, free coupon envelope mass mailed to "resident" addresses will give you nothing more than mass data.

Local Government and School Boards

Local government and school boards keep current census data on file such as property values, business licenses, community residential and commercial profiles, and more.

Media

Newspapers, regional magazines, and business journals often publish profiles for the communities they serve. Look online to tap these data resources.

Visit your local library for the following easy-to-use yet comprehensive demographic data and profile publications. Neither publication offers online data free of charge, but most libraries have the print versions.

- *The Lifestyle Market Analyst:* Focus on the "Market Profiles" section for your metropolitan region or county. Included are basic demographic data per household in a region, such as occupation, education, race, age, income, and lifestyle interests. This publication is updated annually.

- *Woods & Poole Economics, Inc.:* This publication offers similar basic demographic information to *The Lifestyle Market Analyst* but focuses on industry and commerce rather than on households. It also offers a breakdown of retail sales in demographic markets.

The purpose of business is to create and keep a customer.
— PETER F. DRUCKER

TARGET SOURCES

Once you define your target population, you need a *target source,* a starting point.

Your Starting Point

In an established practice, the initial target source is your current satisfied patient/client population. They know you and trust you. Although they may not define your target population for all your services, they are essential to the single most important means of reaching clients: referral.

If you are just beginning practice or are expanding an existing practice, your target source is someone or something with an existing channel of communication to your target population that you can reasonably and credibly attach yourself to for referrals. It bears repeating: referral is the single most important means of building your practice. Referral holds many benefits that no other source for clients can. What is most important is that it provides a basis of familiarity. When potential clients need or want a procedure that involves some amount of risk, is voluntary, and will have monetary, physical, and emotional costs, the first point of contact or reference will always be someone:

- The potential client knows and with whom there is an established relationship of trust

- Who is recommended by someone the potential client knows with whom there exists an established relationship of trust—a family member, friend, or another physician

The link of familiarity and trust is not the only reason referral is the best way to reach your target population. Referral grows as it passes from one source to the next. Referral may be positive word of mouth and a personal endorsement of you. Therefore maintaining a healthy, consistently positive referral relationship is as important as having a source of referral. To achieve this, you should:

- Recognize and extend gratitude to the referral source (maintaining confidentiality where appropriate)

- Continue consistent, relevant communication with the referral source

Without this communication with your referral sources you may be forgotten, and a competitor may succeed in gaining the interest of your sources.

LESSON LEARNED

I encourage the practices I consult with to track the number of procedures performed weekly and monthly and to tie these to specific variables such as age, or for a new patient, to the referral source. One of my clients suddenly had a significant increase in injection appointments, although no promotion or special event had been announced. One month later, it happened again. Everyone was happy about the traffic, but no one thought to find the source.

I was on-site visiting one day and took a patient back for her first injection. She was nervous, but excited, so I engaged her in small talk. "Do you know anyone who has been treated here before? Have you heard of other patients' experiences?"

What I learned in that little exchange was golden. "Yes," she replied, "all the teachers at the high school have been getting injections. My friend was the first who came here, and when we saw her results, we all wanted to give it a try. I'm not the early adopter, but as more of the teachers get injections, we just seem to be a happier-looking group. Believe it, the kids notice. It's my turn. Our secretary's sister runs the medical spa across town, and she is now offering a teacher's discount day on our day off from school. But I wanted to come here. I'm nervous about this, and you treated my friend, and she looks great."

I asked the office manager if and how the practice was tracking referral. They did: the typical magazine, Internet, patient referral, physician referral, and word of mouth were on the list of sources. "Do you ask the patient's name, the physician's name, or the source for the word of mouth referral?" I asked. The office manager looked at me, puzzled.

Had the practice been more careful, they would have realized they had just tapped into a new source for patients, all by word of mouth: teachers. Had they been even more thoughtful, they would have realized the source: the initial patient who opened the floodgates. Had they been proactive, they would have reached out directly to this market and would not lose any of these new patients.

Now that the practice was aware, the staff started offering ideas to help expand this new market. I stopped them all. "Before you decide to grow this market, let's see what other opportunities you have overlooked, or lost, by failing to connect with and collect important information about your patients."

TARGET RESOURCES
Enable Potential Clients and Patients to Find You

Target sources bring clients to you; target resources enable potential clients to find you. Although referral will likely be the core of growth in your client population, there are many potential clients among the target population with an interest in your aesthetic services who do not have a referral source to you. These potential clients will:

- Find you based on your visibility among resources
- Choose you based on your ability to connect on a practical and personal level through these resources

Who you are and what services your practice provides must be effectively communicated to potential patients/clients. This is where lifestyles, interests, and retail purchasing patterns provide the greatest insight to your potential target population, the resources to reach them, and the tone and type of messages to use. Your research will guide your choice of effective communication tools or resources, aid in developing appropriate and attractive messages to use, and help you meet the levels of expectation among the target population. Your messages, resources, and connections can be used to define your identity or brand, build visibility for the practice, and communicate your value.

Effective, targeted communication through strategic resources is essential to make you visible to your target audience—including referral sources. Visibility and appropriate communication, second to referral, are key to drawing a potential client to you first, before that person seeks a competitor's practice. The first provider the person goes to has the advantage in converting that potential client into a repeat client and a patient.

🗡 IN PRACTICE: Moving Out

A plastic surgeon, well-established for 12 years, opened a satellite office just 9 miles from his existing office. The new office was not drawing an aesthetic patient population, nor was it well received in the community. His general market was a large metropolitan area, and the satellite location was in an exurb, where many new homes were popping up on former farm fields. The area hospital was building a $90 million addition, and there was no direct or indirect competition in like providers. The expanding metropolis he practiced in was growing, and this exurb was fast becoming a suburb.

The surgeon communicated his new location to his existing client base through direct mail to new homes in the area and through established advertising channels that had proved successful to him in his home market. He was baffled as to why things were not working in the new location.

I asked if he had researched the growing community's demographics, lifestyles, and interests. "Time not well spent," he replied. "It's just outside my current door; how different can it be?"

Then I asked the doctor to meet me for lunch near his new office so we could discuss the situation. "Well, there's nothing but fast food nearby," he told me. I asked about retail. "There's a Walmart, an Old Navy, and a Gap," he laughed.

"What do people in the community read?" I asked.

"I don't know," he admitted.

The doctor then realized the mistake he had made. He had moved to an area that by all accounts was growing positively in number of households, commerce, and medical services, but he had not researched the population the community was attracting.

In fact, the growth of "luxury homes" involved large homes on inexpensive property that drew first-time home-buyers and families from the inner city hoping to establish a better life for themselves. The new population in this community consisted of hard-working, young, middle-income families who:

- Had little extra income to spend and were deterred by the doctor's projected image of elegance

- Could not relate to his practice identity, which focused on treating the signs of aging

Continued

🪰 IN PRACTICE: Moving Out—cont'd

- Did not connect to his existing patient base, because they had not moved from the next town; they had moved from downtown

- Did not read the publications he advertised in, because these were targeted toward a higher demographic group and were not widely distributed in the newly growing community

The doctor did not want to move, but he agreed to retool: building on the existing practice location, but altering his communication strategy to meet the specific needs and interests of this new population through new sources and communication resources.

For this satellite location, his focus changed from antiaging to youth and vitality. The tone of his message changed from elegant to simple and direct. New communication resources were a problem, however. There were no media targeted specifically to this new area, and the doctor did not want to give too much visibility to his new image in his old market. So we focused on creating a client source, and through a new relationship with the booming OB/GYN practice in town, a successful focus on breast surgery and body-contouring led to a practice that, although not quite what he had expected, has succeeded.

CHAPTER 4

Who Is the Competition?

No enterprise is more likely to succeed than one concealed from the enemy until it is ripe for execution.
— NICCOLO MACHIAVELLI

Competition is inevitable—you cannot deny that competition exists for the services you provide and that competitors are vying for your patients' dollars. Rather than simply competing, your practice must remain competitive: always be one step ahead and better than another practice with the potential to draw the interest and purchasing power of your target population away from you.

UNDERSTANDING COMPETITION

Competition is ubiquitous for the attention, dollars, and fulfillment of services your prospective and existing patients seek. "Competition" ranges from the physician with the same credentials in your building to the designer handbag that your patient may choose to buy instead of investing in aesthetic services. There are four types of competition in business: direct, secondary, extended, and indirect.

Direct Competition

Your direct competition is a provider with the same or similar credentials, providing the same services in a similar environment to a similarly defined target population.

Secondary Competition

Secondary competition involves a provider of dissimilar credentials or in a dissimilar environment who is providing the same services you are to a similarly defined target population. Today franchise medical spas that have no qualified physician involved in patient care are viewed as secondary competition. However, if you have defined your expertise and credentials well, the public will easily distinguish your practice from such businesses.

Extended Competition

Extended competition is more remote from who you are and what you do. With this form of competition, someone or something has the potential to fulfill the personal desires of your target population with a service or product different from those you provide, even if the degree of results is dissimilar. Extended competition reflects the difference between opting for a medical procedure and hiring a personal stylist or wardrobe consultant to overhaul your wardrobe.

Indirect Competition

Indirect competition is the most distant form of competition. This involves someone or something completely different from who you are and what you do, yet is still competing for the interest and spending power of your target population in fulfilling personal desires. Indirect competition is the difference between the life-investing experience of an aesthetic procedure and a once-in-a-lifetime vacation.

WHO IS YOUR BIGGEST COMPETITOR?

Karen A. Zupko

Ask any plastic surgeon, "Who is your biggest competitor?" and typically you'll get a list of names with little or no hesitation.

As to the accuracy of that list, who's to say? The responses are frequently based on external perceptions. "My competitor gets more or better slots on the hospital and the ambulatory surgery center's operating schedule" may be true for one or two facilities. But who knows how full his or her schedule is at a facility you can't monitor because you aren't on staff there? "Her reception room is always filled" might be the case on certain days, but you don't know what's really going on in the office. Sloppy business systems can make even big revenue streams into profit trickles. Or maybe all the people in the waiting room are there for discounted or free services.

Medical community gossip, sometimes fed by company sales representatives, contributes to these impressions. Advertising, media mentions, television appearances, and comments by spouses and patients add to the aura of the leading competitor.

To me this is all hearsay. It's impossible to accurately compare your practice to that of others, yet many surgeons measure their success by such criteria. It's easy to think that if you had his OR schedule, her office location, or his TV show credits, your practice would be flourishing.

In my opinion, competing with yourself is the only race that counts.

Looking over your shoulder at competitors provides a false perception of what others are doing and increases the likelihood that you'll miss what's going on in your own office. The fact is, you can't control what the plastic surgeon upstairs does or the dermatologist across the street is advertising he's now doing. But you can control—or should be able to control—your own practice. And heaven knows there's a lot to control right there: from staff attitudes to computerized records to the nuances of your consultations.

Here's an example: The competing physician starts offering free consultations—so you rush to match the tactic. Mistake! The better response is to focus on how you can more clearly articulate your value proposition to prospective patients. This, of course, entails some real effort on your part, such as meeting with your staff, developing a script, and rehearsing and monitoring the results. This targeted method will surprise you; it's a scalpel versus a wood saw approach. When implemented correctly, you'll see fewer patients, but you will actually *improve* your patient acceptance rate and schedule more surgeries. Less hassle, more revenue—what's not to like about that?

Laserlike approaches require time and attention to detail. Unfortunately, instead of investing the required time, many surgeons find it easier to fall into the TWEEID rut. Not familiar with that acronym? It stands for "that's what everyone else is doing." And it means you will never lead the pack, because you'll be in the middle of it. As the saying goes, "If you aren't the lead dog, the scenery never changes."

Successful surgeons benchmark against themselves by monitoring increases of new patients seen over last month, or last year. They carefully monitor not a so-called global conversion rate, but the actual number of patients, *by procedure,* who accept their surgical plans. Smart surgeons regularly review detailed reports and fine-tune daily practice operations. These

Continued

WHO IS YOUR BIGGEST COMPETITOR?—cont'd

"Most Likely to Succeed" surgeons know the number and names of patients who risk their personal reputation by referring family and friends to the practice. They worry and wonder when this number drops.

Successful surgeons innovate, their offices are unique, their consultations are differentiated, and they offer patients more time and better education. They write follow-up letters. They make their patients *feel special*—not just *look younger.*

The best physicians don't compare themselves to others. They've met their own challenges and professional goals by demanding the best of themselves and providing the best service, result, and care to their patients. Plastic surgeons truly interested in being successful realize that their biggest competitor is the one that greets them in the mirror every morning.

EVALUATING THE COMPETITION

It is worthwhile to evaluate all levels of competition. Through competitive studies you can define the competition specifically vying for your clients, and you can recognize potential partners.

To be competitive you must evaluate the competition's identity and operations, customers and business partners, their visibility to your target population, their image and brand, communication styles, endorsements, and promises. Defining target-specific competition doesn't mean going head to head; in any personal service business, especially aesthetic medicine, little good can come from directly attacking the competition in an effort to elevate one's own status or attract clients. Determining what makes competitors unique and attractive, what they offer and actually provide, how and where they communicate, and where they succeed and fail is essential so that you in turn can communicate your own brand and what makes it attractive to the target population. You must determine exactly what sets you apart from the competition to vie for potential clients in a shared target population.

Identifying the competition and comparing this information to your research on your target population are essential to uncover an untapped niche, recognize voids and saturation, model your brand, and recognize a potential partner. The best mutual partner is generally not your narrow competition;

you are too alike. The best partner would come from your secondary or extended competition. With the diversity of clients among different competitors, you are more likely to gain new clients/patients from your best possible source: referral from existing practice clients.

ACQUIRING THE COMPETITION

Daniel C. Mills, MD, FACS

Purchasing another physician's practice can be a smart defensive move, which is what I did early in my career. The retiring owner of the practice was a board-certified plastic surgeon with two offices, one a mile from my office and another 15 miles away. I wanted to avoid having another plastic surgeon come into my immediate area to prevent the further saturation of plastic surgeons in already physician-rich South Orange County, California. If I purchased that practice, it meant that another surgeon did not. My goal was not to go into his practice and continue in his steps; it was to familiarize myself with his patients and give them a chance to get to know me. His patient list was very valuable—it was a group of people who had already shown an interest in plastic surgery and would probably desire subsequent surgeries at some point. He had performed a significant number of breast implant surgeries, and I continue to see these patients as they need implant replacements. I did maintain a presence in his office for a few years as a way to establish a comfort level with his patients in an environment that was familiar to them. One of the most valuable aspects was to own and maintain his existing phone numbers, which I have to this day. Patients still call that number from cards they kept from appointments years ago.

Staying competitive also means I have had to continually evaluate my own practice and workload. I have been fortunate that my practice has grown over the years so that I am normally in the operating room every day. Once I got to the point where my own time limitations were inhibiting scheduling patients as quickly as they would like, it was time to branch out with physician extenders and consider a partner. About the time I started training PAs to perform laser procedures and injections, a medical spa came up for sale nearby, and I purchased that practice for many of the same reasons that I had purchased the plastic surgery practice. This addressed two issues for me: it allowed me to branch out with physician extenders so I could delegate treatment when possible, and it captured the physician's existing medical spa patients to educate them about plastic surgery procedures that they might be

Continued

ACQUIRING THE COMPETITION—cont'd

interested in. Again, as a defensive move it also blocked another physician from coming in and capturing those spa patients.

Adding a partner gave me another pair of hands to accomplish more surgery and provide a more balanced practice. I chose a partner who complements rather than competes with me. In evaluating what physician profile would best round out patient choice, I wanted to add a female surgeon to the practice. This has worked very well for me; there are some patients in Southern California who are adamant about wanting a female surgeon. Having a partner who captures those patients is bringing new patients to the practice who simply would not have considered me as their surgeon. It also brings a fresh, female perspective to my practice. Having a partner allows us to maintain our referral relationships with other physicians for reconstructive cases. My practice had become primarily cosmetic, and I didn't have enough hours in the day to also see all the reconstructive cases. Now we are able to provide both types of consultation and surgery. It is helpful to have economies of scale and share expenses while offering a wider array of choices for patients.

RELATIVE WISDOM: Against Yourself

I am competitive. I never want to let someone else do what I know I can. But there are times you simply should not try to compete.

My elder son Nicholas was 4 years old when he decided he wanted to learn to play football. Growing up with cousins and friends around me who played high school, college, and even professional ball, I was up to the task. My husband had only played soccer, and Nicholas didn't want a round ball; he wanted to learn to throw a perfect pigskin spiral. With my competitive nature, I had to prove I was a real boy's mom. I had to play football.

We had fun in the yard throwing and catching spirals. And then it happened. My prodigy became my competitor. I told Nicholas to throw a bomb, and he did. The result: Mom received a dislocated finger and torn tendons from a football thrown by a 4-year-old.

Relative wisdom: Many providers of aesthetic medicine are competitive in the same way: they never want to let someone else treat the patient they know they can. But if you are going to compete, be realistic about your intentions, subjects, limits, and the potential outcomes. By underestimating something as simple as a game of catch, you may find yourself not the conquering competitor, but the one sitting on the sidelines.

ABOVE THE CROWD

Businesses differ, and in some cases compete on the common variables of qualifications, image, experiences, outcomes, and price.

Qualifications

Qualifications are easily verified and compared; compete on qualifications only when yours are among the very best. There is no way to top having the very best qualifications. In many states, laws require that in advertising and public communications, physicians' qualifications be specifically defined by recognized board certification. But don't stop there: include recognized national, state, and local credentials, and international credentials if yours is an international market.

Image

Prestige, convenience, warmth, professionalism, access, options, complements, and amenities are just a few of the nuances that can distinguish your practice and define your image. You must recognize that your patients are looking for some, all, or none of the variables that define your image, and you have to accept that there are patients who won't relate to or be interested in your image. A wise competitor acknowledges that you cannot be all things to all people.

Experiences

The value of an experience is relative and subjective. Today your patient may be fulfilled by a weekend away with her girlfriends; tomorrow, her desire may be to look the youngest, the best among her friends. You can only compete with an experience if you know what your patients' true desires and motivations are, and if you can consistently meet them.

Outcomes

Demonstrating outcomes and making promises are two very different things. Ethics prohibits making promises about outcomes. Giving your prospective patient all the information necessary to weigh a decision reasonably is the only way to respond to a competitor's statements about outcomes.

Price

Don't compete on price, whether with other providers or yourself. Set a fee schedule and stick to it. Offer adjustments when warranted, such as for multiple procedures or repeat procedures. Define a policy for revisions and stand firm. Every time you respond to or adjust pricing, you set a precedent.

It's important to know who your competitors are, in general and for each specific patient (I don't mean other physicians; I mean other ways in which a patient may choose to spend dollars). It's valuable to know the level on which that competitor may be attracting your patients, or simply making you look less attractive to your patients. But it's not essential to go toe to toe; use competition to shape and define your own strategic moves, to improve your own practice, or to find new avenues to reach your patients. For example, if a corporate-run medical spa opens across town, with the advantages of bulk buying, resource sharing, and pervasive advertising, must you align yourself with the experience, price, or image they have in the marketplace to remain competitive? Not unless you are vying for the exact patient population with the same expectations of qualifications, outcomes, experience, and price. The value of studying the competition is to better understand your own best practices, not to continually look over your shoulder to outdistance the perceived competition.

Unexpected Competition

Restricted access to your services as a result of economic or regulatory forces can also present an obstacle. For example, the vanity taxes proposed in some states or communities on cosmetic procedures could force providers bordering other states or communities to adjust prices to account for the incremental increase, or simply deal with the expense of moving.

Regulation can inhibit or restrict one's ability to practice aesthetic medicine as you have thus far known it. Whether requiring strict supervision of nonphysicians, limiting or defining the scope of practice for nonphysicians, or enforcing stricter safety practices for treatment or surgery, regulation is evolving in the field of aesthetic medicine. If you've followed best practices all along, you should welcome regulation, because it will only inhibit the competition, not you.

IN PRACTICE: Price Wars

I am often asked how practices should respond to patient questions about meeting low, widely advertised pricing on aesthetic treatments, such as Botox injections or breast implants.

I was visiting a practice and a young, nervous woman was booking her surgery. "I really want this doctor to perform my surgery," she said, "but will you match the price another doctor advertises on the radio?"

The surgeon was speechless, so I chimed in: "We are a practice that does not need or accept patients based on advertising. Our practice has a proven and consistent record of outcomes, happy patients, and fair prices. We want to fulfill your goals, and we know we can. Before you make your decision, I want you to think about this: each time you look in the mirror or you are in an intimate moment, do you want to be happy with what you see and who you are, or do you want to risk the constant regrettable reminder that you decided to save a few dollars on your body and your appearance?" The young woman left, and the surgeon was furious with me because he felt he had lost this patient. Two hours later, she called and booked the procedure.

This is a clear example of competing, or trying to, on one simple variable. It is a bad idea, because it not only sets a precedent, it also devalues your entire image.

In that same practice I encountered another breast augmentation patient for whom the practice offered a "referral" discount. I asked what that meant. "She was referred to the doctor by another patient of the practice, so we offer a discount," the office manager stated. Then I asked, "How will that referring patient feel to know her friend was charged less than she was? That's quite a way nasty way of saying 'thank you for the referral.'"

I asked the doctor about the policy of referral discount. "I don't do it all the time; only when it is warranted," he stated. I asked what warranted a discount, and in this case he stated that it was the referral by a prior patient. He still didn't understand.

So I tried to make it relative: "You go to Café Fabuloso once a week and have your favorite meal: drinks, dinner, dessert. It is your jaunt. You have dinner and pay the bill in full. No complimentary dessert, no free bottle of wine. Nothing. You send a colleague to Café Fabuloso, and he calls you with overwhelming thanks. It was the best meal ever. They asked for the waiter you suggested, and the waiter gave them a complementary cocktail because you, his best customer, referred them."

The doctor replied, "That would make me angry; I am the one who has given them loyalty and a new patron. I deserve the perks." Lesson learned: Don't compete on price with others or with yourself.

COMPETITOR OR PARTNER?

Competing entails much more than finding your most successful competitor and trying to do it better. It involves more than providing better service, a better price, a better experience, or greater value. It is all of these things, but it also requires that you remain true to who you are, engage in ethical practices, and make smart business decisions.

Many medical specialties, especially those involving very lucrative non-payor aesthetic services, have claimed ownership of certain procedures. By doing so they have drawn a line in the sand among the specialties as a group and among the individual providers who are members of these groups. But are these different specialties truly competitors, or can they be partners? Consider the plastic surgeon or dermatologist, the cosmetic dentist who is beginning a practice or retooling an existing one. If the physician partners with someone of the same specialty, they can share resources, enhance knowledge and skills, and work together to grow the practice, providing the exact same services. However, this can create direct competition and conflict within the confines of one practice.

Complements

If two complementary (secondary or extended) competitors team up, they have multiple advantages that go beyond the operational savings of practicing in partnership. They have a single, unique brand that is attractive to different levels of clients' desires and capable of fulfilling these desires. Together they are able to attract a larger pool of prospective patients than they might individually.

Patient retention may also be enhanced by complementary partnering. Over time, a dermatologic patient may want more comprehensive treatment through plastic surgery. Following plastic surgery, a patient may wish to maintain the results through skin treatment. In both instances patient retention is established among a complementary team, and the patient benefits through cooperative care that offers convenience, comfort, and familiarity.

Such a practice is more likely to create a client source through someone who is satisfied with, educated about, and willing to endorse your unique brand to others through referral, and this is more likely to broaden the client source to all specialties of the practice.

I did not invent the concept, but I do fully endorse it: build your client base by building your practice with complements—providers who, when not practicing with you, are among your most highly regarded secondary and extended competitors. You need not practice with them; you can network, cross-promote, and refer to each other. So long as the common goal and the rules competition are defined, partnering with your competitors can be a mutually productive endeavor.

SECTION II
What

*Your practice exists for one simple reason—service.
What differentiates you from others is the means,
method, and meticulous manner by which you
extend aesthetic medicine to others.*

CHAPTER 5

What Is Your Identity?

There is nothing worse than a brilliant image of a fuzzy concept.
— ANSEL ADAMS

When a brand and image do not exist, the only thing that differentiates one product or service from the next is price. Competing on price can be detrimental when health, safety, and fulfilling the most personal desires of others are at stake.

Brand, image, and *mission* are three very strong marketing concepts that collectively identify you. These involve those nuances that set you apart from anyone or anything else competing for your client's and your market's attention.

WHAT IS YOUR BRAND?

Brand is the name, words, or imprimatur that labels your practice as unique. Branding also defines you by your specialty, credentials, and the services your practice provides. It includes the following:

- Added professional training, or the skills and services provided. Examples include treating skin of color, treating children, added certification in minimally invasive techniques or laser procedures, research, and training leadership—all the things beyond title and board certification that define you or your staff as medical professionals.

- Special personal training, skills, or interests, such as fluency in a foreign language, philanthropic care, personal experiences, and communication skills.

- Added certification or accreditation of the staff, office, and treatment and surgical facilities.

- Affiliations, memberships, privileges, and leadership among recognized local, regional, and national medical societies, peer groups, educational institutions, and philanthropic organizations.

Your brand is your name as well as all the things that define your business and that people accept about your business. Nike, Lexus, Armani, Starbucks, Tylenol, and Restylane are all names that are so strongly branded that we know these are shoes, cars, Italian clothing, coffee, pain relievers, and an aesthetic injection, even though these brands include no language that defines the product. Bavarish Motorwerks (BMW) is a brand that clearly conveys that this is a German vehicle, yet most of us simply refer to it by its initials.

In the practice of medicine, branding has been called *marketing on steroids.* You probably don't have the resources or the need to build a brand as strong as mass-market consumer leaders do, but you do need to have a defining, consistent name by which you are identified. You need a brand that is consistent in words and design (colors, typestyle, and format) each time and in each place you are identified. Your brand may be:

- *Your name:* Richard Richards, MD

- *A name that defines your services:* Dermatology and Plastic Surgery Associates; Aesthetic Medical Spa; Deluxe Laser Center; Smile Institute

- *Relative to your geography:* Aesthetic Center of Bigville; South Central Associates; Island Aesthetics

- *Any combination of these:* Richards Dermatology and Plastic Surgery; Richards Aesthetic Center of Bigville; Island Aesthetics and Smile Institute

- *Evocative:* Be Beautiful Plastic Surgery; Perfection Medical Spa

- *None of the above:* Auroraborialium

Your brand may need to define several different providers, services, or concepts. It must be strong enough to identify you, to allow people to easily find you, and to endure throughout your career. It must also be flexible enough to evolve with changes in your practice over time, without diminishing the value of the brand or dramatically changing it.

RELATIVE WISDOM: Brand Matters

Changing a business's name will not change its mistakes. A self-professed aesthetic provider was the focus of a television reporter's investigation into providers marketing dangerous and unproven fat-melting injections. The result of this investigation affected not only this provider's business for these injections but also his overall operation, and deservedly put him out of business. He was exposed as unqualified, simply driven by dollars, and his practices dangerous. In a short time he closed his doors.

Four months later, using his wife's surname, he opened his business once again, not only offering the same unproven treatments and poor-quality care, but also marketing them extensively with his very distinct accent that had been heard on radio commercials run for his previous practice, and these were once again airing regularly.

Four months later, his doors were permanently closed, and he moved out of town. There was no business for him to be found anywhere.

Relative wisdom: Your brand is more than your name. It is a definition you will carry with you, no matter what transgressions or transitions you make.

COOKIE-CUTTER BRANDING

There are many opportunities to present your practice to the world. The Internet has become one of the most omnipresent places where practices are showcased and branded. Cookie-cutter branding is a process by which a service (whether a directory, a referral source, or a prix fixe Internet site, among others) groups all participants by specialty. You are simply one of several predefined, equally packaged options and images presented to prospective patients. The only thing that distinguishes you in this type of program is your picture and small phrases or words within the branding package.

Before investing in such services, ask yourself:

- How will I stand out among countless other providers branded in the same way by this service?

- Am I forced to comply with specific practices that influence my image, such as online consultations, free consultations, or preset prices for consultations or services?

- What does the image of this service do to my image?

- How does the image of other providers with whom I am packaged affect my image?

- What is the true return on cookie-cutter branding—will the prospective patients who seek me out through this contact point become qualified, valuable, and desirable patients?

Cookie-cutter branding doesn't stop there: it also entails consultants, services, and programs that don't allow you the flexibility to personalize the very visible images and information that shape the unique identity that should be yours alone.

WHAT IS YOUR IMAGE?

Image involves the nuances that individualize you as a professional as well as your practice. It is a combination of appearance, personality, communication style, values, amenities, and the credibility and ethics you convey. Image is how you are seen by others, and how you are characterized. Image is conveyed by many things, and can be interpreted, accepted, or rejected by your market and your patients simply by how this image is presented:

- Is the phone answered by a friendly voice ready to help, or by an automated system?

- Are your forms and consents generic, revised, or inconsistent-looking copies? Or are they clear and consistent in content, style, and brand? Are they completely electronic?

- Are you dressed in casual comfort, perfectly tailored tasteful business wear, or dated duds? Or do you greet your patients dressed as though you are headed to a baron's ball?

- Is your practice setting quiet and comfortable, sterile and functional, or chaotic and loud? Is it crowded with clutter, art, furniture, equipment, walls of diplomas and awards, and racks of brochures? Or is it tastefully appointed and organized, private and welcoming? Have you built an inviting center with waterfalls, scented towels, valet parking, and private concierges?

- Do you and your staff make eye contact with patients and treat them as individuals, or do you simply listen, reply perfunctorily, and move on?

- Do you follow up with your patients, no matter how small or large their goals and procedures, or do you assume they will contact you if they need to?

Clearly, some of these image-defining details result in significant faux pas in life and in practice. But consider this: electronic forms may be welcomed by a younger, computer-literate population but could be an obstacle to older, less technology-savvy patients or those with no desire to use electronics. In some markets, a casually dressed doctor is too casual; in others, a doctor in a suit may seem intimidating. If parking is a problem at your location, valet parking may be necessary, but in other locations it may convey an ostentation that patients sense will inevitably be part of the fees they pay. Some patients may be knowledgeable enough to know when or if to follow up; others may want and need repeated contact. Define your image by who you are, by your patients' needs and expectations, and by what is accepted in your market.

WHAT IS YOUR MISSION?

The fact that you have the ability to treat patients with aesthetic medicine is essential, but equally important is how you and your practice carry that out. It is important to take the time to compose a mission statement, which identifies what you as a provider expect of yourself. It reflects the responsibility you take and the expectations you set for your brand. It also addresses your relationship to your community, peers, students, and staff. Your mission statement may be a single line, or it may be a detailed credo.

To address your role in providing the personal appearance desires of clients and patients by ability alone overlooks the source for your relationship with your patient: personal desire. Fulfilling a patient's personal desire requires making a direct personal connection. Accordingly, part of your mission must be to make that connection with potential clients or patients. It need not be conveyed in every communication that represents your office, but the tone it sets must be consistent with your image and brand.

 RELATIVE WISDOM: The Sixth Diamond

Consistently meeting or exceeding expectations breeds loyalty, an indispensable asset to any business.

The hotel business has a lot of diversity in service models. But two hotel chains, the Ritz Carlton and Four Seasons, claim the greatest retention among patrons. In fact, after 9/11, when New York hotels rooms were deserted, Four Seasons and the Ritz Carlton kept their normal, brisk pace of occupancy. Why the success?

These branded firms pride themselves on their service models and their mission. In fact, Ritz Carlton offers a training academy for service individuals in other businesses to learn the Ritz way, defined by their credo, motto, the three steps of service, their 12-point service values, employee promise, and more. Although hotels are commonly rated by diamonds, five being the most, the Ritz Carlton reminds the ladies and gentleman who are part of the Ritz Carlton team that there is a sixth diamond: "mystique, emotional engagement, and functional."

Ritz Carlton knows how important every visitor is, from adults traveling on business to families on vacation. Regardless of the economic conditions, the reason for travel, location, or time of year, their service model never fails to meet or exceed expectations.

Relative wisdom: Service is your business; therefore a service mission statement is essential. Your patients may not read it, but they will in fact experience, appreciate, and expect it.

🥢 IN PRACTICE: Mission Accomplished

A physician was determined to bring her practice to the next level, to create an image, a brand that was uniquely personal, private, and accommodating, with a mission to provide an experience that always put the patient's physical, emotional, and social comfort first.

She invested a great deal in the words, policies, and training that shaped her staff and conveyed to her patients the exact identity she was proud to define. These efforts were exceptional. The problem: she simply did not and could not deliver. The doctor called me, unable to understand why her efforts were not working. Aesthetic patients were simply not comfortable, not accepting treatment.

After spending a day at the office I identified the obstacle to achieving the brand she desired: in the mix of aesthetic patients she saw a number of children in need of serious clinical care. A woman wishing to improve an aging appearance might regularly encounter a child with a severe cleft lip in the office. Many people are uncomfortable around someone with a deformity; they don't know how to respond, or even where to look. "I won't give up treating those children," she told me. "I pride myself on serving those in need as much as serving those with wants." I agreed.

The solution: She revised her schedule so that aesthetic patients and pediatric patients were seen on different days, and she had a second entrance put in that was more child friendly. Decorative covered baskets in each examination room contained toys to keep the children busy. Elegant binders on side tables contained aesthetic practice information, and complementary bright binders contained pediatric information. Staff were given the added duty each night to "turn the rooms" with a few minor amenities from pediatric to aesthetic, and staff members even had different dress guidelines for aesthetic and pediatric days. The change and commitment to this new identity were so successful that the doctor's practice grew, and soon there was such demand for aesthetic services that she was preparing to hire an associate and expand her office.

WHAT DEFINES YOU?

Some may find that the most personal and difficult task in developing their business plan is defining their identity: precisely articulating their brand, characterizing their desired image, and drafting a sincere mission statement. This task is difficult only if you set out to create an ideal model rather than a realistic, achievable objective. Even providers fresh out of a fellowship and beginning practice have a basis for brand, image, and mission; they are not starting from scratch. Nuances that help shape one's identity may be learned from mentors, formed by experience, or fully defined by your skills and personality.

Defining your practice must begin with what exists; then you build on your strengths, identify and correct weaknesses, and revamp where necessary. Do not create a model and define yourself by it; define yourself first, then shape a model that enhances and elevates your definition and addresses the needs of those you serve.

CHAPTER 6

What Is Your Model?

In business, a successful model is not one fashioned after someone or something; it is a sincere expression of your desire for operational perfection.

A service model is more than a menu of the treatments and procedures you provide. It involves the manner and setting in which you, or those who work for or with you, provide them and how you address what you don't offer. It's the amenities you offer or the convenience and access you provide for your patients. In short, a service model is the simplest means of defining a complex set of medical and business definitions.

MEDICAL MODELS: DEFINING YOUR MEDICAL PRACTICE

Your practice may be classified by one or a combination of the definitions of medical practices:

- *Core:* You provide the exact services defined by your core training. You are dedicated and limited specifically to the scope of your specialty. There is no ratio of clinical to aesthetic services; you offer them all.

- *Clinical:* Your focus is on the medically necessary services related to your specialty. You are dedicated to physical healing, such as treating skin cancer.

- *Restorative/reconstructive:* You perform medically necessary or reimbursed procedures that enable your patient to restore a more normal appearance or function, such as breast or post-tumor reconstruction.

- *Cosmetic/aesthetic:* Your practice specializes in elective medical services that improve, enhance, or change personal appearance. You are dedicated to medical solutions that address the physical and emotional needs of your patients.

- *Surgical:* A portion of your medical services is dedicated to surgical solutions, whether in your accredited on-site facility, an ambulatory center, or a hospital.

- *Nonsurgical:* You provide patients with treatments that are medical and do not require more invasive surgical intervention.

- *Academic:* You are involved in the teaching and training of others in your core specialty.

- *Research:* You investigate, explore, experiment, and define new procedures, devices, products, techniques, or theories.

- *Military:* All or a portion of your time is dedicated to providing medical service to the men and women who serve in the armed forces and their families.

- *Multispecialty:* You offer related or unrelated specialty medical services.

- *Multiphysician:* Same-specialty, complementary, or unrelated-specialty medical providers practice with you.

- *Multidisciplinary:* A variety of related or unrelated services are blended in the same practice environment, such as aesthetics, bariatrics, and counseling.

- *Retail:* Products that are required or that enhance or extend your services are sold to your patients.

- *Spa:* Services are provided in a luxurious and sybaritic environment. NOTE: You don't need to call your practice a spa to surround your patients with warmth, comfort, and pleasure.

These are the medical models that shape a large portion of your practice, but you are not wholly defined by these options. The medical model, along with your business model, outlines the structure of your practice. It is the mission through which you execute your medical and business model that will distinguish you, attract patients, and fulfill their experiential and aesthetic needs.

BUSINESS MODELS

Business models in aesthetic medicine are changing, but interestingly, it is the traditional models that endure.

Sole Proprietor

You are on your own, and you own your practice. Anyone who works with you works for you. You are, theoretically and legally, the practice/business owner; all liability is yours. This is the most common business model for aesthetic providers today, and with good reason: as the CEO you set the tone, control what you wish, empower others as you see fit, are responsible individually for the success or failure of your endeavor, and can make decisions freely. You alone define the tone and enforce it, create a careful balance between oversight and micromanagement, and serve equally as physician and business owner. Weakness in either area will reflect on and affect the practice as a whole.

Partner

You and one or more providers are joint owners of some portion of the practice. You theoretically and legally share the burden of debt and risk, responsibility, and resources. Because the practice of aesthetic medicine is a competitive field and involves ego for both patients and providers, successful long-term partnerships are rare: few can find the careful definition and balance to work together harmoniously to serve a like population and like needs, unless they complement one another in training and management styles. Defining not only the individual scope of service, but also the individual leadership, management, and resource contributions to the practice is fundamental to any partnership agreement, whether the relationship was entered into from the outset or evolved from an employment or contractual agreement. The partnership model is becoming increasingly popular when the partners are from different core specialties and their practice together enhances the scope of services, such as a plastic or facial plastic surgeon and a dermatologist.

Employee

In this model you work for someone, whether another physician, a university, or a corporation; you do not own the practice. Your authority, responsibility, and scope, fees, goals, productivity, and limits are defined by your employer. An employment situation may find you with an employer who is familiar with and respects your practice in aesthetics, or it could place you in a situation that exploits your credentials. Choose your employer as carefully as you would a partner.

Satellite

Where you practice is the extension of your business model. A satellite offers aesthetic services at a secondary location, such as a fitness club, spa, salon, hotel, resort, or retail site. The primary business location/medical practice, academic setting, or hospital practice fully oversees and sets the standards for a satellite, based on the model and mission of the primary business.

Contractor

Various contractual models exist, but essentially a contractor practices as an independent provider of medicine within another medical practice or another business entity such as a hospital, fitness club, spa, salon, hotel, resort, retail outlet, or consortium.

Time-Share

In a time-share structure, you are in a solo practice or partnership and share resources, such as office space and employees, with another business entity. There was a time when that business entity was another medical practice. Today it may also be a wellness center, hospital, fitness club, spa, salon, hotel, resort, or retail outlet.

Supervision

In a supervisory model, you oversee the services of others as a function of employment. Today there are a number of aesthetic medical centers with owner-operators who are not physicians; physicians are hired by the owners to supervise or direct. Where the physician can and does have absolute control of the legitimacy, safety, and appropriateness to which procedures are recommended and delivered, supervision can enhance a practice. Where it exists simply to lend legitimacy to an otherwise unqualified nonmedical model providing aesthetic services, it is an accident waiting to happen, and you may end up with blood on your hands, despite never having had your hands on the business.

Corporate

You are the employee of a corporation that provides medical services. Today corporate medicine defines a practice of medicine exclusive to the delivery of service to a predefined set of executives in a time, manner, and place that does not disrupt their ability to do business.

Franchise

As a participant in a franchise practice, you are invested in or work for a model that has set principles for brand, image, mission, and providing service. CAVEAT: Aesthetic medicine is a very personal endeavor, whereas fast food models of service are meant for the masses. In this model, startup costs can be high, and you will likely be required to carry certain products and meet corporate quotas of productivity.

Concierge

A new business model for many different service-based industries, concierge models are based more on a delivery model than a medical business model. This model dictates that every need, desire, and whim of the patient be delivered, whether this involves arranging for an elite postoperative recovery experience, or delivery of requested meals, massages, or manicures during the patient's recovery period at home.

༄

Who will decide how you will define, refine, or evolve your aesthetic practice model? Any number of people and conditions have influence: teachers and mentors, spouses and family, peers and competitors, demographic and economic factors, partners, employers, advisors, and employees, and even banks, lawyers, regulators, and insurers. Trends may intrigue you or dissuade you. Traditional models may seem limiting. There is no one answer, but by carefully examining your options and marketplace and defining your goals, you can find an answer that works for today and has the flexibility to endure or readily change for the future.

🌿 IN PRACTICE: What Should I Do? It's Your Decision

I visited a practice that included a 15-year veteran of aesthetics and a young provider who had recently been hired. The veteran was hopeful that the new provider would help provide care to a busy stream of patients. The new provider was energized about the opportunity to hang a shingle and become an integral part of the practice. The veteran asked me, "What should I do?" in terms of defining and offering the young doctor an opportunity to grow into a partnership relationship. The young doctor also asked, "What should I do?" He pondered whether the offer was competitive, good for him in the short and long term, fair, and attainable.

A doctor in private practice for nearly a decade, hit hard by the struggling economy, was offered a chance to oversee a large chain of corporate-run medical spas. "What should I do?" he asked. The money was good, there seemed to be little definition to his responsibility, and a lot of limitation to his ability.

A doctor limited by a large multispecialty group realized that his patients weren't getting the attention he wanted them to have amid a vast array of clinical and aesthetic patients. "What should I do?" he asked. Go off on his own and try to revise operations to meet his aesthetic patients' needs, or simply deal with the situation at hand?

Throughout your career there will be times when you wonder, "What should I do?" Mentors, advisors, consultants, books, and lectures are available to put things in perspective, to offer advice even if it may be unpopular, and to help define strategies and carry out plans. But the decisions that determine how you will apply your credentials and your skills in medicine and in business must be your own.

I've learned from the wisdom of others, and I've asked, "What should I do?" many times in life. Nevertheless, when it comes to decision-making, "What should I do?" begs the following advice:

1. *It's your decision, not mine.* Listen to and evaluate the advice you are given. Weigh the motivation, bias, experience, and credibility of the source. However, you must decide.

2. *Every decision needs a plan.* Advice may help you to arrive at a decision, but how will you carry it out? Define the process by which you must arrive at a decision. Others may help you in devising your strategy, but you must implement and sustain it.

3. *Yes-men are followers, not advisors.* Do not seek the advice of others to qualify your decision. Advisors and consultants who simply agree with you, who won't provoke you to think deeply or play devil's advocate, are not useful to your process. Seek the counsel of those who will push your decision-making to include logical but far-reaching options.

SERVICE MODELS

A brand, image, and mission are useful and successful only when they communicate and honestly embrace the practice's operations. Building or retooling identity and service models congruently has greater value than creating one to fit the other.

Without question, the operations of any medical practice or practice segment must uphold specific standards in safety, ethics, and privacy. Aesthetic practices are characterized by an even greater need for patient privacy and for the added amenities of comfort, individual attention, and positive support. For an aesthetic or cosmetic procedure, treatment is desired, but not essential. Although treatments may create temporary pain for patients, produce stress, anxiety, and even fear, a successfully run aesthetic practice will create a positive, encouraging environment that does not discount these responses. The patient's entire experience as well as the treatment outcome will define a successful aesthetic practice, one where honesty, education, and sensory and emotional comfort are the core of medical and personal services and retail complements.

The Operational Trilogy

Any aesthetic practice must look at operations as three distinct entities:

1. Medical services

2. Personal services

3. Retail

Each facet of the operational trilogy has a distinct function, individual goals in fulfilling patient needs, and a unique contribution to revenue. Although each can stand alone, it is the synergy among the three operational segments that creates the greatest value.

MEDICAL SERVICES

The medical treatment a practice provides, who the providers are, and where treatment is provided characterize medical services. Your skill and care and that of your clinical staff and supporting staff represent the character of your clinical operations. The office, surgical facility, and postoperative care provided represent the comfort of your operations. In an aesthetic practice the focus of care rests on ability as much as on the basics of character and comfort:

- How and where do you conduct consultations?

- Who is your patient support advocate?

- Where are diagnostic tests performed and how?

- What is the consent protocol?

- What is the preoperative protocol?

- Where is the operating room? Is it under your operational control, or are you using space in a larger facility?

- Who administers anesthesia, and who provides preoperative, surgical, recovery, and postoperative care?

Fully examine all facets of clinical operations, in your office and off-site. You should find congruence in your brand, image, and mission. How you deliver services to each patient progressively builds an expectation that you must meet or exceed, not just for one treatment, but every time he or she is treated. Quite simply, aesthetic medicine is not a linear process, where the relationship begins when the patient engages you for desired treatment and ends with a positive clinical outcome. The relationship is cyclical for two distinct reasons:

- Nonsurgical treatments, what is commonly called *cosmetic medicine,* must be repeated to produce or maintain results, and this may lead to a request for aesthetic surgery as the individual continues in the patient cycle. If you cannot fulfill or maintain the treatments, you have broken the cycle and you will lose the patient.

- Happy patients are your best source for success and growth. Keeping happy patients in an active cycle maintains your visibility with them and reminds them of the value of your services. This will bring the patients back to you for different or added services, or they will refer others to you who will keep your relationship and the service cycle growing.

THE EVOLUTION AND IMPORTANCE OF COSMETIC MEDICINE

Renato Saltz, MD, FACS

Seismic changes are shaking up the field of cosmetic surgery and cosmetic medicine. The globalization of beauty, changing demographics, cultural preferences, patient demands, and advances in technology are converging to shape and transform a burgeoning aesthetic marketplace. For plastic surgeons these developments are having a major impact on the way we practice. We face a changing patient population as baby boomers increasingly seek cosmetic enhancements. We are also subject to a number of pressures from the media, the cosmetic industry, and from patients who want optimal results with minimal downtime.

These trends mandate change. They require us to reevaluate the way we do business and to grasp the big picture. Today the number of nonsurgical

Continued

THE EVOLUTION AND IMPORTANCE OF COSMETIC MEDICINE—cont'd

cosmetic procedures performed is experiencing explosive growth, far out-pacing that of traditional surgical procedures. Aesthetic surgeons can no longer afford to ignore the growing importance that nonsurgical cosmetic procedures play in aesthetic surgery practices. All our surveys and industry statistics indicate the importance of recognizing and adapting to the new trends that are sweeping our specialty. For plastic surgeons practicing cosmetic surgery in today's competitive environment, cosmetic medicine offers exciting options for practice growth and patient retention. By incorporating cosmetic medicine into our practices we can appeal to a broader range of patients over the long term. We have the professionalism, training, and ability to be the entry portal for patients seeking cosmetic treatments and the data to substantiate safe outcomes through our services.

The key is to view aesthetic surgery as a continuum in which nonsurgical cosmetic treatments provide an opportunity to establish a relationship with a patient that will lead to more invasive surgical rejuvenation as the patient ages. Thus it is crucial for us to understand the forces that are shaping our specialty, to plan the best way to embrace them, and to find a way to incorporate cosmetic medicine treatments into our daily practices. The only question is how to accomplish this goal in an efficient, effective, and financially viable manner.

RELATIVE WISDOM: Luxury Brands

The principles of luxury marketing state that once consumers are introduced to and satisfied with a certain level of service or quality in a product, they will become loyal. Luxury marketing has little to do with labels or a high price; it requires value, satisfaction, and consistency.

I have a difficult time buying shoes because my feet are narrow. Salespeople have always tried to convince me that something will fit, even though regular sizes don't. Several years ago a patient salesman suggested that I consider buying Prada, a little better quality and pricier shoe that he believed would be the right fit for me. It was perfect. I loved the style and fit. And I quickly learned the lesson of luxury loyalty: from that point on I always turned to Prada, or that salesman, for my shoe selections. But it didn't stop there: I also looked to this brand for other products that would offer the same quality.

Relative wisdom: Prada is a luxury brand, and your brand is also a luxury brand; it defines a nonessential service and a want fulfilled. Fill you customer's needs and wants precisely, give them the right fit, the right style, and the right result—consistently. Give them value, every time, every visit, every purchase. Start small with an injection or skin care service and they will consistently come back for more. They will expand the services they trust you to provide. They will bring new customers to you. All the result of complete satisfaction.

When I wrote the first edition of this book, nonsurgical procedures and treatments were burgeoning. Since that time they have continued to evolve, serving as an entry point and introducing consumers to aesthetic medicine. If you look carefully at the models of aesthetic medicine today, you will find:

- Purely surgical practices are rare; generally these are highly specialized and limited in the range of surgical procedures performed.

- Aesthetic surgical practices nearly always offer cosmetic injections. According to a 2008 survey by the Physicians Coalition for Injectable Safety, 69% of aesthetic surgeons (board-certified plastic, facial plastic, or oculoplastic) perform injections in their practices themselves.

- Nonsurgical procedures are outnumbering surgical procedures nearly 4.5 to 1, according to the 2008 annual statistics of the American Society for Aesthetic Plastic Surgery.

- The increase in popularity of and demand for nonsurgical procedures and the nature of their delivery has created the need for physician extenders: licensed physician assistants, nurse practitioners, registered nurses, and aestheticians who administer treatments prescribed by the physician.

PHYSICIAN EXTENDERS

Clinical staff play an important role in your practice, but whether these individuals will support you when you provide treatment or carry out the treatments you prescribe is something you must carefully determine. In doing so, you must take into account the regulatory requirements in your community or state and the liability definitions and restrictions defined by your risk-management insurance carrier while respecting the practice and ethical guidelines of your specialty.

Internally, you must also define specific service requirements of your physician extenders:

- Training in technique and your practice's method of delivering treatment, communicating with patients, maintaining records, and providing follow-up

- Supervision requirements

- Restrictions and covenants to your extenders' ability to practice outside your medical practice and to prevent them from taking your patients' private information if they leave your practice

Physician extenders can be a valuable addition to your practice model when carefully selected, trained, and integrated into your team and when given clear protocols and guidelines. Physician extenders who act autonomously within your practice or outside it are clearly not beneficial to you or your patients.

DEFINING THE RULES AND ROLES FOR PHYSICIAN EXTENDERS

Marian D. O'Hagan, RN, BSN

The success of any practice hinges on all staff members understanding and respecting their jobs. It is therefore essential that the nurse/technician have a job description and understand it. Education and understanding are cornerstones to professionals correctly performing aesthetic treatments.

While performing laser/light treatments for a successful dermatologist, I have gained an excellent understanding of how the interpersonal dynamics and logistics should work in a well-oiled office. In addition, as the senior clinical training specialist for a leading laser/light company, I have observed many offices across the United States and Canada. Offices that are affiliated with dermatologists and plastic surgeons generally have a clearer understanding of lasers, intense pulsed light (IPL), and skin physiology. They are also generally on-site when patients are evaluated and when treatments take place. This understanding of the technology and physiology helps their patients attain the results they seek.

Physicians who act as off-site medical directors should be present when treatments are performed. This helps build trust among patients, correctly diagnosis the problem and discuss treatment options with their patients. It allows them to discuss realistic outcomes to their patients. When this information is passed on to skilled professionals, the patient benefits and the practice grows. In all offices, doctors need to be available for questions that the nurse or patient might want to ask. The nurse/technician must have a clear understanding of physics and not be afraid to ask questions. Dialog and open communication are essential between professionals.

It has been my experience that the more successful practices have physicians and nurse/technicians that work as a team, both respecting the other's importance. A nurse/technician can help build that trust by performing treatments with excellence and compassion and thereby contribute significantly to the growth of the practice. Doctors need to choose physician extenders who are willing to follow protocols. Professionals need to be willing to listen and learn about the technology they are entrusted with using. Ultimately, the physician and his nurse/technician must work together to have a successful relationship for the good of their patients.

Physicians must have confidence in the nurse to perform the treatment they prescribe. This confidence has to be passed on to the patient. At the same time, the nurse needs to have a strong understanding of the technology being used on the patient. It is his or her responsibility to become more educated about the equipment and technology. It is also important for the physician to encourage and financially assist the nurse to attend informational meetings and workshops.

I have also been in offices in which the physicians believe they know everything about the technology and don't really listen to what I, as a trainer who has used laser/IPL technology for 12 years, have to say. Once they realize I'm educated in the field, they are the first ones to want further information. They should have that same confidence in their own nurse/technician. Office dynamics plays a very important role. I believe doctors want what's best for their patients. An educated, supervised nurse/technician can be a great asset to any office.

🐝 IN PRACTICE: Just My Friends

He was a very high–profile physician with multiple offices and a constantly full schedule. He was in demand for injections, laser treatments, and skin care, and with good reason: his results were excellent, he had great rapport with patients, and the practice setting was an upscale clinical but comfortable environment. He was so busy that it was time to hire an extender, because patients were having to wait too long for appointments. He hired someone from the outside, because he considered his current staff to be too valuable assisting him. He didn't want to train any one of them to perform injections and then have to hire a new person to assist him.

After months of the "right" person on board, a woman who had performed injections at a medical spa for some time and claimed a following of her own she could bring to the practice, he noticed his injectable business was steady, but his purchases of neurotoxins and dermal fillers were disproportionately high. After careful accounting, in fact there was a great disparity. Product was either being wasted or stolen, because the numbers just didn't match. After investigation and questioning, the nurse-injector admitted, "I've been taking product home to inject at my home, but they are just my friends." Stunned, the doctor did not how to respond. I did.

The next day the nurse-injector arrived at work to find the police waiting to arrest her for theft. She had been stealing medical product. Later, she would be charged with practicing medicine without a license: none of the "friends" she had been injecting were patients of the practice, nor did she obtain informed consent, and she did not maintain charts on them.

The lesson here: Lay down the law with physician extenders. Most are ethical, responsible individuals who understand their value and role in your practice.

NEVER ON A SUNDAY . . .

The physician's busy core practice was adjacent to her busy skin spa. Her office was open Monday through Thursday; the skin spa was additionally open on Friday, Saturday, and Sunday. The office had one phone number, the skin spa another. On Friday, Saturday, and Sunday, if a prospective patient called the practice, that patient had to leave a message to be returned on

Monday. The physician was eager to grow the traffic to her office and new skin spa, but strangely, this arrangement didn't seem to bother her or her staff, nor did they realize the impact it had on potential new patients.

I asked the physician about her staff: were they unique to each entity, or were they familiar with and working in both the practice and the skin spa? "We are fully integrated," she told me.

"How often do people call the practice and get transferred to the skin spa?"

"Every day."

"What happens to the people who call the practice Friday, Saturday, or Sunday wanting to reach the skin spa?"

"They leave a message."

"When are the messages reviewed?"

"Monday."

"How many spa messages do you get?"

"Almost none."

I offered an experiment. For 1 week, staff were to forward the practice calls to the skin spa when the skin spa was open and the office was closed. If the call was not related to the skin spa, the patient was to be connected to the core practice's voice mail. If the call was urgent, the staff member was to act on the patient's needs (staff were fully integrated). If it was related to the skin spa, the staff member was to act accordingly and keep a count of precisely how many calls went to the practice, intended for the spa on Friday, Saturday, and Sunday.

One week later, the physician called me, beside herself: "We had 22 calls come in on Friday alone that were intended for the spa that were going to the practice. I need better yellow pages ads, I need clearer information on my website, and I need to advertise that the spa has its own number."

"No, you don't," I told her. "The people calling the skin spa are calling because they know you and the reputation of your practice, and they have connected to it. You've created a strong brand for yourself, and the skin spa is related to your brand. You don't need more messaging to distinguish the two; you need consistent service that serves both."

The physician disagreed with me but agreed to use her staff resources already at work rather than expend more resources for marketing for 2 months; then she would report back to me regarding the traffic. Two months later I heard nothing. Two weeks after that, I called her. "Sorry for not following up," she told me. "We are so busy at both the practice and the skin spa that I didn't have time to let you know it's working beautifully, and it didn't cost me an extra dime."

*I think it's very important that whatever you're trying
to make or sell or teach has to be basically good. A bad product
and you know what? You won't be here in 10 years.*

— MARTHA STEWART

Personal Service

You are a physician. The services you provide are of a highly personal nature. In some cases, you may even provide nonmedical personal services. No matter which model you use for your practice, however, the principles followed in personal service industries are essential to your patients' experience and overall satisfaction. Personal services are reflected in the way you deliver treatment:

- Using clinical means to arrive at a physical outcome without the experience feeling medical

- Practicing medicine with a team of talented, dedicated individuals who practice the ethics of delivering medical service with the principles of delivering personal service

- Delivering an experience that is wholly based on personal fulfillment

TAKING THE "CLINICAL" OUT OF YOUR MODEL

You provide a medical service. In aesthetic medicine, that service is based on a need to fulfill personal desire, not a medical need to improve one's health or life condition. Therefore, although clinical operations must uphold all of the highest clinical standards of care and practice management, your clients/patients must not feel as though they are in a clinical setting or an operation that fulfills need, not desire. With any practice model, if you expect your aesthetic services to thrive, you should operate as though aesthetic services are the primary or the only function of the practice.

The nuances that differentiate an aesthetic practice, the true personal service elements, must be consistent and present in all cases.

- If your office needs a face lift, will a patient feel you are the best choice to perform one on her? If your staff members are unkempt, will a potential client feel you understand the value he or she places on personal appearance?

- If you conduct consultations in a clinical examination room, will your client be comfortable and candid about his or her goals? Will he or she feel the setting appropriate to the fees paid for elective services?

- If you expect your clients to fill out paperwork, do you expect them to wear or sit on paper while doing so? Does your office provide the paperwork on a clipboard with a pen attached by a metal cord? Do you fear that the loss of a pen will have an impact on your bottom line?

- When a client leaves with paperwork, is it generic, or does every item consistently carry your brand? Is a sheaf of loose paperwork handed to the patient, or is it compiled in a branded folder or envelope? If not, your image may come across as being loosely organized.

- When clients/patients call with questions, how long does it take you or a patient counselor to respond? Is that more or less time than it takes that individual to contact another provider?

Analyze these things, then think about the expectations the client may have based on what he or she is paying for your services. Know that unless the clinical outcome of what you can provide is vastly and evidently superior to the competition, your best advantage is a vastly and evidently superior operation.

NONMEDICAL SERVICES

Some aesthetic practices don't simply apply personal service principles to a medical practice; they enhance the medical practice by adding true nonmedical services. Many practices can and do thrive without them, some offer but don't distinguish them, and still others make a point of calling attention to the personal services provided.

Personal services such as cosmetics, massage therapy, concierges, or the Town Car that delivers your patients home after a procedure are nonessential. Additionally, personal services:

- *Have an impact on revenue:* They may generate revenue or add to your cost of operations or investment in inventory. They may occupy space and require utilities, insurance, marketing, or other essential expenses so that they may be provided and appreciated.

- *Enhance your mission:* Cosmetics were introduced in medical practices to help individuals disguise birthmarks, scars, acne, or telltale posttreatment signs such as pallor, redness, and bruising. They have evolved with science and improved formulations to become an integral part of the aesthetic practice, not only for correction and camouflage and for completing the full aesthetic experience for your patient, but also for maintaining results, protecting the patient's rejuvenated, youthful appearance, and nurturing the skin.

- *Create opportunity:* Whether to improve your patients' experience or your ability to serve them or to invite a new audience to your service business, nonmedical services must create opportunities for you to grow without having a negative impact on your resources, your image, or your patients' experience.

- *Nurture ongoing relationships:* Whatever the personal service, whether it is brow waxing or biofeedback, personal services that by their nature will be repeated by a happy customer keep your core services continually visible to that client/patient, thus creating a greater opportunity for your single greatest source for clients: referrals.

RELATIVE WISDOM: Tattoo You

It made no sense. The physician was known for his genius with lasers and his ability to remove tattoos, not from gang members but from future spouses, ladder-climbing executives, and maturing young adults who realized that a visible tattoo on the neck would not be easy to explain to a future employer, lover, or child. On the flip side, the physician's medical spa offered permanent cosmetics: tattoos for eyebrows, eyeliner, lip liner. However, he didn't know this; his spa manager had decided to contract out for these services. This bifurcation made absolutely no business sense.

Relative wisdom: The trend in adjunct services to nonpayor practices is growing so much that many of these practice segments develop a brand and identity of their own. What is critical is that missions remain congruent. The clinical side of the practice and any adjunct personal services must have a circular relationship in which the motives and messages are shared, even when brand and identity take on individual characteristics.

Moreover, when an adjunct personal service becomes fully independent, it is no longer a complement, but rather an outside resource. The connection between clinical operations and adjunct personal services must be visible, logical, and must be relative to everyone: doctor, staff, and patients. When missions are congruent and consistent, the success of one entity feeds the other, thus building revenue and success.

CONCIERGES

It's a big term in medicine these days: *concierge.* What it means in the world of medicine is that the patient pays a provider an annual fee for all necessary services and referrals, potentially with additional charges for specific treatments, and the provider agrees to enhanced service: house calls, after-hours care, no wait times, added privacy, and a fully personalized experience in which the patient does not feel like a medical case but a true individual. In aesthetic medicine, providing concierge services is evolving as a concept. It is the ultimate in personal service to assist your patients in every aspect of the aesthetic experience.

But in reality, concierge services simply reflect common sense and common courtesy:

- Your patients should never be kept waiting long. This is not a concierge practice; it is a best practice.

- House calls or preoperative in-person checks on your patients who recover at home are appropriate, especially when patients may not want to be seen in public or have limited means to travel.

- For patients who travel distances to see you—whether you are the closest geographic choice, the preferred choice, practicing in a choice destination, or simply *the* choice, regardless of where you practice—providing them with information about getting to, staying at, and enjoying your location is simply good hospitality.

- Assisting patients with travel arrangements, whether for the day of treatment, after surgery, or to come in for postoperative follow-up is a gracious additional service.

- Coordinating postoperative needs, whether these are for skin care, garments, amenities, or a place to recover, is good practice. It is inappropriate to perform a laser treatment on a client's skin, then send that person home with instructions stating, "Apply baking soda compresses and a coating of petroleum jelly for 4 days." Either provide the instructions far in advance so the client can plan accordingly, or send the client home with the items he or she will need for their postprocedure comfort.

You may feel that concierge practices are excessive for most of your patients or are simply not right for your model. However, don't overlook the value or need some patients may have: keep on file referral to a concierge service willing to learn your business, know your expectations, and serve your patients.

IN PRACTICE: No Pain, No Vain

It's a common sight: Patients grasping the hands of nurses while tears stream down their faces and physicians do their work. Women leaving the aesthetic physician's office with ice packs, living for days with visible bruising. Patients who say, "I'll never do that again; it hurt like hell."

I was visiting a practice where all these scenarios were played out. When the physician and I sat together, I asked: "Why don't you do more to keep your patients comfortable?"

"That's the price of vanity," he told me.

"Why don't you allow them some extra time to relax after treatment with ice in the examination room rather than shuffling them out the door?"

"They are busy, they want to get back to life, and I need the room," he told me.

"Do you advise them of the potential posttreatment effects and how to avoid things like bruises when they call to book a treatment, or on your website, or at any time before you actually perform the treatment?"

"They won't pay attention, and bruises are par for the course. Plus patients appreciate their outcomes better if there is some really unattractive time in between," he said.

I could not believe what I was hearing, but then, I was not surprised when I looked at the physician's retention levels and spent some time talking to his staff. Retention was low, and the staff were well aware that he was known as the "painful provider." I couldn't disagree; his manner proved it.

At the end of the day, the physician, staff and I sat down together to discuss things. I don't like putting people on the spot, but this time, it was warranted. We discussed the lack of retention as a service failure; we discussed how the physician was perceived among his patients, and thus in the community; we discussed the means to make it better. Pain was not essential to the outcome or the experience, we all agreed—except the physician.

Several months later, he called me. His practice was down, a provider from across town was opening an office next door, and he needed help. He was in search of an aggressive marketing blitz to fix his apparent problem. My advice to him: marketing could not correct his lack of understanding and service for his patients. He needed to fix his service model, which might eventually repair his reputation, achieve a better retention rate, and make him the provider of choice in his market. I never heard from him again. The word is that he is now painfully retired.

Retail

The goods that your practice sells to complement, support, or enhance the services you provide must be tied to your service model, but also have some very independent characteristics: retail requires appropriate accounting and inventory, including the collection of sales tax. In some practices, retail goods are the only "sale" on which commissions can ethically be paid. They require an investment in inventory, typically carry a 100% markup, and require close inventory monitoring (as any retail function does) so that stock available for client/patient demand can be accounted for and maintained in sufficient quantities. Retail product sales are enhanced by display, but they invite theft. Products can be sampled or tested, whereas the procedures and services you provide are often very difficult to present in an experiential format.

Choosing Products

Although retail practices have distinct differences from your service sector, retail items must be integrally and intimately a part of your service model if you are going to include them in your practice. Clinical skin care or cosmeceuticals are products that your patients/clients purchase from your practice based on:

- Exclusivity—they cannot be purchased except through the physician.

- Expectation—the products you sell provide a distinctly better or different result than products purchased elsewhere.

- Science—the research behind the product is consistent with medical research standards, testing, and approval.

Products must be chosen based on quality, unique properties, clinically proven benefits, ease of use, safety, brand reputation, and vendor support.

Retailing in an aesthetic practice involves much more than a patient's simply choosing a product; it requires that the physician or physician extender recommend the correct product to treat or prevent skin conditions, protect healing or healthy skin, prevent or reverse the effects of aging, and encourage renewal. Today even products sold in the drugstore tout these benefits and more. As a medical practice striving to satisfy your patient, if you cannot confidently sell a product that can accomplish what is promised, you should not sell it. If it is sold in a drugstore or department store nearby, make certain you can compete for dollars before you invest in inventory.

Once clients use and are satisfied with retail items, the expectation is that they will continue to purchase them from you. This creates an ongoing revenue stream and brings them back regularly as a customer to purchase more products. These repeated visits to your practice are opportunities for maintaining visibility and continuity of your relationship with the client.

Retail can be a vital service complement and business component in an aesthetic practice, but for those who sell or recommend it to patients, training is as critical as training for the procedures offered in your practice. Designate specific personnel to staff your retail operations or fulfill the retail function in addition to other roles. For the retail side of the practice to succeed, you must encourage and insist on staff education and training in both product knowledge and sales technique. Putting product on the shelf and expecting that the client will ask about it is ineffective. Practitioners must find opportunities to recommend products; sales support staff must expand on this recommendation and suggest complementary products as well.

Selling Skin Care

Today selling skin care in your practice does not begin and end in your practice. Many practices are focused on e-tailing—selling product on the Internet. If you are going to franchise a site you can design to match your own brand, a turnkey operation you can build to be your own, or choose to build a retailing endeavor from the ground up and in your own in-house retail operations, heed these caveats:

- Do not sell prescription-strength products unless you have a patient record, an in-office visit, and a prescription on file for the patient.

- Do not sell products you are not familiar with or would not recommend to patients to treat a specific condition or fulfill a specific function.

- Do highlight products by problem and solution and by product type and brand, and do list complementary and conflicting products. Don't sell someone a product that results in distress instead of a solution.

- Do highlight brands. Consumers look for recognized and well-known names.

- Do collect data on those who purchase online and compare these with data collected about customers who purchase in-office. If online sales are cannibalizing your in-office sales, you are losing a valuable asset of retailing: the traffic that brings people into your door for products *and* service.

Skin care, cosmetics, and at-home devices, whether mechanical or light based, are all valuable extensions to your practice, but they cannot sell themselves, and if they are misused or misguide your patients, they tarnish your image rather than creating value.

SKIN CARE IN THE AESTHETIC PRACTICE: To Sell or Not to Sell

Gene Colón, Esq.

A patient walks into a dermatologist's office for a combination laser-peel-injection regimen. After the procedures are completed, she leaves with specific postcare instructions and a small bag of targeted skin care products for home use. Sound familiar?

Gone are the days when a "one size fits all" aesthetic procedure filled the bill. Today savvy consumers with less time on their hands demand a more global and personalized approach to younger-looking skin. The trend is clear: people want minimally invasive treatments that are skin-type specific, including the relevant ancillary tools to maintain those in-office results at home. Patients are also now taking a more active role in this search for youth. The longer they can make the results of the procedure last, the better.

Given the trust, knowledge, and convenience established in the physician-patient relationship, who better to provide these relevant tools to achieve optimal results than the doctor who is performing the initial in-office procedure? Dispensing products has become a natural extension of the practice. In fact, these aesthetic physicians have already been dispensing other kinds of products (services, advice, prescriptions, surgeries, and so on) to treat their patients. It is only logical that skin care would follow as an acceptable product to be dispensed.

While I am far from advocating a carte blanche capitalistic attitude regarding this business model, I do believe certain tenets must be maintained to ensure the ethics of this strategy. First and foremost, the best interest of the patient must always be the paramount concern. Avoid a coercive sales atmosphere in the office. Second, there should be good science to support the product's benefits. With so many options available today, patients should expect credible clinical data behind the products recommended by their doctors. Finally, any financial interest should be disclosed. For good measure, I would recommend maintaining reasonable pricing and offering a money-back guarantee.

In today's culture, patients expect a one-stop shop (consultation, aesthetic treatments, and home care products). As long as the well-being of the patient comes first, there is no reason that dispensing skin care product cannot remain an important and valuable part of this dynamic. Everyone wants a happy patient. Consistent and longer-lasting results are essential. And in today's economy, selling skin care products is the prudent thing to do.

WHAT'S MY LINE?

Private labeling of skin care products has become a trend in aesthetic practices. Some physicians have put their names on and have been a part of the research for mass-marketed product lines sold at Saks Fifth Avenue and Nordstrom, and now at CVS and the corner grocery. Every physician seems to want a bottle or jar to label his or her own. Hotel chains have long had little bottles of shampoo and skin care products privately labeled with their brand so that patrons who have forgotten to pack these items have them to use and take home, reminding them where to stay again. In medical practice, however, the goal of choosing generic products and putting one's own brand on the label negates the entire point of offering skin care in your practice: products are sold on the premise that they have scientifically proven value and greater benefit than mainstream or generic products. Putting your name on a product implies that you have been a part of the development, and science behind that product. Putting your name on a generic skin care line is nothing less than deceptive, nothing more than self-serving.

🦋 IN PRACTICE: Model Data

It's a familiar model: a solid aesthetic practice with only those restorative procedures that ultimately have aesthetic goals, with an added nonsurgical skin care complement and robust retail offerings. Many practices have this all in one location; others have satellites to extend nonsurgical and skin care services further into the marketplace.

On visiting a practice in a bustling suburban area, the physician-owner was concerned: his three practice segments, surgery, cosmetic medicine, and retail, seemed disconnected. In fact, a review of practice data showed that skin care services and retail were frequented by clients who were not a subset of his surgical patients, and the surgical patients rarely were patrons of the skin care services.

I met with the physician and staff to discuss the problem, the source of which I could fully predict. The physician did not know what skin care was offered, so he did not recommended any. Aestheticians abided strictly by his "no pushy sales" rule and did not discuss treatments they did not administer. The nurses performing laser and injection treatments were "so busy" they did not have time to engage their patients in a discussion of other services, even if the patients expressed a desire for them. This was a disconnected practice with a lot of excuses, so I laid out a very specific multistep plan:

- The physician received a briefing on all the skin care products offered and services provided by the aestheticians. He received a "prescription pad" listing all of these services to keep in his pocket, recommend, check off, give to the patient, and pass them along to the skin care staff to complete the service and the sale. If the physician recommended it, patients would buy it.

- Aestheticians were given an in-service session on client education, not solicitation. They were taught to query the interests and goals of their clients and to mention the opportunities the physician provided to fulfill their cosmetic goals beyond skin care. They were given appropriate, practice-branded literature that defined a service in layman's terms. They were given access to the physician's patient coordinator, if she was available, to meet with a client who was interested in a procedure, or to schedule a complementary consultation with the patient coordinator if she was not available at the moment.

- The too-busy nurses were given some direction and were made aware that they were, in fact, the missing link that connected skin care services to the physician, and the physician to skin care services. Each nurse received a prescription pad like the one given to the physician, and all were required to attend the aesthetician in-service session. Preprocedure and postprocedure protocols included two very specific things that took the nurses only a moment: asking what the patient's specific goals for appearance were, and asking whether all needs and questions had been addressed. As I told the nurses, "What can we do for you?" and "Is there anything else we can do for your or recommend today?" are very polite and simple practices.

A few months passed, and that data began to show a strong connection among the practice segments. The doctor was happy, the staff were happy, the patients were happy. But several months later, data again demonstrated a disconnect. It didn't take long to discover the reason: the prescription pads were ineffective because the skin care product offerings had some changes. The doctor stopped using them, and the nurses stopped using them. The doctor introduced some new services, and the skin care practice added aestheticians. No one thought to train, retrain, or update. Everyone lost enthusiasm.

The moral here is simple: Model data do not self-perpetuate. Model behavior, model enthusiasm, model updates, and model communication must continue and evolve to remain effective.

RELATIVE WISDOM: Must You Add a Medical Spa?

My son Andy loves to fish. It's his undying passion. No matter where we go, no matter the weather, if you ask him what he wants to do, he wants to go fishing. One summer day Andy and his babysitter decided they were going fishing. When they arrived at the favorite fishing hole in our neighborhood, Andy encountered an older gentleman fishing with worms, not lures. Andy, respecting the older man's maturity, began to dig for worms. He gathered some, fished with them, and caught nothing. Andy returned home and put his fishing rod and bucket on the patio and headed inside to wash for dinner.

The next morning I was chagrined to discover that there was bird poop all over the glass patio doors, all over the patio. Andy's worms had been fodder

Continued

RELATIVE WISDOM: Must You Add a Medical Spa?—cont'd

for the birds. As my young fisherman and I were cleaning the mess, he looked at me and said, "Mom, I guess this is one of those lessons that you don't need to do what everyone else is doing."

Relative wisdom: Your practice model should not be dictated by what everyone else is doing. You should do what suits you best, works well for you, your patients, and your market. You don't need to build a medical spa because everyone else is building one. Including the service touches, the right amenities, and desirable services can happen in your practice, and with a multitude of model and brands. If you try to follow someone else without researching the options, you might end up with no one taking your bait, and a mess to clean up later.

CHAPTER 7

What Do Your Patients Expect?

*A successful practice is one with the ability
to fulfill need and nurture realistic expectations;
it does not distort or build expectations, and it
must not deny them. A practice weak on accepting
this reality is indeed a weak practice.*

You and your practice are defined. You have identified your targets and recognized the competition. Your identity is clear and consistent in image, brand, mission, and operations. Now you must find a way to link all of these factors to the needs and expectations of those you serve or potentially may serve. What do your patients need and expect from you, your practice, your medical services, and your service model?

In the practice of aesthetic medicine, client/patient needs are based on the personal desire to enhance appearance. Patients may expect that this enhancement in appearance will also enhance their confidence and perception of self and that improved image and confidence will have a positive impact on their lives. What is variable is just how their lives will be enhanced and to what degree. However, your patients' needs and expectations are not simply for the services you will provide, the manner in which they are delivered, and their expectations for outcomes. Needs and expectations are far more complicated.

Interest

Interest is essential to bring a prospective patient to you. Interest occurs outside the practice, when the subject is a target audience member who is drawn to you by your own external marketing efforts or as a referral from another physician, a professional connection, or one of your patients. Interest may also return a current patient who wants additional or different services.

Education

Education about potential medical solutions to a prospective patient's goals, about your practice, your credentials, services, and the nuances that differentiate your practice from others occur at multiple points. Externally, education occurs through resources such as your website, other patients, physicians, or professionals who know and will speak candidly about your services. Internally, education occurs through initial conversations or correspondence and ultimately a consultation. Patients need and/or expect to be educated before making a decision.

Comprehension

Comprehension is essential to formalizing the physician/patient relationship. Thoroughly and honestly evaluating how well your client comprehends his or her own needs and expectations allows you to make the appropriate recommendations for treatment to achieve those goals, and to what degree. Comprehension allows the patient to confidently accept your recommended course of treatment and all the attendant experiences, obligations, and potential positive or adverse outcomes that may result.

Comprehension is best achieved though objectivity, sensitivity, listening skills, and candid, careful dialog between you and those within your practice who will be involved in this patient's administration, care, or decisions.

Influence

Influence comes in many forms, may be apparent or latent, and can affect a patient's interest, education, and comprehension at varying levels. Influence can be healthy or toxic to your relationship with the patient; it can come from family, friends, and other providers. Influence may strengthen or alter the patient's decisions. Media news or features and social media such as blogs and ratings can shape the patient's decisions. Social status and social pressure can be persuasive. Such influences cannot be controlled or prevented, but through a strong and forthright relationship with your patient, positive influences can be reinforcing, and negative influences can be diffused.

Your Market

As interest, education, and comprehension are essential to the process of treating your patients, so too is understanding precisely who you must attract. Your market can generally be defined by one or more of these categories, each with special needs:

- *Medical:* Medical patients come to you for a cure for a disease such as skin cancer, for treatment of an anomaly, or for some other need that is not solely based on improved appearance. Patients may come to an aesthetic practice for medical needs because they trust a particular provider, are influenced by others, or hope that the aesthetic provider can produce a more aesthetically pleasing result.

- *Restorative:* Patients may come to your practice in need of restoration to a more normal appearance or function after an injury, a trauma, or disease such as breast or skin cancer. In recent times restorative needs have also been defined as those that return a patient to his or her former appearance, such as a face lift to restore a youthful appearance. The most important distinction to make is that one category of restorative procedures is recognized and generally reimbursed by health care insurers; the other is purely for cosmetic needs. Correction of a constricted scar or reconstruction of a breast lost to cancer is restorative. A face lift, although it restores a more youthful appearance, is purely cosmetic.

- *Cosmetic:* Cosmetic surgery reflects the patient's desire to improve, refine, refinish, renew, or restore some aspect of appearance. Whether this involves a simple facial peel, an injection of a filler, laser hair reduction or skin resurfacing, a face lift, breast enhancement, or body contouring, the desire and the outcome are purely for improved appearance.

- *Child or adolescent:* A prospective pediatric patient has needs and expectations similar to those of an adult patient and requires the same attention to interest, education, and comprehension. However, all of these factors are at far different and divergent levels based on age, health, maturity, and even the condition for which the patient has come to you. Influence by parents in these cases can range from demanding to encouraging to forbidding treatment. Legally, you must have the consent of the parent or guardian to treat a child or adolescent. Ethically, you must have the absolute best interests of your patient in mind at all times.

- *Adult:* Legally capable of making their own decisions, adults can be your easiest or most difficult patient population, because their needs and expectations can be straightforward or highly complex, unyielding or highly inconsistent, and wholly self-motivated or highly influenced.

- *Senior:* In the growing senior population, there are some with spending power, some without. Some have explicit needs, while others have unrealistic needs. Treating seniors requires the same level of caution as for treating any other patients: carefully discuss interests, educate them, and ensure that they completely comprehend the procedure, its potential, and its pitfalls.

- *Indigent:* You may have patients who are unable to pay for treatment. These patients may come to your practice of their own volition, or you may invite them or travel to them as a result of your personal philanthropic endeavors. Indigent patients deserve respect and proper cautious care, and they to require interest, education, and comprehension of their options and opportunities. However, you may choose not to mix this population with your general patient population.

- *Critical:* Critical may mean life or death, or it may mean *now.* You may encounter patients who need your services immediately, even if that time is inconvenient for you. Response to complications must be swift. If this is your patient, it is imperative that the response be immediate for a trauma or injury, or the patient should be promptly referred and cautiously followed. Consider a patient with disrupted sutures, one with a laceration from an accident, and one with a ruptured implant. All deserve immediate attention from you or someone you trust to treat this patient.

- *Difficult/demanding:* Dealing with difficult or demanding patients requires a very special set of variables.

  - *Observation:* Observe patients early in the relationship to assess which individuals may become difficult or demanding; sometimes it is simply best to avoid them in your practice.

  - *Removal:* Remove the patient from negatively influencing anyone else in your practice, but don't engage the patient alone; always have a staff member present and silent.

  - *Inquiry:* Ask specifically what has transpired to cause the individual to be upset, on edge, or in despair, and listen.

  - *Resolution:* Offer a solution if you have one, offer your apologies if you don't, offer a refund if you must. It is better to avoid the difficult or demanding patient and to diffuse the difficult or demanding situation than to expend valuable resources of time, energy, and identity in trying to "win."

- *Ineligible:* Some patients simply are not appropriate candidates for treatment. Whether they are poor candidates for emotional, physical, or financial reasons, you have the responsibility to decide and communicate when it is either not possible or not appropriate to treat a patient.

  - Do not accept a patient who you know may risk severe financial hardship to pay for cosmetic procedures.

  - Do not accept a patient with an emotional disorder that indicates the need to deny treatment.

  - Do not accept a patient with unrealistic hopes or expectations that a procedure will be the miraculous life-changing event this person needs to save a marriage, attract a spouse, or become a movie star.

INTEREST

The only means of linking your practice to an outside target audience member is effective communication, which may be direct, or linked through sources and resources. Outside your practice, the interest of your target audience is defined through research. (Sources for researching your population are provided in Chapter 3.) Knowing the interests of your target patient base is essential to helping members of that audience uncover or heighten awareness of their own needs so they can act on this need by coming to your practice.

Interest does not define communication, but it does shape external communication strategy by attaching the content of your message to what interests your target audience. To be effective, you must keep your tone consistent with the tone of other lifestyle interests of the target audience. For your message to be received, you must deliver it directly through media that are readily accessible and effectively used by the target audience or through sources and resources that you trust will carry your message forward and maintain the integrity of the message. In blending what you learn about the interests of your target audience and the needs that prospective patients may have and by conveying your identity and your services, you have three specific goals:

- *Visibility:* You want to reach a larger pool of potential patients or individuals who may be referred to you. Then, if they are interested, people must be able to locate you.

- *Awareness:* You want to communicate information about your services to a broader potential patient population and to previous patients who may have become inactive in your practice. You must also inform current patient referral sources about the services you provide, giving them the opportunity to pass along information.

- *Consistency:* Every time, every place, through every referral source or resource your practice has to reach prospective, existing, or inactive patients, your brand, image, and mission must be consistent.

Research garners the interests of a target population, not an individual. Once an individual enters your practice, communication is based on that person's interests. His or her interests are specific and personal and require:

- *One-to-one communication:* Patient to practice, practitioner, or staff—essential to learning the interest not just for a particular service, but in general for this patient. Learning the patient's service interests is essential to making qualified recommendations to fulfill his or her goals. Learning the general interest of this patient helps you know more about his or her lifestyle and intentions, as well as more about the population of people interested in your service. This valuable research can help you improve and expand your outreach to your target audience.

- *Consistency of intent:* To be certain the interests of the patient are sincere and strong. People have been known to act on a whim to fulfill a fleeting interest for a cosmetic procedure. Aesthetic medicine is not a fleeting interest; its results can be permanent.

- *Consistency of service:* Each encounter your patient has with your practice will shape his or her experience and can strengthen or weaken his or her interest in you as a provider.

If a patient loses interest, there may be a variety of reasons:

- *Anxiety:* Anxiety is a perfectly normal reaction to the unknowns of an aesthetic procedure. Through education the patient's anxiety can be alleviated but will never resolve completely.

- *Medical conditions:* Whether temporary or not, illness can supersede a person's desire to undergo an aesthetic treatment. When illness does not impair the ability to fulfill treatment at a later date, the patient's interest must be kept fresh through communication.

- *External influences:* Family, friends, media, and money can all work against patient desire, and you cannot control these influences or may have no knowledge of them. The strength of your patient's desire and internal influences—your effective education and the patient's comprehension—will determine whether external influences or personal desire prevails. If the patient is a minor, parents or legal guardians are not external forces; they are essential to your relationship with the patient. In any other case, your obligation is to your patient.

Interest can wane when too much time passes between points of communication with a patient. Ongoing communication between your practice and a patient who is a good candidate and demonstrates a sincere interest in treatment is critical to this patient's accepting treatment.

Growing interest is shared interest. Patients excited about fulfilling personal desires share their excitement with those they know. Patients with excellent results lead others to develop a desire for their own fulfilling experience. Female patients are more likely to share the joy of fulfilled desire than male patients are. Men tend to be much more private about their interest and needs; they will rarely share their interest, and when they do, it is only with a very few close friends or family members. The value of growing interest is that when it is nurtured and maintained by you and your practice, it can translate to your single greatest resource for new clients: referrals.

In the Interest of Marketing

Marketing by definition is the process required to price and package your goods or services, attract a market, and sell to them. That may include a number of strategies, of which advertising is just one. Advertising, a website, a seminar, cultivating referrals, or any other marketing tool to help attract an interested audience is an ethical and valuable tool for your practice.

- It is unethical to make false claims, whether through advertising or on your website. If you are the best, you'd best prove it. If you are a "top doc," you'd best not have paid for that title.

- It is unethical to entertain a group of people in an informal, nonmedical setting and on that same occasion, to provide treatment to individuals in that group. A proper process of interest, education, and comprehension requires a consultation and informed consent. And there is no "two-drink limit"; ethical providers have a zero tolerance policy for treating individuals who have been drinking or are under the influence of any recreational drug or drink.

- It is unethical for a physician to pay for referrals, whether from patients, hairdressers, or image consultants.

It's appropriate to show gratitude; it is not appropriate to have patient-funneling referral fee arrangements with anyone. Pharmaceutical firms' rules don't allow representatives to incentivize their relationship with you by paying you to recommend or prescribe their product over another. Act by the same rules. There's been a practice of websites recruiting physicians who will "pay per lead." Don't do it, unless you know that lead was genuinely interested, appropriately qualified, and did more than simply go shopping. In a November 2008 article in the *American Medical News,* published by the AMA, attorney Steven Harris wrote: "The American Medical Association's Code of Medical Ethics provides that a 'payment by or to a physician solely for the referral of a patient is fee splitting and is unethical.'"

The conventional wisdom is to follow the ethics of your profession and of your specialty such as the codes of ethics of ASAPS, ASPS, AAFPRS, ASDS, AAD, ΛΛOPRS, or any other qualified professional organization to which you belong or endeavor to belong.

What you do as an ethical provider/proprietor of aesthetic medicine to gain patients is to communicate your brand, image, mission, and the services you provide. You do not tout your services; you educate clients and patients about how you can fulfill their personal desire for appearance enhancement. A patient's decision to come to your practice for a treatment confers on you the responsibility to ensure that the patient fully comprehends the service you will provide, how treatment will be administered, and at what monetary, physical, and emotional cost.

🦋 IN PRACTICE: Interested?

I was visiting a practice when a sweet elderly woman came in for a consultation. During her visit, she pulled an ad she had clipped from the local paper; the headline read, "10 Years Younger in 10 Minutes." Clever marketing.

The ad was not run by this physician's office, but by a medical spa at the busiest mall in town. The sweet lady didn't like going to the mall; it was crowded and busy, and she felt pushed around, so she came to this physician, recognizing his name as the one who was treating her daughter with cosmetic injections.

The physician was earnest in his response to her interest; he educated her so that she could fully comprehend that no treatment could result in her looking 10 years younger in 10 minutes. She weighed her options, looked a little sad, and before she could say anything more, he said, "Call me with any questions you have, but please don't visit this spa; they will simply be taking your money." As she reached for her wallet, he stated, "There is no charge for this visit."

I commended the physician for his actions. Taking her money for a consultation was pointless, and could harm the relationship he had with the woman's daughter. Then, being who I am, I grabbed my bag, my coat, the ad (which also touted the most natural and undetectable results), and asked one of the office staff to point me in the direction of the mall.

For a woman in her forties, I am pretty well kept. I have had my share of injections, peels, and laser treatments. I walked into the medical spa with the ad in hand and asked, "Hi, who could I speak to about looking 10 years younger? I've got 10 minutes."

The girl behind the desk was eager to introduce me to Stella, a woman of 22 with a healthy shellac of makeup and long fake nails. First Stella asked my age. "How old do I look?" I asked. She giggled and promised me that instead of looking like 30, I'd look like 20. This place was awesome; by just walking in the door, I looked 12 years younger.

Within 10 minutes, Stella had recommended that I have a particular type of thread lift (with a product no longer on the market), a skin-tightening laser procedure, skin bleaching, and a series of injections to fill out parts of my face, melt the fat in other parts of my face, and vitamin injections that would "fool my blastocysts into forming more collagen." This is what Stella offered to make me look 10 years younger. "Wow, all of that will make me look 10 years younger? In 10 minutes? What's the price tag, and how soon can I sign up?" I asked.

Stella promptly told me she would have to see how much time the nurse had on her schedule, because this stellar package would take about 2 hours.

"Your ad says 10 minutes! I don't have 2 hours."

"I know," Stella told me. "You really didn't believe that, did you?"

"I did," I told her. "This is false advertising."

Stella went to get the nurse, who came and offered me a 10% savings because of the misunderstanding if I had the treatments that day. She had time now. "Shouldn't the doctor examine me?" I asked. "Will I need someone to drive me home? Are you qualified to perform surgery, because wouldn't putting threads under my skin mean incisions of some kind? Are there risks? Side effects? Can I head back to the office, because I just ducked out for lunch and wanted to look 10 years younger in 10 minutes."

"You ask a lot of questions," the nurse told me. "You must not really be interested."

When I returned to the office, I shared my findings with the physician and we filed a complaint with the state medical board. I called the city licensing department to learn whether this business was indeed licensed to perform medical procedures in this town. The physician called me 3 weeks later: the medical spa was closed.

The lesson here: Be careful about the interests you attract, the promises you make, and the manner in which you do business. At worst, you'll be exposed; at best, inevitably or quickly, people will lose interest.

You know, nothing is more important than education, because nowhere are our stakes higher.

— ARNOLD SCHWARZENEGGER

EDUCATION

The stakes are high in the practice of aesthetic medicine; therefore the means by which you educate your patients and the effectiveness of that education are critical to success in your practice. Outcomes are important, as is educating your patient on every option, every aspect, every expected result and potentially adverse event of the treatment. Motivation is important, but not as important as your learning about your patient's motivation for the procedure. Service is important, but not as important as knowing your patient's expectations for service and defining what you can and cannot provide.

Interest is essential to reaching people; education is essential to influencing a person's decision to select you to perform one or more services.

Educating Your Market

The education you provide your target population or prospective patient is an education about you (your image, brand, and mission). It defines you by the basics: credentials, services, affiliation, and geography. It also provides procedure-specific knowledge. The conduit may be advertising, your website, directories, referring physicians or patients—the sources are unlimited. It must always convey your image, brand, mission, and tone. If you use inconsistent messages and materials to educate those who do not yet have a one-to-one relationship with you, you will only confuse them and inevitably lose credibility.

Educating the Individual

The most significant education occurs in direct conversation with a prospective or current patient and your referral sources. Patient education lasts indefinitely, from the moment the individual contacts you until you or the patient elects to discontinue the relationship.

Individual education can be simply defined:

- Begin with a personal introduction to the practice that affirms your image, brand, and mission.

- Follow with a general discussion of the options your practice can offer to fulfill the patient's wants or needs.

- If the patient decides to proceed with the recommended treatment, thoroughly explain the procedure and experience, his or her obligation to follow the guidelines provided preoperatively and postoperatively to optimize health and avoid complications, and the expected and potential outcomes.

The first two areas of education—personal introduction and general education—must be concisely addressed at the initial points of contact. An initial phone call should do more than schedule a consultation; it must:

- Answer general questions that enable you to better screen the prospective patient, or schedule a subsequent call to accomplish this two-way educational experience

- Provide encouragement to facilitate the consultation process: what the patient is to expect and what is expected of him or her

- Define the policies and parameters of a consultation and the practice, if the prospective patient schedules or inquires about scheduling a consultation, including the length of time a consultation typically takes, the cost involved, directions to the office, and collection of necessary patient data (whether completing forms or logging in)

When initial contact does not immediately result in the prospective patient's scheduling a consultation, the response must still connect the individual with the practice:

- An offer to provide practice background or specific procedural information

- Direction to resources, such as a website, and specifically what on the site is relevant to the client's initial interest

- An invitation to contact the office at any time with further questions

- An offer to follow up with the prospective patient (after a short but reasonable length of time) to ensure that the information provided was adequate and understood, to allow the individual to ask further questions or express additional interest, and to extend an invitation to schedule a consultation

❦ RELATIVE WISDOM: Never Say "No"

How many times have you called or entered a business and inquired about a specific product, such as a specific vintage of wine? You call the local cellar, enter your favorite wine store, or sit down at your favorite restaurant wanting a particular variety, label, vintage, and the sommelier says, "No." He doesn't ask what you like about that variety or label or why you prefer the specific vintage, does not offer you something equally crisp or simply more valuable. He just says "No."

Relative wisdom: How many times has someone called your office asking if you provide some unusual (or even common) procedure, and a member of your staff simply says "No." If you and the staff take the time to answer questions with questions, you may be welcoming a new patient, and the patient will appreciate that your office took the time to offer a newcomer the education that led to a satisfying result.

Consultation

The greatest component of education is consultation. At this stage, the individual already has some knowledge of you, your services, and your mission—knowledge that contributed to this individual's electing to consult with you. If the individual does not have some knowledge of you, the practice has missed the mark on education when scheduling the consultation.

Patients are savvy; they may have some clinical knowledge of the procedures that are appropriate to fulfill their goals. This knowledge may have been gained from media, other providers, or even a referral source. Their information may be valid or not; it may drive the patients' expectations or not. For the provider, a consultation is commonly the first opportunity to gain knowledge about patients and what brings them to you. After sincere greetings and introductions, perhaps breaking the ice with a little small talk, the consultation should quickly focus on the patient's personal desires and his or her expectations of your fulfilling his or her goals. Although most patients are eager to discuss their personal desires and the outcomes they hope to achieve, it remains essential that the provider directly ask about the following:

- The patient's personal desire or intention for aesthetic medical treatment

- The patient's expectations for the physical outcome of aesthetic medical treatment

- The patient's expectations for personal outcomes (how he or she expects this procedure to affect his or her life)

- The patient's preferences for treatment, such as surgical or nonsurgical

- The patient's limitations in resources or time, or, if appropriate, any health limitations

- The patient's questions

The answers to these questions will allow you to determine whether the individual's goals and motivations are sincere and well defined, that his or her physical expectations can be safely achieved, and that personal expectations are rational. This information will allow you to determine whether you should pursue the relationship and recommend a specific course of treatment and alternatives to meet this patient's goals. Next you can progress to a general review of health. Health history further qualifies a good candidate for a procedure based on individual physical characteristics and general health. At this stage a health history may only disqualify a patient for a particular procedure; it is not used to qualify the patient. You may now confidently make recommendations about the procedure or procedures you recommend, the options to your recommendations, and the differences among the options.

INFORMED CONSENT

The next phase of consultation, which may or may not occur at a subsequent meeting, is the process of informed consent. Education in this phase is clinical, and should detail the following:

- A physical assessment of the client's condition and goals for improvement, including an evaluation of general health

- The procedure and special techniques you recommend to achieve the patient's stated goals

- The preoperative expectations you have of your patient, including medications, following a pretreatment regimen, and avoiding certain activities, such as smoking, sun exposure, antiinflammatory medications, and so on

- The physician's and patient's expectations and preferences regarding surgery, including location, anesthesia, time, comfort, and immediate recovery

- The recovery involved, including how soon the patient will go home, his or her obligations for posttreatment care and behavior, the important signs of complications, and precautions necessary to ensure proper healing

- How results are expected to present or develop and the time necessary for final results to be evident

- Potential adverse events, how these can be identified, how the patient must respond, and the options to resolve those events

- How soon the patient can resume daily activities and feel comfortable in a public setting

- Important aftercare if treatment requires multiple stages or to maintain and preserve good outcomes

When the patient has accepted treatment based on this comprehensive education of every detail involved in fulfilling his or her personal desires to improve appearance, the educational phase of the consultation has been effective. If the patient chooses not to undergo treatment after this detailed education, you may allow the patient more time for consideration, encourage the patient to ask more questions, follow up accordingly, or simply accept the patient's decision.

However, education does not cease when an individual becomes a patient. Information will be communicated frequently between the practice and patient and the patient and practice. Following a procedure, you will want to learn about the patient's perceptions of and satisfaction with the treatment experience. This information is essential to measure quality and to progress in patient care and operations.

Beyond fulfilling patients' specific desires, the practice must maintain communication with every patient by providing educational updates about the practice and its providers, innovations in treatment, and overall health concerns. Such communication will maintain your visibility with a satisfied patient and will offer two very significant resources to grow your aesthetic practice: new or repeat services to this existing patient and the potential for referral of new clients. It is a message that cannot be repeated enough: referrals are your single greatest resource for new clients.

PHOTOGRAPHS AND FEES

There are two uncomfortable moments in the patient's pretreatment experience in your office, whether during a consultation or in a preoperative visit, that are nevertheless essential to your ability to fulfill a patient's needs and expectations. These are the need to obtain clinical photographs and to discuss fee quotes.

Taking preoperative photographs heightens the patient's vulnerability: the patient is documented, potentially unclothed, for the very concern he or she has come to you. Be sensitive to this. Carefully explain the need for photographs, both for you and for the patient: these images can be used to show computer simulations of the results that may be achieved, and photos will later allow the patient to see the progress or result after treatment. Do not ask robed patients to parade down a hall to a photo room. Let no one make flippant remarks or use humor to break the ice; use compassion. Do not show patients preoperative photographs unless they ask or unless you feel this will assist in explaining potential outcomes or procedural options. Do give every patient a consent form and allow him or her to elect whether photographs can be used for the education of other patients and other physicians, for media use, or any other purpose. Follow up before you use those photographs with a consent specific to the occasion and use. If you cannot reach the patient for consent to this specific use, do not use the photographs. Fee quotes are the moment of truth for many patients.

Never should the physician define the fee; this is a business transaction that should be conducted by a qualified support person with whom the patient is familiar. This staff member should sit down next to the patient, not across a banker's desk, and review all fees, associated policies, the means for payment, and answer all the patient's questions specifically. This is a critical moment where all attention must be on the patient, not on ringing phones, office disruptions, pressure tactics, or small talk. Fees must be communicated after consent is obtained and before treatment is performed. Patients may be nervous, but if they are hesitant, they must not be pushed. A patient should be allowed all the time he or she needs to consider the fees. The fee quote should be dated and the time frame for which it is valid specified. The patient is invited to follow up at any time, and a team member should make contact with the patient after a short but appropriate time frame.

RELATIVE WISDOM: Feeding the Children

The year 2008 will long be remembered as the year of the mortgage crisis. As the result of more than a decade of free and easy loans, tens of thousands of loans were going unpaid, and banks were closing as a result of these defaults.

We were having dinner with friends, a family who for years owned the bank in the town where I grew up and where we now live, when the subject of loans gone bad came up. Cautiously, our friend, now running the bank his great-grandfather founded with multiple successful branches, proudly stated that at their bank there were no bad loans, no foreclosures. Business was solid. When I asked his strategy for this success, he stated solemnly, "My grandfather taught us all that banking was a relationship business, that you must never make a loan that will prevent someone from feeding the children. To this day, I teach my loan officers to review credit histories, consider down payments, but get to know the people you will lend money to, and never make a loan that will prevent someone from feeding his or her family."

Relative wisdom: Patient financing options abound for anyone who truly desires an aesthetic procedure. My dear friend, Mary, who has spent more than two decades with her patients in her husband's practice, once told me that it is important to get to know your patients completely and never to agree to schedule a procedure when you know that paying for that procedure will prevent someone from feeding the children.

FREE CONSULTATIONS

I do not believe that physicians should provide consultations free of charge. Your time has value. If the case were a medical case, you would bill the insurer. If the case is aesthetic, you must charge the patient. Consultation fees serve two purposes: (1) They tactfully eliminate clients who are not yet ready to commit to aesthetic medicine but are still "shopping," and (2) they attach value to the time a provider spends in clinical review with a client.

There are exceptions, and you must define those based on your practice limits and preferences. Complimentary consultations to friends or medical colleagues who you know are serious and complimentary consultations to existing patients are just two examples of situations in which you may elect not to charge the patient for the consultation.

When business is slow, services are new, or the physician has time, complimentary consultations by the physician are still a poor choice. My preference is for a nurse or patient coordinator to handle the consultation; this person can effectively screen and educate a prospective patient free of charge, rather than the physician's spending hours in consultations that take time away from other productive services and do not generate revenue. However, no one—no one—but the physician who will prescribe the treatment and perform the treatment or delegate it to an appropriate extender must ask for and accept the consent of the patient for treatment. For surgery, it is the physician who must ask for and accept consent for any patient on which he or she will operate. Furthermore, one physician must not accept patient consent for another physician who will perform the surgery.

There are no cookie-cutter solutions; there is no set formula defining consultation scheduling or charges. Defining a formula that is right for your practice must maximize the time a provider has available to provide services and generate revenue, and balance time in consultation with that variable. Consultation fees may vary based on the services sought by a patient, an established relationship with the client/patient and the type of consultation (initial or comprehensive). However you choose to structure and charge for consultations, your policy will be defined by:

- The abilities and preferences of staff who provide support in conducting consultations. A physician who is impatient or difficult to understand when educating patients will need a strong individual to conduct consultations.

Continued

FREE CONSULTATIONS—cont'd

- What is acceptable practice for *your* market—not the geographic region where you practice or what the doctor down the street practices, but what is acceptable for your practice, time, and your patients' expectations.

In addition to policy that defines the structure and fees of a consultation, your practice must define appropriate protocols for every type of consultation. Identify and assign consultation responsibilities to staff, but do not dilute the patient's experience with too many people and contacts. Empower others to take responsibility for specific nonclinical items of the consultation agenda to make the most of provider time.

IN PRACTICE: Whom to Educate

This is a lesson for every kind, personable, and skilled provider of aesthetic services. Referral sources are your best means for growing your practice, but only when they are properly educated.

I was visiting a very busy cosmetic dermatologist whose days were so filled that patients gladly waited at length to see her. Nothing seemed to run on schedule.

The physician insisted on performing her own consultations—perfectly acceptable. It was only when I sat in on several that I learned her downfall.

A lovely lady of 70-plus came in with horrible sun damage to her skin. She had been referred to the physician by another dermatologist in town who only handled clinical cases. My client listened carefully as the woman explained how she disliked the spots on her skin. My client explained carefully that she could be treated with lasers, a peel, skin care, or a combination of procedures. The dermatologist explained what each entailed, the benefits and cautions, and the cost. The patient was puzzled. "Won't my insurance pay for this?" No, the physician told her. These are cosmetic procedures.

The patient proceeded to ask a lot of questions, take a lot of notes, and then toward the end of nearly a 25-minute visit asked, "Will my insurance pay for this visit with you?" The physician told her not to worry, there would be no charge. Then the physician moved on to the next room, and on and on as her busy waiting room recycled patients waiting longer and longer to see her.

The physician and I sat down late that evening to discuss the day, and I asked about the many people referred by the clinical dermatologist's office and how many of them actually accepted treatment. The physician stated that this was her best source of referrals, so much so that she often treated his wife free of charge. So we ran a referral report, only to find that in the past 6 months, of the nearly 200 patients referred by the dermatologist, only six had accepted treatment. Moreover, because these prospective patients were referred by a colleague, my client rarely charged a consultation fee. I had more questions: When was the last time the clinical dermatologist visited my client's practice? When was the last time she updated him on technologies and opportunities she had to offer his patients? When was the last time she visited the clinical dermatologist's practice to see what he offered?

Several weeks later, the physician called me. She had visited the clinical dermatologist and together they sat down over lunch. She began to educate him about her newest procedures, but he stopped her. "Those are all cosmetic; they are not important to me." But they were the reason he was referring his patients to her, or so she assumed. "No, I don't refer them to you because you offer cosmetic procedures. I refer them to you because I know you have the patience to meet with them."

When she explained to him that these no-cost consultations were costing her a lot of time and money, he was surprised to hear that his patients were not accepting treatment. "When I refer my patients, I don't tell them these are cosmetic procedures that insurance won't pay for. I want them to go see you and be happy. I expect the cost is not much more than their deductible, anyway."

The lesson here: It is as important to educate your referral sources as it is to educate each individual patient. Keep your referral sources up to date, and keep an eye on the reason, validity, and value of the referrals they send you. You may find that those referral relationships are costing you a lot of time, patience, and money.

COMPREHENSION

Interest is what you use to communicate with your market and to maintain a relationship with patients. Education is what is necessary to convert interest into action—the willingness of an individual to undergo an aesthetic medical procedure in your practice. Comprehension results from effective communication and education and ultimately leads to happy patients, based on outcomes and the entire treatment experience.

Measuring Comprehension

Measuring comprehension at the interest stage is relatively basic:

- *Qualitative analysis:* Are clients who come to you clear on your brand, mission, and the services you provide?

- *Quantitative analysis:* Where do patients originate from? How are they referred to you? What are the patient's goals?

The education process affords another opportunity to measure comprehension:

- Is the patient at ease and confident with your practice and recommendations for treatment?

- Does the patient elect treatment? Is the elected treatment consistent with the patient's stated goals? Is the treatment consistent with your optimal recommendation? Why or why not?

A lack of patient comprehension in any instance is a failure by the practice to fully educate patients and thus is a failure of quality care. A patient's dissatisfaction with a course of treatment because of discomfort, side effects, or achieved versus stated outcomes demonstrates a failure by the practice to communicate effectively or a failure to ensure patient comprehension. Similarly, disbelief or lack of acceptance of complications or adverse events demonstrates a failure by the practice and provider to fully disclose all possible complications or risks or to ensure that the patient understands.

Failure of Comprehension

A lack of comprehension, whether from inadequate communication or a failure to ensure that the patient accepts what has been communicated, is measured:

- *Qualitatively:* In the patient who is unhappy in either outcomes or the process necessary to achieve outcomes

- *Quantitatively:* In the patients your practice is unable to retain, and who will not refer or recommend you to others

If you believe that client-to-patient conversion and the number of procedures you perform in any given period are the only data necessary to measure your success, you are mistaken. To remain competitive, you must not only convert clients to patients; you must also convert clients to happy, fulfilled patients who have been fully informed of the total experience, including potential pain and discomfort, the recovery process, and results. Patients who were informed of what to expect, accepted this from you, and are now happy with their outcome will recommend you to others and will maintain their relationship with you.

Patients whose experience as a whole is flawed because they were not taught to expect the things that typically occur during or as a result of treatment, such as bruising, redness, or discomfort, or patients who simply are not satisfied and regret undergoing treatment are service failures. The data you can collect from these patients are essential to assessing your practice's success at providing aesthetic medicine.

You should practice with the expectation that happy patients are a great source for referrals and that referral is the single best means of growing your practice. Consider the impact of unhappy patients: they will vociferously share negative experiences and find opportunities to discredit you, whether deserved or not, more often than patients who share their good experiences and refer others to you.

Implement procedures to measure comprehension quantitatively and qualitatively at every stage. Review this regularly. Look for trends; look for strengths. Identify and immediately correct any weaknesses. In doing so you will achieve a consistency for meeting your needs and expectations: you will readily attract prospective patients who are willing to accept the services you provide, and you will develop patients who are fully satisfied with the total experience of your care, who would do it again even if the experience included discomfort or unexpected, yet disclosed, potential adverse outcomes.

🦋 IN PRACTICE: Who's Fooling Whom?

I love watching the experts in action. You learn so much. Sometimes even they learn a little from their actions.

A young woman was on her final visit to the office the day before her breast augmentation surgery. The physician made it a practice to meet all of his patient's postoperative caregivers if the patient elected to recover at home. He did this because he believed he knew his patients well—and young women in particular didn't take the instructions they were given seriously. "Where is your driver, your caregiver?" the patient coordinator asked. The young woman quickly replied, "My mom can't take that much time off work, but she'll be here tomorrow."

The physician instructed the patient coordinator to speak with the patient's mother and review all the vital information for the following day. "My mom can't take calls at work," the young woman stated. "Here is her cell number; call her after 5 pm tonight." The physician and staff accepted the young woman's sincerity and later that evening he made the call. No one answered, and the voice mail was a generic greeting with only a telephone number. The physician called the young woman and told her that her surgery would have to be rescheduled at her expense if he did not hear from her caregiver before surgery.

The day of surgery arrived, and so did the patient, alone, to the surgical center. "My mom dropped me off and is just out shopping. She's totally familiar with what she needs to do. She's not worried at all. She'll be back at 1 o'clock. You told me I'd be released about that time, right?"

"Well, I am sorry," the physician told her. "But unless your mom is here so I can discuss all the requirements for your recovery with her before you go into surgery, you are not going into surgery. It is part of our practice policy, you signed that you understand this, and you will have to bear the cost for rescheduling."

Distraught, the young woman called her mother, who quickly arrived at the surgical center, quite upset. The physician recognized her as one of his patients, someone he had treated several times. "I'm angry," said the mother. "I am your patient, and you know how difficult my work schedule is and the demands on my time. You know me, and you know I am competent to take care of my daughter today. Why must you insist that I be here before her procedure? I certainly planned to be here to take her home."

"I didn't recognize your name on her caregiver form," the physician stated. "I am so sorry."

"I remarried last year," the woman stated. "Who do you think referred my daughter to you?"

The physician thought the patient was fooling him, that she did not in fact have someone to drive her home. The patient thought the physician was fooling her; he would never postpone her surgery. And the practice team were fooling themselves into believing that they knew their patients well, but they certainly didn't know how this patient had come to them.

PATIENT NEEDS AND EXPECTATIONS

Interest, education, and comprehension are essential to attracting and serving your patients in the most general sense. How do you look at specific populations and assess whether you are meeting those needs and expectations?

Prospective Patients

Data are key to discovering how your patients are introduced to your practice. It's more than simply asking, "Where did you hear about us?" on a form with "Check all that apply." Talk to your patients and learn exactly what motivated them to want a procedure, what compelled them to seek your practice, and who or what provided them with the contact information that resulted in that first call, email, or visit. Review the prospective patient's educational process: were there many questions, insecurities, inconsistencies, or contradictions between what the patient thought he or she could achieve and what you might provide? Accurately track patient recruitment, conversion, lost opportunities, and recovery.

- Recruitment occurs when the prospective patient engages you for a consultation and actually appears for the consultation.

- Conversion occurs when the patient accepts treatment from you: distinguish whether conversion is for the recommended treatment, or an alternative, or a service unrelated to the initially stated goals.

- Loss occurs when there is no contact, no reply, or no desire from the prospective patient to engage your practice.

- Recovery occurs when a prospective patient you have documented as a loss, returns for further education or to accept treatment.

Patients

Individuals who have consulted with your practice in person and who have accepted treatment (or not) are your patients. The ability to recognize where you have met needs or expectations or had service failures is derived from a combination of data and experience.

- Interest is met when the patient demonstrates the trust to pay for your expert opinion to meet his or her goals.

- Education is successful when the patient confidently chooses (or does not choose) a course of treatment and can explain his or her reasoning.

- Consent is valid when the patient not only agrees, but is also compliant and prepared for the course of treatment and tolerant of a less-than-perfect experience or outcome.

- Feedback is essential to know your patient's true feelings about your practice, the outcomes achieved, and the experience.

- Referral is a positive means of knowing that whether this patient accepted treatment in your practice or not, that individual respects and trusts you.

- Retention demonstrates that a patient is loyal, accepts the value of your services, and will return to you rather than try a cheaper, newer, different service option.

Lost Patients

Your best lessons in service failure are lost patients. Although we learn by positive experiences, we grow by the lessons that sometimes are hard to accept:

- Tracking enables your practice to truly deem a patient "lost" in interest and from your practice.

- Recovery enables your practice to revisit the patient you considered lost.

- Dismissed patients are those you must formally inform you cannot serve. The reason may be one for the record, but where a patient is at risk, or represents a risk detrimental to the health, safety, and success of your practice, you must dismiss that person.

IN PRACTICE: Case Dismissed

She was known by everyone in the practice as the difficult patient. Whether she was scheduled for an injection, a peel, her child's acne appointment, or for any other reason, she was generally late, failed to arrive and didn't call, and became belligerent when there were no appointment times to suit her demands. She wanted to try everything in the practice's menu of services, was happy with nothing, but always seemed to return asking for more.

One day, in typical fashion she showed up more than an hour late for a "quick injection," an appointment she had already failed to arrive for 2 weeks earlier. A member of the staff politely took Ms. Difficult aside and told her that she would have to wait until the physician could see her. "Sure, I'll wait until she's done with her current patient." No, she was told, she would have to wait until there were no patients waiting, because she had missed her scheduled appointment time. "It's just a quick procedure, and I need it now. I'll be leaving town next week, and I don't have time to reschedule, and I am not going to sit here and wait. If she wants my money, she'll see me now."

The staff member pulled the physician aside between patients to tell her what was transpiring. Suddenly a loud voice was heard in the reception area. Ms. Difficult was complaining to another patient, "I don't know why I come

Continued

✍ IN PRACTICE: Case Dismissed—cont'd

to this practice, because they don't respect my schedules. They are always happy to recommend the latest, greatest, most expensive treatment, because they know I have the means to buy anything I want. So I'm a little late, and they expect that I'm going to wait?"

The physician told the staff member to bring Ms. Difficult to her office, and to wait with her there. When she arrived, the physician handed her a letter and told her firmly, "I am discharging you from my practice. We pride ourselves on providing patients valuable treatment and experiences. It is clear we can no longer fulfill your needs, nor can we meet your expectations. Please let me show you out."

Suddenly Ms. Difficult was silent, ashamed, and didn't know what to say. She left without a word.

Later, I asked the physician if she wasn't worried that her actions would backfire, that out of anger the woman would badmouth her to others. The physician confidently replied, "Anyone who knows her and believes she is right to be angry with me is no one I want in my practice. Case dismissed."

CHAPTER 8

What Defines Risk?

Life is never without risk.
To disregard the potential for risk in practicing
aesthetic medicine is to risk life.

In medicine you can never fully predict or control what might happen. Minor complications simply make the treatment less than perfect. The greatest risk is either loss of life or impairment that is more significant than the original condition for which treatment was sought. In aesthetic medicine there is an added risk—that of unfulfilled goals or dissatisfaction with outcomes, which in turn can become a risk to your practice's image and success.

Red flags are cautionary indicators that arise from the words or actions of a patient alerting you or your staff to matters that should concern you, or from your own words or actions alerting a prospective or current patient, or even a colleague to a potential problem. Whether the source for risk is the patient or your practice, recognizing and minimizing unnecessary risk are the responsibility of the physician and the practice.

PATIENTS AT RISK

Health conditions can place patients at risk. Unhappy or misguided patients put your practice at risk. The key to avoiding risky patients is to be selective about accepting patients, thorough in patient education, and vigilant about patient compliance to all the obligations and instructions necessary to avoid complications.

In consultation, the provider learns about an individual and his or her goals for improving appearance. The three essentials to discover during consultation include:

1. The patient's desire or intentions for aesthetic medical treatment

2. His or her expectations for the physical outcome of the treatment

3. The patient's expectations for the personal outcomes of the treatment (how the physical outcome will affect his or her life)

Realistic goals involve much more than a physical state that can be reasonably and safely achieved. Determining these three factors is essential to avoid the patient's having unrealistic expectations or dissatisfaction with the experience and outcome of a procedure. Although a patient coordinator or nurse can ask the patient about these factors and should document the responses, it is you, the treating physician, who must ask and accept that a patient's answers are sincere, because inevitably you will assume responsibility for the patient, agree to treat the patient, and define a course of treatment.

You must learn to read your patients, to recognize when they have underlying personal or psychosocial influences or potential mental health issues that influence their ability to accept reality. You must look for the warning signs that indicate that a patient is unable to let go of impossible aspirations. Question each patient to affirm comprehension and avoid misunderstandings about goals and expectations.

REALISTIC GOALS

For the provider, the key to detecting unrealistic goals lies in understanding what constitutes realistic goals. Fortunately, this is relatively simple:

- Realistic goals are safely attainable.

- Realistic goals do not produce extremes, or push extremes.

- Realistic goals come solely from the patient and are not the result of an outside influence.

- Realistic goals are not based on an expectation for dramatic or instantaneous life alteration.

- Realistic goals are what emotionally healthy individuals want to achieve to improve their appearance.

The most egregious of errors occurs when a provider does not respond to the patient's unrealistic goals. As a provider in aesthetic medicine and as a medical doctor, you are ethically bound to identify patient goals that are not attainable. Although you may decline to treat a patient who cannot grasp reality, do not dismiss a patient with unrealistic goals. You must respond to unrealistic goals, educating your patient and proposing achievable aesthetic outcomes so that he or she can determine in which reality he or she chooses to live. Be candid and honest and expect the same of your client. Negotiate if you feel there is room to negotiate, but always qualify *why*. It is better to have a client understand why you cannot or will not fulfill his or her goals than for that individual to take those unrealistic goals to a less ethical provider. Although you may not convert a client to a patient, you will affirm your credibility.

Any improvement in an individual's appearance—new clothing, a new hairstyle, or an aesthetic medical treatment—can produce a short- or long-term change in posture, confidence, and self-assurance. With clothing or hair, the extreme is reversible. In aesthetic medical treatment, the extreme is not so easily reversible. Unless you want to be known as someone who fulfills patients' requests for extreme alterations, you should not fulfill these goals. You will brand yourself as extreme. No significant other or parent should influence the patient to undergo aesthetic medical treatment. They may, and certainly should, support the goals of the individual, but they should not be the compelling reason that someone seeks treatment. It bears repeating: aesthetic medicine fulfills personal desire.

When a battered woman, a child with a birth defect, or an individual with a disfiguring injury undergoes treatment to restore appearance, this is a personal goal. This can be life changing, and it certainly encompasses appropriate goals. But when patients state that they want to enhance their relatively normal features in the belief that this will significantly alter or improve their daily lives, you must search for the underlying message. Will softening ethnic features reduce the bias and discrimination the patient may have encountered? Will an improved figure restore a failing marriage? Will a younger appearance lead to career advancement? The provider's sound judgment is essential when the patient's expressed goals include a life-changing experience. The likely reality of that change is a part of qualifying risk.

Determining that a prospective patient is emotionally healthy is as much a matter of observation as of judgment. Although the provider expects that the patient will honestly answer questions about medical conditions, including emotional health, an emotionally unstable individual probably cannot provide objective self-evaluation. This person can represent a significant source of risk to your practice. The more you and others in your practice observe a patient whose emotional health is questionable, the more likely you will arrive at a confident decision regarding whether to treat this patient.

REALISTIC EXPECTATIONS

Realistic goals are what a client wants to accomplish by undergoing aesthetic medical treatment; realistic expectations involve the fulfillment of goals as well as satisfaction with and acceptance of the process. Although you may have a patient whose goals are fulfilled, he or she may still be dissatisfied because of the experience or the process necessary to achieve those goals. After you have determined that a client's goals are sincere and attainable, ensuring that risk remains low requires that you fully explain the process necessary to achieve those goals. This includes:

- Pretreatment or preoperative expectations and patient obligations

- The discomfort, anxiety, and pain involved

- The time commitment, including recovery, down time, and the period necessary for results to be attained

- Posttreatment or postoperative expectations and patient obligations

- The potential for unfulfilled goals and possible undesirable results

- The potential for and definition of adverse events

- The patient's financial obligation

To make certain that no aspect of the process is overlooked, a consultation agenda form should be created that assigns responsibility for each segment of the process. Use this agenda as a checklist to ensure that nothing is overlooked during consultation, that the patient completely understands and accepts every element of the process, and that the patient has been given all appropriate forms and instructions. Following a checklist reduces the risk of failing to fully disclose the process or to provide essential documents. Question your patient's comprehension of all that is communicated; don't assume that your message has been thoroughly understood.

Realistic expectations also require that the patient grasp the potential for adverse outcomes or less than ideal results. Physical risk should be minimal if you have carefully qualified the patient as a good candidate. But if he or she does not comply with preoperative and postoperative instructions, the results may be less than optimal, and you could be held responsible. If you fear your patient won't quit smoking before a procedure, won't stay out of the sun, or will misuse pain medication, don't take chances. As part of informed consent, have the patient sign an acknowledgment that he or she accepts the practice's policies and procedures defining the patient's responsibilities, and the financial or physical consequences of noncompliance. Provide valid data about what can happen if the printed instructions are disregarded. Emphasize that these are not scare tactics, but are for the patient's own safety and well-being for which you ultimately take responsibility, and that you can and will deny treatment if the patient is noncompliant.

RELATIVE WISDOM: Blueprints

It's common knowledge—no remodeling plan goes without alterations. The problem, according to most home remodeling contractors, is that clients decide to make alterations to their plans but don't comprehend the cost or the time considerations that changes generate. However, according to those of us who embark on remodeling projects, sometimes you just really want things to be perfect. Where the two meet is the place called "timing is everything."

We decided to remodel our master bath after what began as a discussion about new towels and a coat of paint evolved into a plan for new cabinetry and tile and resulted in a room stripped back to the studs. When I had finally selected the right marble, granite, mosaic, and wood, we realized that the existing spa tub simply would not complement the new layout. The new spa tub was a different dimension than the old, which would allow for a larger shower. The larger shower featured steam and rain, which required more hot water, and thus the need for new plumbing. The need for new plumbing required running some pipes into the ceiling, and thus provided the opportunity to raise a dome above the tub. The raised dome allowed for a chandelier above the tub, and hence the need for new wiring. There were no circuits left on the board, so now a new panel had to be pulled into the house.

In every family there is a familiar story of remodeling and a project that never seems to end, and when it does, the final bill is astounding to the homeowner and no surprise for the contractors.

Relative wisdom: The desire for an aesthetic procedure often begins with a patient's straightforward wish for little changes—they are easier to accept, and it's more likely that the goals are realistic and the experience will be favorable. As a result of a favorable outcome, the patient may define new goals and desire new services.

For your patients to remain happy on their journey of self-remodeling, you must remain meticulous. Don't overlook the discussion of goals and expectations with each new treatment simply because you are familiar with this good candidate. Don't mistake new goals as realistic because the patient has proved realistic in the past, or assume motivations are sincere because the patient is known to be straightforward. Always follow your blueprint for minimizing risk and you will not only avoid risk, you will retain happy patients.

INFORMED CONSENT

As a practitioner and proprietor, you accept the importance of informed consent; it is essential to risk management. Informed consent is so varied and comprehensive based on the individual procedures and clinical preferences of physicians and practices that it must be customized. As a legal tool, thorough informed consent must contain the following:

- The clinical definition of the procedure

- The definition of the condition for which the procedure is being performed

- Alternatives to the procedure (where they exist)

- The defined benefits or outcomes of the procedure

- Definitions of the risks associated with the procedure

- An explanation of the unknown factors associated with the procedure

- Verification of the patient's competence in voluntarily accepting treatment

- Verification of the patient's state of health and ability to undergo treatment

As a vital measure of the success of your aesthetic practice, informed consent must be more than a legal tool. It must be a document that verifies by patient signature that the individual willingly accepts treatment and understands the process involved, all clinical implications, and any potential risks.

In addition, informed consent is a means of demonstrating trust between provider and patient. It communicates that the patient has chosen this provider based on confidence, is willing and unwaveringly wants to undergo treatment, agrees to be compliant with all preoperative and postoperative instructions, and that he or she is not being influenced by anything or anyone other than a personal desire to undergo treatment.

I am not a lawyer. My job is to help ensure the success of your practice. You don't need to be a lawyer, and you don't need to hire a lawyer to tell you that even with informed consent, the potential still exists for risk, for an unhappy patient, or for adverse events or unexpected outcomes. What a lawyer will not tell you, however, is something essential to your success: informed consent is not only a valuable a risk management tool but also a measure of patient satisfaction.

If you have done your job in communication and education and the patient is candid and unwavering, commitment in writing to the points discussed and the traditional elements of an informed consent should not be an issue. Informed consent works in your favor with educated, informed, and confident patients. You are disclosing everything fully to your patients and asking that they fully disclose all of their intentions for treatment and compliance. Patients will respect the fact that as much as you need to honestly disclose information for their understanding before treatment, you expect the same of them. By doing this, you are helping to ensure that your patients respect your responsibilities and accept their own.

Applying Informed Consent

There are numerous publications and standards that define the law and letter of informed consent. It is so vast a topic, with so many variables, that in itself it is a comprehensive guide to an essential component of the success of your practice.

Recommended resources for informed consent include publications of the medical societies of your specialty. Most pharmaceutical and medical device companies provide sample informed consent documents and releases specific to their products. Ask your sales and practice-support representatives for these documents. Most sources will offer single documents or compendiums of sample informed consent documents. Your best option is to request software containing these documents, allowing you to personalize forms to your individual practice needs. Reasonable standards in informed consent documents are best set by someone other than you. You define standards that apply to a particular case, but you do not define all of the standards that exist across your specialty or for a particular procedure.

Personalize informed consent by including vital practice branding information on documents. Track these documents in an overall checklist of patient information. Keep these documents organized, update them as needed, and track your updates in a personal compendium of practice forms.

Take as much time as necessary to explain and present informed consent documents to your patients. Take the time to question the patient's comprehension of documents. Take more time to explain documents to patients with questions. Have a witness present. Let the patient know that informed consent is not simply a means to protect yourself or your practice, but is for the benefit of the patient, to verify that he or she fully understands what may be very comprehensive variables and outcomes of treatment.

CHECK, PLEASE

It's an all-too-common scene: The patient coordinator who was warm, inviting, and attentive during the earlier consultation suddenly, in presenting the informed consent form to the patient, begins reciting in a rapid-fire, robotic manner, scribbling checkmarks down the side of her document as she rattles through her list, looking up briefly after each point for a compliant nod.

Consider the image you have just painted for your patient, who has been nurtured and attended by your staff, and now that he or she is ready to accept treatment, is rushed through the informed consent process.

Processes exist for good reason. Take the time to give your patient proper attention, in this and every phase of your relationship. Your continued success in practice depends on it.

🌿 IN PRACTICE: What a Girl Wants

She was a tiny thing, very nervous about consulting with the physician about breast augmentation, with her boyfriend standing guard. I sat quietly through this bizarre consultation, where the boyfriend expressed images of what he expected she would look like, and where she said little unless directly asked by the physician. The surgeon did all the right things: he reminded the man that the woman was his patient and he needed to focus his attention on her wants, needs, and questions. He tried hard to get answers from her about her wishes, but she always deferred to her boyfriend. When it came time to measure her for implant size, the boyfriend was vocal—nothing could be too big. The surgeon clearly defined what he felt was the largest size appropriate for this tiny woman's figure and safe for him to implant. The boyfriend questioned the limits. The only thing that anyone was in agreement about was that breast augmentation would, in fact, benefit this woman's figure if that was what she truly wanted for herself.

Finally, I chimed in. I asked the man if he would please join me in the next room where I might show him different implants and photographs of the resulting appearance. The physician could do the same in the examination room with his patient, and we would see if there was consensus. I took the time to show him photographs of horrific large-volume implant results, which can readily be found online. I told him if he really loved this woman, he would never allow her to do this to her body or her life. And then I did one more thing: I turned the tables. I asked if he would ever allow her to dictate what he would do with his body. I then led the boyfriend to the reception area and asked him politely to wait.

The patient coordinator was stunned and shocked. She thought that I had crossed the line. No, I told her, what I did was educate someone who was heavily influencing a patient in the practice. It would have been easy at this juncture to dismiss this case and these two people, but the boyfriend would readily find a surgeon somewhere who would listen to him and maim her.

In the meantime, the physician had some quality time with his patient. He learned that she had previously been in an abusive relationship. Her current boyfriend truly loved and cared for her, and while she wanted the implants and wanted to please her boyfriend, she was indeed nervous. She didn't want to be disfigured; she didn't want her disapproving family to censure her further for something that would look unnatural or obvious. She was worried about surgery, because she was a single mom and afraid that if something went wrong, she would not be there for her child.

The physician and I met in the hallway, and he looked at me with anguish. What now? Should he dismiss the case? Should he refer her for counseling? He was a seasoned surgeon, but flustered by the events at hand.

I advised him to follow the process that never fails.

We met the boyfriend and the patient, spelling things out clearly: She was a good candidate for augmentation. The surgeon explicitly stated her safe and reasonable augmentation options. He defined her experience, obligations as a patient, anesthesia options, the outcomes, and potential adverse events. He followed all the proper procedures. He told this couple there was a waiting period required for her to consider her options, and that she was free to call back or come back at any time. He then looked at the man and offered his hand and said, "Every man who truly loves a woman, whether his girlfriend, his daughter, or his mother, will give her what *she* wants." He put his hand out to the woman and said, "Only you can decide if this is what you want."

When they left, we were all sure we would never see either of them again. Two weeks later, the doctor called me. Guess who had arrived in his office, this time with her boyfriend's mother? After the two women sat through the entire consultation together, she booked the procedure precisely as the surgeon had recommended.

WHEN TO SAY NO

There are no absolutes as to when you must say "No" to a patient. In every case it is inevitably your judgment and the judgment of your staff who also have a perspective on the patient that will influence your decisions. However, there are common warning signs that a patient might not be one you elect to treat:

- A patient with unrealistic goals

- A patient with unrealistic expectations

- A patient with emotional disorders

- A patient who is not self-motivated

- A case in which results cannot be safely or reasonably achieved

- A case that might put an individual's health at risk

- A case in which the patient clearly does not comprehend the procedure, the likely outcome, or potential adverse results

- A case in which the patient is clearly not going to be compliant

Body dysmorphic disorder (BDD) is well documented in mental health studies, particularly in relation to aesthetic procedures. BDD is a condition whereby one has an unhealthy obsession with perceived or minor flaws in appearance. The growth of cosmetic medicine, including nonsurgical treatments, has increased the number of elective procedures available and the number of conditions that individuals seek to treat. It has led to a population segment that some have described as "appearance obsessed." But there is a difference between patients who are frequent consumers of cosmetic medicine services and those who have a diagnosis of BDD. BDD involves more than an active interest in cosmetic procedures; BDD patients undergo those procedures without ever achieving satisfaction. Additional indicators of BDD include extreme grooming habits, such as overplucking brows or picking skin, avoiding mirrors or constantly looking in them, and the use of excessive makeup or clothing selected to camouflage imagined defects.

Unfortunately, many of these signs are subjective. As there is no absolute variable for saying "No" to a patient, there is no absolute variable for determining when the patient's desires for improvement are unhealthy without evaluation by a qualified mental health professional. Your instincts and judgment will ultimately help you determine whether you can treat the patient or must refuse care. Refusing treatment is not simply a means of protecting this individual from unnecessary or unwarranted procedures; it is essential for protecting your practice from exposure to a troubled patient who will never be satisfied with the results.

Saying "No" has its negative consequences. A truly unhealthy patient may feel anguish, anger, or despair, and will blame you. Your decision to refuse treatment must be cautiously determined and your message carefully delivered. Although it may be reassuring to a healthy person to hear, "You are beautiful, and I would not change a thing; I never mess with perfection," to an unhealthy person this is simply not acceptable or comprehensible.

RELATIVE WISDOM: The Very Best Customer

In every designer boutique or specialty store, and even in some auto dealerships, there are customers who buy everything, and return everything. Whether shoes, dresses, handbags, or sports cars, the customer takes them home and a few weeks later returns with an explanation that the items don't fit, don't match, aren't good enough, are too good, and countless other excuses. These chronic shoppers cost your business time and money, but in good times and bad they are there buying, and eventually they do keep some of their purchases. In their minds, these people feel they are your very best customer.

Relative wisdom: Aesthetic procedures are not like retail goods that can be tried on (experienced) or returned if the customer changes his or her mind. They are not like a bad hair color that can be corrected, or a bad lipstick that gets wiped off and tossed away. They are not a bad entrée that can be sent back to the kitchen, or a bad landscape design that can be uprooted and planted again. If you have patients who regularly elect services, are chronically unhappy with the outcomes, and often negotiate revisions, you do not have your very best customer—you have a significant potential for risk.

THE IMPORTANCE OF PATIENT SELECTION

Jack P. Gunter, MD, FACS

Although Dr. Gunter focuses his practice solely on rhinoplasty, the measures he uses to identify good candidates apply to any aesthetic procedure.

One of the key factors in obtaining a successful result is patient selection. The ideal patient is one who has realistic expectations. The patient must understand the difficulty of the operation and know that the goal of the surgery is a significant improvement and not perfection. Perfection in rhinoplasty is seldom, if ever, achieved.

He or she must also understand that the ideal nose is one that looks natural, is in balance and harmony with the other facial features, and has normal function. A nose that looks good on one person may not look good on another who has a different bone structure, different skin thickness (thick skin will not drape as well as thin skin), and different spatial relationships of anatomic structures—the eyes, brows, lips, and mouth.

Continued

THE IMPORTANCE OF PATIENT SELECTION—cont'd

Although all of these factors may seem obvious to a surgeon, they are not always that apparent to the patient and sometimes, after a lengthy explanation by the doctor, the patient still may not understand. One of the main reasons for this is the information the patient has been bombarded with over the past decade. Television shows such as "Extreme Makeover" and various plastic surgery marketing efforts (all the gimmicks the media is highlighting) have led many people to believe that plastic surgery involves just a "nip and a tuck" and that you can go in that morning, have a complete makeover without any risks, with very little bruising or swelling, and be back on the street in a week or so looking marvelous. There is more to it than that.

Although the risks with plastic surgery are low, there are risks with every type of surgery, and patients should be made aware of these. The complication I worry most about is for the patient to be expecting me to give him or her a better result than is possible. When this happens, it is usually because I didn't prepare the patient adequately or the individual didn't listen or didn't take my remarks seriously.

When surgeons feel their patients do not understand the information set forth, and they've done their best in trying to explain it, they should inform their patients that they are uncomfortable performing the surgery because they are concerned that they may not be able to achieve the result the patients are expecting.

There is nothing more difficult to take in hand, more perilous to conduct, or more uncertain in its success than to take the lead in the introduction of a new order of things.
— NICCOLO MACHIAVELLI

INVITING RISK

Your market and prospective and current patients are not the only sources for risk. Your practice may invite added risk.

Medical research, when conducted ethically, properly, and with the right motivations, leads to improved treatment options and outcomes for patients. Valid studies and the resulting findings deserve to be shared with other physicians in journals and at symposia. The patients who elect knowingly to participate in such research must be fully educated; research is the origin of informed consent. If you are not conducting research, there is no acceptable reason to invite added risk to your practice, but there are unintended ways that it happens.

WARNING SIGNS

You evaluate your prospective patients as good candidates; likewise, others are evaluating you to confirm that you are a good provider. This includes patients, staff, peers, and referral sources. This assessment is ongoing; it occurs through every phase of an individual's relationship with your practice.

What defines a good provider? It is someone who is qualified, reputable, and meets the standards that a patient would expect. Being a good provider does not necessarily mean that you are this patient's best choice; it means that you are a valid and viable option. You and your practice may be unintentionally raising red flags through inappropriate messages, attitudes, outlook, and clinical issues.

Maintaining a positive client/patient relationship throughout the patient's cycle and succeeding in practice requires that you constantly monitor for and recognize any warning signs—and correct them quickly. When you do not recognize the red flags that others perceive in your practice, you risk being labeled for your shortcomings, and you may be disregarded as a potential provider, discontinued as a provider, or remembered as less than a good provider. As time and trends change the needs of target populations, clients, and patients, your practice must evolve to meet those needs. Continuing to be alert for red flags is as important as continuing to evaluate changes in your market and the consistency of patient satisfaction.

Inappropriate and Risky Messages

Sometimes a message, born of aggressive marketing or consultation strategies, is perceived as inappropriate. Other times unintentional or poorly thought-out messages from your practice invite risk or signal your market and patients that you and your practice are risky business.

An inappropriate message is generally defined as one that either implies guaranteed results or violates taste and ethics. This can occur with messages inside or outside the practice, whether they are verbal or printed or come from the actions of a provider or staff member. They are counterproductive to your success. Your market, patients, peers, and possibly even your staff will question your credibility.

The greatest potential for disseminating an inappropriate message occurs when a provider compels rather than interests, sells rather than educates, and convinces rather than measures patient comprehension. Catchy phrases that draw attention to the practice and call individuals to act on their existing interest are perfectly acceptable. What is not acceptable is pressure, gimmickry, and manipulative messages that play on emotion.

PRESSURE TACTICS

Pressure tactics urge individuals to act based on conformity, taking advantage of their insecurities and creating a sense of urgency. Pressure is the message that everyone is doing it, and you must not be left out. Those who use pressure tactics view each patient as a sale rather than recognizing patient interactions as a privilege of one's vocation. Pressure is urging someone to do something before an opportunity expires, or before there is an unpleasant result.

GIMMICKRY

Gimmickry is using a catchy phrase or cliché to persuade an individual to act. It involves such tactics as a sale, a bonus, a special deal, or special feel, or even bait and switch. Gimmickry used in an aesthetic practice puts volume and revenue above patient satisfaction. It involves an unsubstantiated promise with an unattainable result. It is claims made about a magic potion or device with no credible supporting evidence, endorsements by self-proclaimed celebrities, and seals of approval by obscure professional organizations. Using spurious credentials and false board certifications or credentials that are not recognized by the American Board of Medical Specialties is deceptive, and in some states illegal to use in advertisements.

MANIPULATIVE MESSAGES

Manipulative messages twist facts and data to make a provider appear more credible or to elevate a deceptive value. They may use terms and descriptions that are contrived and cannot be validated. Manipulative messages take advantage of naïve clients; they do not generate fulfilled patients. These catchy phrases promise a "miracle lift," "face lift in a jar," "face lift without surgery," or they claim to "erase your wrinkles forever" or make someone "look 10 years younger in 10 minutes." Like gimmicks, they are deceptive and unethical, because you simply cannot deliver on them.

🔖 IN PRACTICE: Not Me

The physician had purchased the newest, hottest device in aesthetic medicine. The company was spending a great deal of money on advertising and promoting this as a nonsurgical alternative that mimicked surgery. I asked the physician why he would offer such promises to his patients, and he carefully told me, "The device has merit, and with proper patient selection and good education, we have happy patients."

When I reminded him that his message was not the only message his patients might encounter about the device, he repeated, "The device has merit, and with proper patient selection and good education, we have happy patients."

I sat in on a consultation with him and a patient who was specifically interested in this device. He focused on her goals: What did she want to achieve? As he explained that this would not produce what he thought she expected, she seemed dismayed. As he explained what she could achieve from this device compared with what she could achieve from other treatment modalities, namely surgery, she really became upset.

"Doctor, you advertised that this device could give me the same results as surgery, without surgery, and now you tell me that you cannot accomplish this. That is false advertising."

The physician said that he had never advertised such a thing. Other doctors may have, the device company may have, but he had not.

She reached in her handbag and pulled out a magazine. The physician denied that he had ever advertised in that publication. She opened the magazine with the device company's ad marked, and his name and practice location were listed in the ad.

The lesson here: The message projected by those you do business with must be congruent with your standards, ethics, and business practices. Never allow anyone to advertise on your behalf, and make it clear that no one should ever use your name without your express permission. Cooperative advertising with device or pharmaceutical companies is beneficial, but only when you are aware of and approve the message, and to whom and how it is delivered.

Appropriate Messages

Appropriate messages build image and credibility. They carry longevity in your market, with your patients, and all of those in contact with your practice who pass them on and thus generate referrals.

ATTITUDE

Your attitude as a provider of aesthetic medicine may change during your business life cycle, just as the attitudes of your patients are likely to change somewhat over very long cycles. Attitudes are how you view your practice and patients at the moment, relative to how you view your commitment to practice and fulfill desire. Attitudes may be conscious or unconscious and are visible not only to your target population, patients, staff, and peers, but also to known and unknown sources and resources.

When noninvasive treatment of the aging face was first being offered, perhaps you were skeptical. It may have taken some time before you accepted such treatment as appropriate to your practice mix. Once you accepted this as a component of your practice, did you regard these noninvasive procedures with less seriousness or candor than invasive procedures that carry greater risk? Of course not—all treatments, all patients should benefit from a consistent attitude of goals, education, and comprehension.

Regardless of the treatments you provide and the reasons for which you provide them, your attitude and the attitudes of your staff members must be consistently focused on what your patients and your market would expect of a skilled provider and a high-quality practice. When you are fulfilling the personal desires of another person through medical treatment, your attitudes must:

- Center on the individual patient
- Respect the patient's desires rather than imposing your personal views
- Demonstrate your commitment as a caring provider by acting with serious conviction in every case
- Be consistent inside and outside your professional life

The nuances of your attitudes are what define your identity and brand. The core of attitudes, as listed on p. 140, is the basis by which others will judge you.

Although some patients may come to you acting on a trend in aesthetic medicine, they still are trying to fulfill a personal desire (if not, they are not good candidates). You must, in every case, focus on that individual and his or her desire; not the trend, not your desire, not your preference, not even your expectation, but on the individual you are face to face with.

If a patient comes to a physician to eliminate the spider veins on her legs, he or she should not suggest taking care of the lesion on her nose as well, unless she expresses that desire. The lesion might not bother her, but the veins do. Addressing something other than the personal desire the patient has approached you for, even though it may be relevant, may not be appreciated.

The exception to respecting individual desires lies in extremes. If a patient's desire is extreme, you have the right to decline providing treatment. Extremes have their opposites. There are cases where a patient's desire may seem inconsequential to you. However, if the individual has taken the time to engage you to fulfill desire, it is not inconsequential to him or her.

You took an oath to treat human life with dignity. But you do not practice life-saving medicine; you practice life-enhancing medicine. Whatever the treatment or procedure, whether it involves a minor or major improvement, you must still treat the patient's desire to enhance his or her life with conviction and respect for the patient's need. In doing so, you will demonstrate your commitment as a caring provider. You should require that those on your staff support you in demonstrating this commitment.

Do not think that your attitude and the attitudes of those who work for you are only relevant within your office. My grandmother used to say, "Ears and eyes are everywhere," and from personal experience we know there is wisdom in those words. Always demonstrate respect, consistency, and dignity in your role as a physician, no matter how private and confident you may feel at any moment. You never know when an offhand, flippant remark or an unconsidered act may resurface. Such a transgression can reflect badly on your status as a respected, dignified provider of aesthetic medicine. You must be one who upholds the privacy and highly personal nature of his or her profession in every way, at all times.

CASES OF ATTITUDE

Consider these brief incidents and you will understand the need for monitoring red flags and attitudes.

The trend for Botox therapy is an indication of how quickly populations interested in aesthetic treatment can act. Regardless of the millions of people who have become Botox devotees, all good candidates who seek wrinkle reduction by injection are doing so out of personal desire. Perhaps they are influenced by the current trend, but they are not acting on the trend. (If one is acting solely based on a trend, he or she is not a good candidate for treatment.)

I was shocked when I heard a provider in consultation tell a client, "Welcome to the club."

Just because everyone is doing it, do not depersonalize it. A patient wants to undergo treatment to attain his or her own personal goals. Always focus on the individual.

Respecting individual desire requires finesse to make a distinction between respecting individual desire and fulfilling personal goals. For example, many breast augmentation patients are women who have completed their cycle of child-bearing and want to restore breast volume lost from pregnancy. These women may very well benefit from a tummy tuck also. Believe it or not, I know a surgeon who made it a policy to recommend some other form of body contouring in conjunction with any aesthetic breast procedure. He believed in up-selling.

Up-selling is fine, and it is a way to grow your business, but it will backfire when a client comes to you with one very specific desire and you, uninvited, offer other suggestions for improvement. When you fail to respect that individual's desire, you heighten your patient's sense of caution. Clearly identify desire in consultation, and your attitude and ability to respect individual desire will be perfectly clear.

If you trivialize anything, you and your practice may be viewed as uncaring. This applies to your staff as well. For example, an assistant to one of the kindest, most caring providers I have ever known went to inject a patient with local anesthetic. She basically took a stab and stated, "bull's-eye."

In another instance, a patient came into an aesthetic provider's office. While in the waiting room, the patient had an asthma attack. Rather than offering assistance, the receptionist asked the individual to wait in the hallway, so as not to disturb other waiting patients with the coughing and wheezing.

In yet another example, a postoperative patient was devastated at the initial appearance of scars following her face lift. When she expressed this concern to the provider, rather than suggest appropriate cosmetics or offer caring assurance and reiterating the aftercare and time necessary for wounds to properly heal, the provider simply responded, "Don't worry, they will fade in time."

These are among countless examples of inappropriate attitudes. They may seem rather harmless to you, but they can quickly bring into question your mindset as a provider in a practice committed to the highest quality of care and experience in every case. If you and your staff approach the care of every patient with an attitude that conveys commitment to the individual at all times, there is little likelihood that red flags will wave.

You must project a consistent, caring attitude both inside and outside your professional life; this is something that many people overlook, not just in aesthetic medicine. The way you speak of your practice and the service you provide must remain constant. The way you regard and speak of patients must always remain focused on protecting their privacy and their trust, even when they allow you to use their likeness to educate others.

Whether you are out to dinner, playing golf, at the grocery store, or at little league, someone may recognize and overhear you if you are indiscreet, and they may pass along what you say. The person who overhears you may be connected to the patient you are speaking about, or may be a prospective patient.

RELATIVE WISDOM: Process of Elimination

My mom called one day to tell me that a friend of hers had been diagnosed with breast cancer and was researching the surgeon her physician had recommended. My mother was well aware that I knew the man personally, and she knew how I felt about him. But being the good mom she is, she didn't want to convey my words for me, so she had her friend call me.

"Marie," the friend asked, "what do you know about this surgeon?" I replied that I knew he was board certified, on staff at the hospital, and had been in practice 16 years.

"But what do you know about him? Your mom tells me you are acquainted."

"Yes, we are," I responded.

"So tell me about him."

I didn't know what to tell her about him. Quite honestly, he could be a brilliant surgeon, but my personal opinion was that he was pompous, arrogant, and self-absorbed and didn't give the courtesy of a hello when he passed someone he knew at church, at the club, or at school. He was above it all and rude.

Relative wisdom: How do the people in your community view you, inside your practice as well as outside? Your behavior may be the source of your being eliminated from consideration without your ever knowing it.

OUTLOOK

A good outlook is one of reality, candor, and compassion; it emphasizes the positives first and respects the personal desires of others. The practice of aesthetic medicine is about enhancement, not change. Likewise, the outlook of your practice can be enhanced, but it should not change. You don't believe the glass is half full one day, and half empty the next. You don't use a low-key approach one day, and aggressively market your business the next. You don't change a tasteful private practice one day to a franchised storefront drop-in clinic the next. Why? Because change implies that something is wrong, and something that is wrong is a red flag. You will alienate the people you have served and confuse the people who seek your services.

Your outlook should be:

- **Realistic:** Do not promise something you cannot achieve, whether in clinical outcome or in a life-altering change.

- **Candid:** Do not omit details for any reason; fully inform your patients and never gloss over the realities, such as pain, risk, and possible unfavorable outcomes.

- **Compassionate:** Demonstrate that you possess emotions; are here to help and to endure. Failure to care for your clients and patients, their quality of experience, their satisfaction, and their quality of life, could be a warning sign.

If your outlook is focused on anything other than the personal desires of the individuals you educate and treat, you raise a red flag. Your goal may be to generate revenue, your brand may emphasize new high-tech modalities, your image may be upscale or holistic, but your outlook must still project your commitment to fulfilling patients' desires.

I always wonder about the people behind the practices that project flashy, inappropriate messages suggesting "the best results," "your dreams come true," and "we can change your life." One of my favorites was found in a telephone directory: "A substantial discount will be offered on all services, and together we will stimulate the economy." The author of this statement was merely stimulating his imagination.

Providers disseminating such messages are desperate to succeed; they are short on ethics, and their outlook is barren. They will use any gimmick or buzz to get people in the door. They are less than frank in discussions with potential patients, then deny culpability when the results fall short of expectations. If you do not believe that these people invariably fail, pay attention to how often such messages appear and disappear, much like these practices do. They constantly change, because they do not work.

🦋 IN PRACTICE: A Star Is Born

I often invite or recommend physicians for appearances on television programs to educate consumers about aesthetic procedures. I carefully screen these physicians, educate them about the expectations of participation, and offer assistance to coach, rehearse, and support any phase of the agenda.

I was preparing for a segment of *The View* that had come up very quickly, and in my haste to pull it all together, I did not have the chance to carefully interview a replacement physician who had been recommended by a technology company to demonstrate their device. This doctor, I was assured, was well versed and experienced with television. Little did I know that she was also relentless in her desire to become a star.

As everyone arrived in the dressing rooms, the physician began to question not only her contribution to the segment, but she also questioned the whole segment. She began to speak of alternative procedures, and had the audacity to bring a competitor's product, suggesting she should present it as well. Rehearsal began and the physician not only missed the mark—she left her manners and her common sense elsewhere. She disrupted the crew, the lighting, and the staging. She questioned the candidacy of her patient, whom she had personally invited to demonstrate the procedure. While we were rehearsing, her sister, mother, four friends, and her young son all arrived on the set, without ever asking or informing anyone of their arrival, and then told the crew she expected they'd have front-row seats. Finally, I had to act—I told her that her portion of the segment was being cut because we simply did not have time.

Later that day someone back in the green room came to me and said, "She's one doctor I'll never go see."

The lesson here: No matter where you go, what you do, your attitude, your outlook, and the resulting red flags accompany you.

Clinical Issues

Your credentials and your experience are of little value unless your patients are satisfied, and patient satisfaction is in clear jeopardy when clinical issues raise red flags. Clinical issues are those where you fall short in the expectation or image of a compassionate physician.

DISORGANIZATION

You are being trusted to fulfill the personal desire of another through medical treatment that is finite, delicate, and possibly irreversible. If you or your staff are perceived as disorganized in handling paperwork, process, or in any other way, it is likely the patient will question your attention to detail in the treatment process.

LACK OF PREPARATION

Patients expect you to be prepared with the knowledge and tools necessary to respond to their needs. It is as simple as your staff knowing to whom to direct a question. If you are not prepared to respond to a simple question, how can a patient expect you to be prepared for the unexpected during treatment?

QUICK JUDGMENTS

You may need to make a quick judgment in the event that something unexpected occurs, but what is the perception when you make a quick judgment of personal desire or recommended treatment? The perception is that you regularly make snap decisions and this may be a warning signal to a prospective patient. Aesthetic medicine should not involve instant judgment, just as it does not involve triage.

POOR PRACTICES

What do you convey when you fail to wash your hands before touching a patient? This says that to you, hygiene is not important. Fail to knock on the door before entering a room? You are indicating that HIPAA (and common courtesy) is irrelevant to you. These may seem like minor offenses, but they are indicators of major transgressions.

RECKLESS PRACTICES

A red flag of any kind will not be forgiven or forgotten, and is rarely isolated. Most practitioners who fall victim to these danger areas are practicing recklessly. In the practice of fulfilling individual, deep, personal desires, you must focus on what is positive, fulfilling, and most advantageous. You do not fix or correct because there is technically nothing wrong. You improve and you enhance—make this your first objective, and then be candid about pain, risk, possible unfavorable outcomes, and where alternatives may fall short.

☙ IN PRACTICE: Reporting Risky Business

I received a call from a physician who was clearly distraught about a woman who came to see him. She had received cosmetic injections from a qualified provider. She had horrible complications that included necrosis, and she wanted help. When the physician asked if her treating physician had addressed her complications, she stated, "Not really. He told me these were the potential outcomes we discussed, and he has stopped taking my calls." Biopsy revealed the woman had not been injected with the brand she was told would be used; she was not even injected with a recognized substance.

The doctor was calling me because the physician who had treated this woman was a colleague, clearly practicing recklessly by using an imported or illegal substance, and the doctor wanted my opinion on whether this physician should be reported to the state medical board, to the hospital where they were both on staff, and to the state and national medical societies to which they both belonged.

He was very upset for the woman, but equally upset that someone he considered a close colleague would act so recklessly. The problem, he told me, is that those who report the dangerous, illegal, or unethical practices of others are often treated as whistle blowers; they become pariahs. Those who offer expert testimony in clear cases of negligence are blackballed, and those who take the high ground often suffer repercussions from their actions. He knew what was right, but he wanted to stay anonymous.

Here is the advice I offered him and that I would give anyone in a similar situation: I am not a lawyer. I would suggest that you give the woman who presented in your office the information she needs to contact the FDA, the state medical board, the hospital, and your professional organizations to report her adverse events. In addition, I would ask you to weigh what you feel is more important: preventing this physician from harming anyone else and potentially damaging the reputation of the specialty in your community, or being hopeful that somehow, some time, some way these practices will come to an end. Consider your oath to the practice of medicine, the ethics you accepted when you were accepted into membership of your professional societies. Then only you can decide if you too wish to report these actions.

UNDERSTANDING RISK

Judgment and an inherent sense of ethics are the greatest defense against inappropriate messages; observation is the greatest enforcer of this. While you observe messages around you and identify those as inappropriate, others are also observing you and your messages. Through this observation, you realize that even the smallest questionable element can bring irrevocable damage to an image.

Take a moment to look at your practice from the outside in: observe what you and your practice do and the messages you convey. How do you define and maintain your image, identify the needs and expectations of your audience, and recognize risk? These factors cross over in an intricate weave of different people, communication styles, and perceptions. The result of that weave is your success. When elements are tightly woven with little variation, your practice is strong. When elements are loosely or inconsistently joined, your practice is weak. Weakness in any one area is a weakness that will permeate the practice and threaten your success.

Observe everything and everyone in your practice on a regular basis through the eyes of your patients. Role play, as uncomfortable and elementary as that may seem. Be the patient with unrealistic goals; position yourself as a consumer reading one of your ads or visiting your website. Sit through the process of informed consent with your patient coordinator and make him or her sit through the process too. Sometimes we all need to walk in another's shoes. As you look for potential red flags, look too for opportunities to improve, grow, and evolve.

SECTION III

Where

Where is more than a place. The "where" of your practice requires a journey, and a connection to the place you travel to. The physical location where you provide services is an important reflection of your image and an element of your patients' experience. Where you practice is the end to a means. The means—the journey and the connection—are found in the marketing and media messages vital to bringing patients, and ultimately success, to your door.

CHAPTER 9

Where Will You Practice?

*I was going to have cosmetic surgery
until I noticed the doctor's office was full
of pictures by Picasso.*

— RITA RUDNER, COMEDIAN

You practice medicine and perform elective procedures that focus on self-improvement, self-enhancement, and self-fulfillment. Your patients choose these procedures to make themselves look and feel better about themselves. The medical treatments you provide may result in pain, discomfort, and anxiety and test the limits of the patient's humility. Where you practice, including the physical location, the furnishings, and the functions of your facility, must be an appropriate, safe medical location as well as an inviting, comforting destination. Whether you are just starting your practice, remodeling or relocating, considering adding additional locations to your practice, or simply evaluating how well your practice is performing or what you might improve, it is essential to recognize that where you practice is an important aspect of your image.

RELATIVE WISDOM: The Road Less Traveled

Vacations are easy to plan, with all the pictures, videos, reviews, and ratings available online. Yet going to a new destination always evokes two key feelings: excitement and caution.

We were heading down to a remote resort for some quiet time away from the world. The destination had fabulous reviews and was recommended by trusted friends. When we arrived we were thrilled: the service, the site, the opportunities to relax or to recreate were just perfect for us. We spent a few days lounging on the beach, fishing off the shore, watching the sunsets, and just enjoying every moment of our R&R—until a crocodile found his way onto the beach. We were on the Pacific Coast of Mexico, and it was suspected that the croc had somehow wandered out of the jungle to the north, down a river, and into the ocean. Now he was on the beach, and panic erupted. The staff of the resort quickly cleared the beach and closed it, and the authorities circled to remove the crocodile. Two hours of violent crocodile-wrangling spectacle disrupted a quiet vacation for many, but the breach of our peace did not end there. Vacationers were afraid to walk the beach that night. They were afraid to walk on the beach or fish the next day. They were afraid to hike through the jungle—who could blame them? What had been the perfect experience in paradise quickly and unexpectedly turned to a paranoia that marred what should have been a perfect vacation.

Relative wisdom: Regardless of how well you research your location, how perfect the office you build, how capable and gracious your staff are, the unexpected can and will occur. It won't be crocodiles on the beach, but it could be a fire in the building, a hurricane that destroys much of the community, or a teetering economy that panics patients and potential clients. Ice on the sidewalk can cause spills, upset patients can disrupt the office, or a distinct odor may waft from the restaurant next door. Always expect the unexpected, and be as prepared as possible to meet the challenge.

LOCATION

There is so much more to your practice facility than its physical address. Today site selection for an aesthetic practice is not limited to medical buildings or hospitals; aesthetic practices are found in locations other than hospitals and medical buildings. These include storefronts, malls, quiet row houses, skyscrapers, hotels and resorts, and fitness clubs. Your site may be selected for its architecture or amenities, but whatever location you choose or its appearance, you must carefully consider access, utilities, image, light, privacy, neighbors, hazards, and restrictions.

Access

How will patients reach your office? If they are driving, there must be parking. If they are taking public transportation, there must be close proximity to transportation stops. If they are handicapped, the office must be barrier free. Access also requires that your office be clearly marked, but without garish signs that prompt your patients to seek a back door for entry. Broken curbs or icy sidewalks, untrimmed shrubs or bougainvillea hanging over the door, heavy and hard-to-open doors are all little things that inhibit access.

It is also essential to consider access to your target market. If you are located in a distant part of town in the belief that your patients will appreciate the quiet, make certain they are willing to make the trip. If you open an office adjacent to a fitness center to capitalize on the market, make certain your patients aren't required to mix and mingle with muscle men just to get to your door.

Access from your office to adjacent offices, medical spas, or a surgery center or hospital are also important to your equation. If you operate away from your office, you have two locations to introduce and appoint appropriately to invite and serve your patients. Consider access in case of an emergency: how readily can emergency services reach your patient, and how distant is the hospital? An urgent situation can result from more than just the care you provide; it can occur any time, any day, and with people who are not your patients.

Access inside your office is imperative. High, narrow stairs, long waits for elevators, dark basements, and even a location on an upper level in a high-rise building can inhibit access for patients who have physical or emotional obstacles to overcome.

Consider too that access to communication and technology is a relevant factor today. If your office is paperless, do all your patients accept this? Are they able to use the technology? Do you provide alternative methods for those who cannot?

Utilities

Electricity and water are essential, and backup generators for power failures are vital. Telephones, the Internet, security, and for some offices, satellite or cable communications are required utilities. Just as important as having access to these utilities is evaluating the condition and source for these utilities. Is the infrastructure up to date and ready for future growth, or do you need to invest and upgrade?

Water must be fresh, clean, tasteless, and odorless, or your office restroom could smell like a landfill. The water quality must be appropriate for your laundry and sterilization requirements, or you will have to budget for bottled and distilled water. Electricity must be consistent, up to date, and sufficient to support all the technology and medical equipment you will have. Overloaded circuits or dated wiring can damage expensive equipment. Outlets that are in poor locations or not grounded can cause service failures. Consider whether your location is wired properly for phone and high-speed Internet service. Check wireless service availability and quality; if cell phones don't work consistently, you might have unhappy patients. Moreover, you could have limited access to your own staff and physician extenders.

Image

The site you choose will project its own image, one that may reflect, complement, or contradict your practice's image. If you are in a medical center, what do the messages and the people your patients come in contact with convey? If you are in a hospital, what is the proximity to other providers, services, and patients? Are these practices concordant with your own?

Image is reflected in the building's architecture and design, and in the views or lack of views. If you establish your office in a nonmedical location, consider the image of the site, as well as of the surrounding businesses. Locating in a strip mall or quaint shopping corner is advantageous for your retail services, if that center attracts people in your market and your patients. How exposed will your patients be when they come to your office? Will they feel vulnerable when they walk out of your office, somewhat bruised and buffeted after an injection? Will they be apprehensive when they walk into your office that they might be seen by acquaintances who frequent nearby businesses?

One current trend is to practice in or near resorts, spas, and salons. But can such a location impair your image by making aesthetic medicine look less professional, or completely nonmedical? Does the image of your location appear too up-market, thereby discouraging potential patients? Or is the location too unfashionable, thus disappointing patients who expect a more elegant setting?

Light

Consider the natural light or lack of it in your location. There is nothing more welcoming, warming, and flattering to the appearance than the ambiance of soft natural light. If you are located in the desert, however, the hot sun beating through your windows all day will be too harsh and uninviting. Window coverings and softening landscaping may be an option. Consider the contrast of lighting; you don't want your patients to feel they have walked out of a dark theater into daylight, or vice versa.

You might not be able to control the lighting options in common areas, but consider the overall illumination of your site. Hallways, elevators, and vestibules as well as driveways, parking lots, walkways, and front and back doors should be well lit during all hours of business operation.

Privacy

Although your office may be in a public area, you must provide privacy for your patients. Does security require that your patients identify themselves before entering the parking lot or building? Can neighbors watch through storefront windows to see who is entering the plastic surgeon's office? Some patients may not be concerned about walking through a main entrance and being seen by others; some may ask for a private entrance that should be accessible and appropriate. What does your patient see or experience through that back entrance? For example, if your private entrance is the back door next to a janitorial closet, make certain the closet is always closed, unmarked, and without odor.

Consider the function of common areas inside and outside your office. Do they foster privacy, or expose your patients? Do walls of glass expose the people in your reception area, or inside treatment rooms? Light and glass are beautiful and welcoming when they are obviously screened for privacy.

Neighbors

My great-uncle Peter used to say, "Choose your neighbors carefully. You must live with them every day." There is wisdom in these words, but you may have little control over who your practice's neighbors are, or more unexpectedly, who may become your neighbor. For example, if there are vacant lots near your office location, find out what that land is zoned for and what it may be used for in the future. If there are adjoining offices, spaces, or stores for lease, it is wise to consider who might move in. A physician once signed a 5-year lease on a storefront space and began to build a beautiful medical spa, only to have a drum store move in next door. Although you may not have the ability in your lease to preapprove new neighbors, make certain you have a nuisance or business disruption clause in your lease. Likewise, you may wish to have a competitor clause so that in your location you are the only permitted provider of your specialty. A physician once called me, furious that the spa he had made an agreement with had invited a competitor to practice in the spa on the day he was not there. Don't let this happen to you.

Neighbors are also important to privacy and safety. Consider the people your business neighbors may attract. Consider the times your business neighbors are open for business and what they are doing when you are not on-site.

Hazards

Your location may have obvious hazards that can be easily rectified, or latent hazards that you discover only in a dire situation. Snow and ice must be cleared from walkways; handrails should be convenient and up to code. If you are in a fire-prone area, a hurricane alley, a flood plain, or the highest point in a lightning-prone valley, make certain you have the right safety precautions and procedures in place.

The equipment you use daily may not seem like a hazard, but in the wrong hands such devices can be deadly. Strict policies and practices must be in place so that dangerous drugs are locked away and devices are disabled when not in use. For example, a laser that is in an unattended room and has a key in its lock is a hazard. Needles and scalpels in the unlocked cabinet of an examination room where a distracted parent sits with small children is an accident waiting to happen.

Electrical cords that cross the floor, low-hanging medical lighting, open cabinet or closet doors, and medical waste are additional perils. Expired fire extinguishers, dated emergency phone numbers, and even broken ceiling tiles or clogged toilets must be corrected. Have procedures in place for rectifying these matters to prevent trouble before it occurs. Regularly inspect your property inside and out for hazards.

Restrictions

It is essential to know what is and is not permitted for your office location based on your lease, landlord, neighbors, zoning, and local and state regulations or covenants. Restrictions may include the hours of operation as well as the types of procedures that you may or may not be permitted to perform on-site. Consider also issues that can restrict your ability to grow or downsize your physical space if necessary. Must you relocate and rebuild, or is there flexibility to expand or scale back?

ACCREDITATION

Although it is not required of every office or every aesthetic specialty, accreditation for your office is very important. Whether the American Association for Accreditation of Ambulatory Surgery Facilities (AAAASF), Accreditation Association for Ambulatory Health Care (AAAHC), Joint Commission on the Accreditation of Healthcare Organizations (JCAHO), or Medicare, accreditation demonstrates to your patients that this location meets specific standards for human safety. Don't simply prepare for inspection and review; live the guidelines and practices every day, and in the event of any untoward event, your office setting will be secured, your staff prepared, and your patients in the best possible conditions for their safety.

ACCREDITATION

Alan H. Gold, MD, FACS

Although aesthetic surgery can have very positive and life-altering benefits for our patients, it is not without risk. We discuss those risks and benefits as an integral part of our consultations, and these matters are appropriately of great concern to our patients.

To be successful in the highly competitive environment of aesthetic medicine and surgery, it is critical that you not only demonstrate your aesthetic vision and artistry through your surgical results, but you must also provide the best possible patient experience in an environment that demonstrates your commitment to patient safety. With most aesthetic surgery now performed in office-based or ambulatory surgical facilities, the best way to ensure the safety of your patients and demonstrate that commitment to them is through accreditation.

The critical importance of facility accreditation has long been recognized by plastic surgeons, and actually led them to develop the American Association for Accreditation of Ambulatory Surgery Facilities (AAAASF) in 1980. Increased public, organizational, and governmental acknowledgment that accreditation was critical to ensuring the highest level of safety and quality in all aspects of the outpatient surgical experience led to an expansion of that organization's focus as the American Society for Accreditation of Ambulatory Surgery Facilities, to include oversight of the facilities of all specialties. Other national accrediting agencies, such as the JCAHO and the AAAHC, also began to focus efforts on ambulatory facility accreditation. In 1996 California became the first state to mandate accreditation for all outpatient facilities that administer sedation or general anesthesia, and professional organizations, such as the American Society for Aesthetic Plastic Surgery and the American Society of Plastic Surgeons, soon mandated that their members operate only in such accredited facilities. Unfortunately, as of this writing, only 26 states mandate some sort of accreditation, and the vast majority of ambulatory surgery facilities remain unaccredited and operate independent of any peer review and inspection process.

To be successful in your aesthetic medicine and surgical practice, you must make a commitment to lifelong learning and modify your techniques or learn new ones to provide the best possible results for your patients. Similarly, you must appreciate that maintaining safety and quality in your ambulatory surgery facility is also a dynamic process. While the basics of practice and surgical care may remain constant, it is critical to incorporate advances in technology and changes in standards of care into your practice to reflect the current state of the art and to ensure the safety of your patients. The most reliable way to do so is through accreditation by, and ongoing compliance with, a recognized accrediting organization that has developed the systems to effectively monitor and implement the latest advances in outpatient care delivery that directly benefit you and your patients.

There are many factors that can contribute to the success of your practice; a visible and demonstrated commitment to patient safety through accreditation is a critical one.

ACQUISITION

Today there are as many opportunities to acquire your office location as there are practice models. At one time leasing and purchasing were the most prevalent options; today the alternatives include office condominiums, timeshares, and arrangements whereby you do not pay for space, but are contracted to pay a percentage of your fees for the ability to use space. You must be cautious about laws that regulate ownership in surgical and diagnostic centers. Whatever acquisition arrangement you pursue for your location, there are three essential variables you must not overlook: feasibility, legal review, and financing.

During the acquisition phase of any location, the physician-owner should consider not only the practice's immediate needs, but must also look to the future. Goals and a business plan for 1, 2, 5, and 10 years into the future are essential to formulating a decision that will favor the practice's success and will ensure the ability to secure the funds needed to acquire a location with an image that best suits your practice and your patients' comfort and expectations.

Feasibility

Before committing to any location, you should retain the services of an architect to assess the feasibility of the location, specifically the square footage appropriate to your needs; access appropriate to local and state regulations for medical facilities; utilities; and construction. You may discover that a location you are considering cannot support your utility requirements or would necessitate expensive alterations to bring the site up to code for a medical office.

Legal Review

Never sign a lease, purchase, time-share agreement, or any arrangement without a proper legal review by a real estate attorney. Your attorney should look at the details of the transaction as well as the liability, restrictions, and covenants that are defined within. Landlord and tenant improvements and allowances must be clearly defined, along with assessments, taxes, restrictions, and countless other vital details. It may take weeks and several versions of the legal agreement to secure an acceptable arrangement. Communicate regularly with your attorney, and never hesitate to ask questions.

Financing

Financing must be arranged not only for the purchase or build-out of your location, but also for all the furnishings and equipment that will go into that facility. Whether you are building, remodeling, or simply redecorating, be careful how much you invest in cash at the outset, how your loan or lease payments are defined, and what cash flow will be required to cover acquiring your facility as well as keeping your practice operational. Because interest rates, borrowing opportunities, and investment opportunities fluctuate, it is impossible to define a set formula for investment and leveraging. You must work with an accountant, banker, and investment advisor you trust, to collaborate to find the best possible arrangement for you. You should also be aware that you may be asked to secure loans with your personal assets. Although this is a common practice, it puts not only your practice but your private life at risk if you extend yourself too far.

DESIGN

Design encompasses much more than a color palette, artwork, and decor. An effective design must take into account the space you will need, how you will integrate the space, the way in which your practice will function in each area, and what you want the entire facility to look, feel, and sound like. Beware of design for design's sake: marble floors are lovely, but they are loud, cold, and can be slippery. An elegant but inflexible layout can hinder opportunities to grow and adapt within the same footprint. I applaud no-waiting-room concepts, but only for practices that already have the ability to control schedules, ensure patient privacy, and effectively use time.

The design should respect all the essentials of your location—access, utilities, image, light, privacy, neighbors, hazards, and restrictions. It must also project the image of an inviting, appealing setting that will draw patients to you for aesthetic services. Design can be the most individualized aspect of your entire practice, but depending on your business model and location, it may also be the most restrictive.

I won't tell you what color to paint your walls, but I will tell you that your design must:

- *Focus on your patients:* There should be no distractions in sight, sound, or smell. You may like Picasso or Warhol, the smell of gardenias, or the sounds of salsa music, but consider how these things may relate to the individual tastes of your patients.

- *Reflect your image, not your life:* Pictures of your family remind you of those you live for and love, but they should never be visible to your patients, for the sake of your family's safety. You may be an avid golfer, but if your waiting area looks like a stop on the PGA tour, your patients may feel they must be golfers to communicate with you. You may love sleek, minimalist modernism, but asking your patients to sit on low, molded acrylic chairs might be a little off-putting. Find a happy medium that is functional, stylish, and comfortable.

- *Preserve privacy and support modesty:* Patients should never be shuffled from room to room in various states of undress through the corridors. Clinical photography may be essential for your purposes, but realize how uncomfortable this is for patients. Give them robes to wear, not paper gowns and drapes. Don't wheel patients on gurneys or in wheelchairs though public spaces. Design an environment that gives patients a sense that you value their privacy and that their visit will be handled with discretion.

- *Account for safety and upkeep:* Soiled linens and medical waste should be properly handled and kept from patients' view. Stainless steel sinks and counters are sleek and easy to disinfect, but the water stains on them are ever-apparent and hard to clean. A waterfall and koi pond in the entry may be lovely and peaceful, but if it requires constant water testing and filtration to kill the algae or attracts the fingers of visiting children, it is a distraction.

- *Exude comfort and warmth:* Warming blankets on leather examination tables in the depths of January are relaxing. Soft terry robes to cover a patient in any stage of undress are comfortable, warm, and luxurious.

- *Be consistent and dynamic:* Design should never make every room in your office look unrelated to the next, or to your patients. But design must also be flexible to allow multipurpose options and growth for new uses or technologies.

- *Endure:* Your design should have a life span of at least 10 years. Avoid the use of trendy colors and styles that will quickly appear dated.

Location and design may have far less importance than the clinical outcome of your procedures, but they contribute to your patients' experiences and to the nuances on which you will be measured and recalled. You select the people on your team for their ability to connect with your patients and provide treatment and service; you must accept a design for your practice that can connect with and provide comfort to your patients.

DESIGNED FOR SUCCESS

No location, no practice can succeed if it does not have an emergency action plan specifically tailored for the location and the people in the office. Whether you encounter an emergency of a clinical nature, a natural disaster, an accident, or an act of violence, you must ensure the safety of all persons on your premises, of others who enter your practice in the event of an emergency, and of all data specific to your practice.

Weather forecasting has made it feasible to predict hurricanes, ice storms, and tornadoes, but unanticipated emergencies can arise. You should develop a plan that specifically defines:

- Who is accountable for patients and what actions are necessary to protect their safety and privacy

- Who is accountable for all other individuals on the premises, whether they are staff or visitors, and for contacting law enforcement or emergency services

- Who is accountable for data and backups and how these will be managed and used in the moments, hours, or days following an emergency to contact patients; who is accountable for the emergency contacts for any individual who may become injured or disabled

- Who is accountable for medications, equipment, and other items that can be readily stolen or accessed if your premises is not secured

- Where individuals must be relocated, whether immediately, for a few moments, or until your office is operational again

- Who determines where it is safe to seek shelter on a moment's notice, or when it is safe to return

In addition, you should regularly check the operability of safety equipment, such as fire extinguishers, generators, alarms, and data backup systems. Scheduled safety checks of the premises for hazards or obstacles such as windows that are stuck, emergency exits that are blocked, or equipment that overheats must be conducted and documented. Periodic safety drills, whether fully executed or simply a virtual experience, will ensure that staff are prepared for any eventuality.

Without the very best safety practices in every facet of your practice, you simply cannot and will not succeed.

🌿 IN PRACTICE: Plan for the Future

A newly formed practice partnership was planning to open a truly comprehensive facility dedicated to aesthetic medicine in the center of town. The site was near the hospital, adjacent to a quaint hotel, and with all the necessary infrastructure; the physicians were thrilled with the location they had found. There was a back entrance that was easily accessible for patient privacy, a beautiful view of the city from every window, and fabulous boutiques and shops at the street level below. They were so eager for this golden opportunity that they did not want to waste a moment. They disregarded advice they were given to secure a letter of intent, perform a feasibility study, hire a lawyer, and take the time to follow all prudent measures. Instead, they immediately signed a 10-year lease with additional options.

The physicians designed a beautifully appointed practice center. No expense was spared in design or amenities; the facility was stunning. However, shortly after they moved into this grand new location, they found themselves with one very serious problem: the quaint hotel was sold and razed, and in short order a mammoth skyscraper was under construction. The physicians were faced with enduring months into years of closed sidewalks, trucks blocking their building entrance, and heavy construction noise, only to be followed by a building that would block their every view.

They weighed the substantial expense of breaking their lease and having to relocate or trying to sublease the facility. Unfortunately, their landlord was not willing to negotiate, and their lease would not allow them to sublet. To add further unwelcome news, they learned that they were so highly leveraged that they could not afford to move. They continued to lose patients, because no one could get to the building as a result of construction traffic or into the building without passing the construction crews. They tried to endure at this site, but as the building next door went up, their patients stopped coming. The practice filed for bankruptcy, and the physicians went their separate ways.

The moral of this story: Be careful where you cut corners. Your resources must be used for the practical as well as the pretty. Investing in a feasibility study would have revealed what was transpiring next door, and investing in a lawyer to protect their interests would have uncovered the limitations of their lease.

OPERATIONS

In addition to the physical location where you practice, there are a multitude of operational considerations to your location that contribute to your success. You must approach these operational elements with solid research, a feasibility review of the options, and careful consideration of your present and future patients and practice.

Equipment and Supplies

From sterilization autoclaves to copier paper, a vast array of day-to-day supplies is essential to your practice, and taxing to your resources. The trend toward conservation and consideration of carbon footprints is responsible, but more important is your time, money, storage, and efficiency and your patients' experience. For example, avoid using latex gloves or be diligent about asking patients about an allergy to latex.

Information and Technology

You will require business systems for data storage, practice management and scheduling, and daily accounting. Some doctors also require dictation equipment. The use of electronic medical records (EMRs) and electronic prescriptions (ERx) is growing, and these systems are essential for the future. Make certain your business technologies are integrated, appropriately updated, and that all staff members receive proper training to maximize the functionality of your investment. Whether you send information electronically to your patients is your choice and theirs, but make certain that your networks and data are secured, protected, and backed up daily.

Telephone

The best telephone system in the world has little value unless the people who use it do so effectively. Voice mail is essential but is not a primary means to communicate. Yours is a personal service, so don't let automation rule your phone system; live people must answer the phone. Nothing is so off-putting as being parked on hold indefinitely, listening to the looping message, "Your call is very important to us. . . ."

Heating, Ventilation, and Air Conditioning

A top-quality heating, ventilation, and air conditioning (HVAC) system is essential to maintain steady temperatures and provide silent airflow. An inefficient system can cause drafts from a vent above an examination table or carry the sounds of your operating room into other areas of the office. HVAC must be efficient and unobtrusive.

Security

Alarm systems only work when they are enabled. I am shocked at how many offices with expensive supplies of retail goods, drugs, and medical devices simply have a lock and key. Security is important, whether the office is vacant or in use. Panic buttons and preprogrammed numbers to local authorities and key providers in your office are essential, and all phone numbers must be current.

Clinical Safety

Do not overlook the importance and function of sterilization and sanitation equipment and procedures. No one should leave medical waste at the back door overnight and expect that the service will come by to collect it. Always have a Banyan Stat Kit, an automatic external defibrillator (AED), and properly trained staff on-site. If someone has a cardiac event in your office, you must act first as a doctor who saves lives.

Equipment

Lights, lasers, scalpels, sinks—all equipment must be current and properly functioning, stored, and serviced.

Garments/Uniforms

Office apparel sets the correct tone for your practice. Provide strict guidelines for dress and set the example yourself. Never wear soiled scrubs; always have spare clothing. Never greet a patient with your mask, cap, or gloves on. Greet them outside the sterile perimeter; let them see your face and your smile and feel the warmth of your handshake. Name tags and uniforms are at the discretion of your practice, for which you may or may not have authority. The people in your practice who interact with your patients should be so personable and attentive that name tags are not needed for them to be memorable. The purpose of a name tag is a reminder for the patient, not a crutch for the staff. You want staff to be remembered for their kindness and service more than for their fashion choices.

IN PRACTICE: By Design

The things that I see in physicians' practices never cease to amaze me. A physician invited me to her new office, which had an on-site OR, on moving day. I had not been to her prior location nor worked with her previously. I was curious to see this grand new facility she had built. The staff were there, as well as the designer (the physician's daughter) and the moving men, and deliveries were coming and going. In came the men to deliver nitrogen tanks. In came the men to deliver the autoclave. Out came a lot of questions, and subsequently tempers flared.

It seems that the designer-daughter had no medical experience, nor did the architect (her daughter's friend). Thus they had made no plans for the utilities to support necessary medical equipment, such as the liquid nitrogen and the autoclave, nor were there designated areas for properly storing this equipment.

The nurse stepped in and found some counter space near a sink at the nurse's station where the autoclave would have to go. Problem solved, until the designer-daughter walked by and shouted, "Who put this on the counter? No clutter. No clutter. That thing is hideous!"

The nurse walked into the preoperative area to compose herself, only to find a lovely side table, a soft upholstered chair, an area rug, and a bamboo plant. She walked out and asked, "Who put a cloth chair, a rug, and a plant in the preop area?" The designer replied, "I did. We are employing feng shui, the Chinese law of aesthetics and balance. There must be calm and warmth everywhere."

The scene got uglier. There was no cabinetry in the examination rooms, only pedestal sinks. Where would supplies, trash, and waste go? The designer brought out lovely mother-of-pearl decorative trash cans for each room. Lovely glass etageres were delivered and placed next to the sinks for which there were fingertip towels, lovely tissue boxes, orchids, and a shiny handheld mirror.

Continued

✌ IN PRACTICE: By Design—cont'd

I watched in horror, wondering how the designer would survive the wrath of the office manager, who had no file storage space, nowhere to place her printer, fax machine, or even a Post-it note on the lovely glass table that was to be used as her desk. Her desk held an orchid, a cordless phone, and a cordless laptop computer. The office was supposed to be paperless, the designer insisted, so there was no need for storing anything.

This was a clear case in which the architect and designer had no concept of function, and the physician had provided no oversight nor sought input from her staff on layout issues.

The lesson here: I am the very first person who will insist that your office be as attractive as it is functional, efficient, safe, and appropriate. But if you cannot or do not want to be part of the design process, make certain your design preferences and your clinical needs are conveyed to qualified experts in the planning process.

CHAPTER 10

Where Will You Connect?

*A weird combination of isolation and connection
and disconnection; discomfort and awkwardness.*
— ROBIN WILLIAMS, ACTOR AND COMEDIAN

Communication, your ability to connect with others, is the key to success in any business or relationship. Your clinical outcomes and your ability to connect and communicate are the most important variables in the success of practicing aesthetic medicine.

Without communication—words that connect you and your message to others—you will not have traffic into your practice. Without traffic you will not attract prospective patients, and without communication in the form of education, you cannot convert these individuals to patients. Failure to regularly communicate with patients to retain them and increase their value as referral sources is the point at which many aesthetic physicians fail to connect and succeed. Timely, effective communication can make your patients' treatment experience a positive one, even when the clinical outcome is less than perfect.

Connection requires more than simply attracting the interest of potential clients, educating them, and retaining them. Inside or outside your office, every connection you make can enhance your ability to thrive. Successful communication requires:

- *Consistency:* In your brand and the expectations you define every time, everywhere

- *Compatibility:* Adapting your message to the audience or situation without diverging from your brand

- *Precision:* Delivering your message with the right words, tone, vehicle, and at an appropriate time

- *Manners:* Even if someone is being unpleasant, or an experience is uncomfortable, one should still communicate politely

- *Truth:* If you cannot be sincere, be silent

Making a connection requires:

- A specific goal, what you hope to accomplish by making a connection

- Using the most effective and appropriate vehicles to get your message delivered and acted on

- Understanding how tone affects your connection, and the call to action your message is designed to compel in others

- Recognizing the cost, both expense and value, that communication has and optimizing this

The most successful practices make and maintain a connection at every opportunity and communicate effectively. Some may say that this is marketing; it is not. Marketing is all the activities necessary to exchange product or services for money, or barter; it includes many variables such as pricing, your brand, and your service model. Some may call it advertising; it is not. Advertising is a paid message about a product or service one is attempting to sell for money or barter. There are, in fact, many successful practices of aesthetic medicine that do not advertise.

Most people get their information about aesthetic medicine from television, magazines, the Internet, and other people. This is not how they find a provider—this is where they get their information. Where individuals find and ultimately connect with a provider varies widely: it can be through referral by a physician, friend, or family member, or through an Internet listing or advertisement. Do you want to be represented among the sources that others read about in the media and connect with? Do you want to be the source your existing clients and patients reconnect with for additional detailed information? Do you want to be the most attractive source in a directory, or the one people confidently refer their friends to? What will it take to accomplish these goals? Quite simply, strategically targeted and appropriate communication that makes a connection that yields results.

RELATIVE WISDOM: Covering Basis

A childhood friend was discussing his business with me. He is a successful pharmaceutical representative specializing in cardiac care drugs. I asked him about the tools he uses to succeed, and add to the success of his clients—physicians who prescribe the drugs he represents. The key to his success, he told me, is no different from that of any direct relationship: it depends on mutual fulfillment of one another's needs.

I then asked how he knows what his clients' needs are. His reply did not at all surprise me; it was indicative of his success. He stated that he discovers his clients' needs through communication—quite simply, by asking. "I regularly and directly ask any client what I can do for his or her practice to improve patient relationships. The answer is consistent and unilateral: patient education."

His clients—practitioners of essential, not elective, medical treatment—see the need to educate their market and patients about their conditions and care as foremost in fulfilling their relationships. The single greatest tool these practitioners need, other than the ability to provide treatment, is the ability to communicate with and educate their patients.

Fundamental to your success is the ability to communicate your abilities, to candidly describe treatments so that patients can make an educated decision and accept that treatment. If you do not ask someone what he or she expects or needs, your relationship cannot advance. If you do not effectively educate a potential patient about his or her choice to undergo treatment, you cannot succeed.

Patients who refuse treatment in traditional medicine may impair their health. Patients who decline treatment in aesthetic medicine may miss an opportunity to enhance their sense of well-being. Although your messages may differ, the commonality is patient education. Without it, no one will choose to undergo treatment, and you will not have the opportunity to fulfill your relationship with those you serve.

MAKING CONNECTIONS

Every message conveys some form of education. To target populations, clients, patients, and others you view as sources and resources to your practice, you communicate essential information about the services you provide so that others may benefit from your skills. For example:

- Advertising or direct mail educates your target audience about what you do that will attract them to your practice.

- Brochures educate about a specific procedure and about your practice. You would be surprised at how many do not include practice information. Without this, what value does the brochure hold for your practice specifically?

- Informed consent educates about the process a patient will undergo, its potential benefits and risks, and statements validating a patient's motivation and your commitment to quality care.

Although the popular media keep the public abreast of innovations in aesthetic medicine, your role is to educate your audience about what you practice in aesthetic medicine, and in some cases about what you do not practice, and why. When a physician refers an individual to you, it is your job to educate this potential patient about how you can fulfill his or her personal desire. A referral from another patient may communicate an endorsement of you as a provider of aesthetic medicine, but you must educate that person about who you are, what you do to validate that endorsement, and how you can specifically fulfill personal desire.

Every message must be a consistent reflection of you, your practice, and your image. To make communication valuable to your success, the contents and efficacy of your message must be sound. The message must have a goal, a defined purpose, an appropriate tone, and a relative call to action. Each message must:

- *Define a goal:* How will the success of this connection be measured?

- *Identify your connection:* Outside or inside your practice, and with what vehicles or methods?

- *Clearly convey purpose:* What is the message designed to accomplish and to whom is it targeted?

- *Garner attention through tone:* Who does this message need to positively attract its intended audience?

- *Present a relative call to action:* How do you want others to respond to this message?

Goals

Before you begin to examine how you connect, with whom, and for what purpose, you must understand the goals of communication. Goals define a target, something we wish to achieve, and an outcome, something that signals we have accomplished those goals. Look carefully at the messages and tools you use to connect with your market, community, peers, patients, staff, and even the messages in your interpersonal relationships. Some messages may have simply and clearly defined goals, some may have multiple goals, and others may have conflicting goals. You must continuously evaluate how well you are achieving your defined goals and making the desired connections.

Inside or outside your office, your connections must have one or more specific or indirect goals:

- Failure to attain a communication goal will result in the failure to connect now or in the near future. (If you don't make your service menu available, no one will know what you offer.)

- Failure to approach those goals honestly creates a false connection. (If you embellish or avoid the truth, you will cast doubt on your veracity as a responsible provider.)

- Failure to communicate goals consistently will result in a failed connection. (Undefined or documented postoperative instructions to the patient may fail to communicate critical variables.)

Goals define what you expect to accomplish through a given connection. Purpose is the intent of your communication.

VISIBILITY

You and your practice must be visible to those with whom you need to communicate. If you do not make the effort to be visible in a directory, on a business card, on a website, through advertising, or at public functions, how will others know who you are and where to find you?

ANNOUNCEMENT

An announcement is appropriate when you have something important to convey, such as a new location, an addition to your staff, new hours, new services or procedures, new policies, or specific rebuttals to misinformation in the popular press. Don't attempt to impress by announcing something trivial, dated, or unsubstantiated. For example, don't claim to be the leading provider of a cosmetic injection or to have some innovative injection technique unless you can prove it.

Announcement with your staff is equally important; for example, share your vacation schedule for continuity in your business and so that plans can be made accordingly. Tell staff if you will be scaling the Himalayas so they understand you won't be readily available. Sharing the cost of your trip is extraneous and distracting.

SOLICITATION

You have something to sell—a service or a product. However, be careful what you solicit, to whom, and how. You may make a connection, but is it truly the connection you need to succeed? Sharing your service menu on a website or with referring physicians is solicitation.

EDUCATION

Every communication should be designed to educate, whether directly, subtly, personally, or to a wide audience. If you don't have at least one key piece of valuable information to share, remain silent. Explaining your service menu to staff, referral sources, prospective clients, and peers should focus on educating.

NEWS

News is of the moment, previously unreported, important information that is of use or interest to others. It is not self-serving; in the purest sense it is a form of public service. If you have valuable news, share it. If you strive to make news, be certain your intentions are for public service, not self-aggrandizement. Responding to a tragedy or sharing an accomplishment that has true meaning to your audience is news.

NOVELTY

A novelty is something new, fresh, inviting. If you establish a goal for connecting based on a novelty, be certain you are well informed about what that novelty can accomplish. You may be enthusiastic about a new treatment, device, or technique, but before you promote these, make certain that what is cutting edge today will endure tomorrow, and that it offers a valid, legitimate benefit for your patients—the Next Big Thing may turn out to be the latest face lift in a jar or the next lipodissolve. You may wish to be known as a trendsetter, but make certain you're backing the right trend. How long will the novel new item last in your practice, and what benefit will it bring to you and those you serve?

COMPLIANCE

Compliance is a message with two very distinct functions. You want to communicate to patients that you are compliant with the highest standards of care and ethics in your specialty, whether with CME or accreditation of facilities. In addition, you want your staff to understand and comply with your office policies and procedures, beyond OSHA guidelines.

You should also communicate to patients that they must comply with instructions that are essential for good outcomes and safety, such as not smoking for 2 weeks before surgery, or for 2 weeks after, or using daily sun protection. Set clear definitions and expectations of compliance, demonstrate your commitment to compliance, and others will understand and respect the need to comply.

PRESSURE

Using pressure tactics undermines credibility. The only time it is appropriate to emphasize urgency is when a clinical condition exists that will affect the patient's outcome and potentially the patient's health. Placing pressure on a client/patient to act now because of pricing or novelty creates a false connection, and will surely lead to a relationship that will fail.

PRICE

Quid pro quo: something for something. Your service has a valid cost. Your employees and the services you provide should be appropriately compensated. Connecting with a potential patient on price is valid only when you know specifically what is desired and appropriate for that individual. Trying to connect on price with unknown variables is like catching butterflies in the dark. If your goal is to advertise the best price, know that you will create a price war with someone.

VEHICLES

The way in which a message is disseminated represents a significant portion of its value: unless a message is received by its intended audience, it is worthless. Dissemination is a means to get a message from originator to recipient with varying levels of efficiency, speed, attraction, and cost. The vehicles used to disseminate information can range from basic to technologically progressive. They can be economical or extravagant, sent at a leisurely or a rapid pace, and serve an individual or a wide audience.

There are three general communication efforts essential to every practice of aesthetic medicine: client and patient relations, outreach, and advertising:

- *Client and patient relations:* Specific messages are directed to active and inactive participants in your practice; they are designed for visibility and education, to retain individuals as active patients, to encourage service and repeat service, and to elicit referrals. An example is the patient education material or core practice material that you personally put into your patients' hands.

- *Outreach:* Outreach refers to no-cost or low-cost messages to your target population that provide visibility and education and generate traffic. Examples include your practice's website and spending time connecting with your referral sources, social media, and networking. You may pay to have such messages shaped, created, and managed, but you do not pay for the message to be delivered or presented to the intended audience.

- *Advertising:* Ads are created specifically to reach your target population, clients, and patients; they provide visibility and education and generate traffic, and you pay a fee to have them transmitted. Examples include directories, magazine or newspaper ads, your recorded message on your telephone system, and even articles that you pay specifically to have placed in a publication or online.

You do not expect your patients to comprehend the intricacies or the physiology of how the service you provide will fulfill their needs. To make an informed decision, however, they must comprehend:

- The basic function or action of the treatment or procedure you recommend

- Any alternatives to the recommended option

- All cautionary information (risks, complications, down time, the potential for undesirable outcomes)

- The active obligations of the patient in treatment

- The physical, emotional, and financial cost considerations of treatment

In choosing communication vehicles, you don't need to understand the intricacies of every medium, but you must make an informed decision about which vehicle has the greatest potential to help you succeed in your communication goals and objectives. You need to determine whether your message must be disseminated externally, internally, or both. You must comprehend the basic delivery function of the communication vehicle and its direct audience, any alternatives, and the differences among them in function and audience, all cautionary information (acceptable standards and ethical obligations), your obligations (submission guidelines), and the cost of using that vehicle.

Critical to the success of your communication efforts is knowledge of how these vehicles can be applied to disseminate your messages so they achieve their objectives with your intended audience. Chapters 11 and 12 define external and internal means of connecting. The vehicles used and the methods and messages may differ, but the constants are your goals and how your brand and image are conveyed. Although the message and the means are separate and distinct forms of connecting, they must reflect one another:

- Your goal is to lead those who receive your messages to become patients. Your messages, actions, and methods must be clear and concise to excite the attention and engender the trust of the individual.

- Current patients may also receive your external messages. If the message is incongruent with their experience in your practice, this can cause confusion, mistrust, and the potential to lose your most valuable assets: loyal patients.

THE ART OF CONNECTING

Even for those who are born communicators, there are moments when we don't know what to say, how to say it, or what type of response we hope to receive. As you establish what you want to say and how you will deliver your message, you must think about how to make an effective connection, prevent disconnection, and avoid awkwardness with messages that make the recipient uncomfortable.

The tone and purpose of your message will influence how it will sound to recipients. How they interpret it can result in curiosity, attention, a response, and a positive action—or it can result in dismissal or avoidance.

PURPOSE

To you the purpose of your message is clear: you are communicating valuable information to benefit your audience while helping your business to succeed. Yet to each recipient, the purpose and content of the message may be perceived in a different way. Because each recipient filters the information through his or her own understanding and experience, all messages about your practice must carry a very clear and common purpose that supports and reinforces your defined image, brand, and mission.

Market Purpose

When you do not know the individual needs of a target audience, you must use characteristics defined through demographic and market research to help determine their needs and interests. This research will help you define the purpose of the messages you send to this group and shape the type of communication you will select. When your message's purpose does not appeal to the interests of your target audience, it ultimately has little value and will not contribute to your success.

There are three distinct purposes for messages directed at your market and prospective or potential patients with clearly defined education and information goals:

- Brief, introductory, or general identity messages. The purpose of these types of messages is to convey your image, brand, and mission and in some cases, provide an overview of the services you provide. Messages such as these will typically appear on the home page of your website or in general directories and often fulfill the goal of increasing your visibility.

- Comprehensive introductory messages. The messages convey your image, brand, and mission, and outline in detail the services you provide, where you provide them, and how they are provided. Messages with this comprehensive purpose result from the individual who answers your phone and include your practice profile, in print or by electronic medium. These messages are intended to increase your visibility and educate your audience by defining who you are, what you do, and why.

- Targeted introductory messages. These messages either provide education about a specific service or element of your practice, or they provide information to a defined target group and elicit a specific response from that group. These messages include conversations, advertising, or media relations that educate others about a specific treatment and give information about you as the provider, patient education about a specific treatment or procedure that contains information on you as the provider, or detailed information on you as a provider, such as from physician-finder services specific to a procedure or treatment (a plastic surgeon's listing on a breast implant manufacturer's website). The goals of these messages may be to convey news, novelty, or in some cases, compliance: you have the credentials and experience to offer a specific device or treatment.

These three types of messages are sent to target populations and prospective patients to generate interest and create visibility for your practice. In many cases, your communication with a target audience will progress through each of these three objectives. Each objective leads you to the goal of direct communication with a potential target or potential patient, thus converting an unknown audience member into measurable traffic.

IN PRACTICE: The Consistent Message

Suppose a practice has a clearly defined identity in its messages to target populations and potential clients. It has developed a good message and communicates it through reasonable vehicles. The same message continues, unchanged, repeating through countless cycles. I see this often, and it truly troubles me. It can last for years.

If you run the same ad consistently in the same media over many years, what are you conveying? If you never update an Internet listing, what and who are you missing? What might be incorrect? Failure to update your messages, especially those that are far reaching to an audience who does not have a direct relationship with you, indicates that you are stagnant, complacent, and haven't changed with the times. This is not something one wants from a medical practitioner.

Today we have many more ways to connect with people than ever before. Your own website is one, and now social media options have become the marketing tool of the future. If you don't Facebook, or if you aren't LinkedIn, are you missing out? Just because these are new options for communication does not mean they are appropriate or valuable for your purposes.

Advances in nonsurgical treatments have introduced a whole new population to aesthetic medicine. If you don't offer nonsurgical treatments, will you still be able to relate to individuals who don't want surgery now but may someday?

Although the image you present in your messages should be consistent, especially to audiences that do not already have a direct relationship by which to judge you, the message must not stagnate. You should review your communication with your target populations and potential clients annually; this means every directory in which you are listed, every ad that you run, your service menu, even your business cards. In addition to confirming the accuracy and timeliness of the message, review the demographics and interests of the target audience and decide whether the message is achieving its objectives. If it's not, it is time to redefine your message.

Patient and Client Purpose

Once someone becomes a patient, you have an even greater need to individualize your message and maintain your image, brand, and mission with this individual. Recognize that something or someone and a specific interest has prompted this person to come to your practice. If your message does not address that interest, you will lose the relationship. If your message does not support the image, brand, and mission conveyed in prior communication to that person, you will weaken the relationship.

But you also have a need for less individualized communication at this relationship level, and this is where most practices fail. General communication with existing clients and patients is crucial to keep your brand, image, and mission visible to them, even when the relationship is not active. This accomplishes two things. First, when the client or patient decides to act, you are a known provider. Second, when that client knows someone else who wants to act, you will come quickly to mind.

IN PRACTICE: Clinical Overload

I was called to consult with a practice that had just done a complete re-branding. They had redecorated to include plasma televisions that blared procedural demonstrations at every public spot in the office. They had built a "presentation room" where physicians conducted seminars and demonstrated procedures, often in very personal detail. The practice had rebuilt their website to include volumes of lengthy descriptions and pictures of nearly every patient who consented to include photographs and a download of the 40- to 60-page informed consent documents for nearly every procedure. The office manager proudly stated that this was the ultimate in education, connecting with patients at every level, at every opportunity.

But the practitioner and staff were puzzled. Prospective patient traffic was not enhanced; it was falling. There were more questions from patients, not fewer. Fewer clients were converting, and more were leaving after a consultation without committing to treatment. The practice manager decided her staff of patient coordinators, preoperative nurses, and schedulers needed better training. She believed the practice was making the connection; these team members were simply failing to maintain that connection and carry through to treatment.

My assessment of the situation was simple: this was a case of clinical overload. Not everyone wants to see what a procedure entails, especially if that procedure is unrelated to the patient's goals. Demonstrations of very personal procedures can make the audience uncomfortable and squeamish. A website is meant to introduce your practice and capabilities. More pictures does not mean better education. Lengthy information can obscure the sole reason someone has visited your site: to find a solution to a personal need. Moreover, an informed consent document should only be presented in person. It serves no purpose to place it in view of those who may not be appropriate candidates, who may not understand, or who may have legitimate concerns and questions.

The office manager disagreed with me; that was fine. The lesson here is clear: Know what your prospective patients want and need and deliver it where they can access it, and where you can connect. Clinical overload occurs when too much information is given at the wrong time, in the wrong place, or to the wrong audience.

Put specific and comprehensive patient education in the hands of those who are interested. Place it in specific areas, such as consultation rooms, or deliver it via email when the prospective patient contacts you with questions or to schedule a consultation.

Don't stop there. Take all of your clinically specific patient education out of the waiting room and off the racks on the shelves and walls for 2 weeks and only dispense it directly to those you and your staff know have an interest. Take all of your magazines out of your waiting room, or at least put them in only one location at a distance from seating areas. In seating areas, place your general communication: newsletters, clinical updates, a practice brochure, a brochure that emphasizes your credentials—things that convey your value overall, what you do, and what is new and interesting to those you serve at large. Do the same for your website: offer general information about your practice, services, and procedures and leave the very specific photographs and details for the consultation setting, where they belong.

Now observe what people are reading, requesting, or asking questions about. Then ask yourself whether this change in the way you present material has lessened your ability to educate, convert, or retain clients and patients, or has improved it.

Resource Purpose

Resources are where your clients and patients find you; sources direct your clients and patients to you. It is essential to communicate with sources and resources; without them you would not have many clients or patients. Although sources and resources both generate traffic and potential clients and patients, they are approached very differently. Communicating using resources requires messages that engage the resources to support you in fulfilling the purpose of communication with your target and potential clients.

Messages of professional outreach maximize your status as a medical professional. Tap the hospitals where you are on staff, the specialty and subspecialty societies you belong to, and the companies who manufacture or supply the treatments you administer, prescribe, or sell. When you engage them, expressing your value to their audience while upholding a consistent and appropriate image, brand, and mission, they will eagerly assist you to use the referral and communication programs they offer providers.

Messages of commerce allow you to engage the services you need to reach your potential clients. Your practice requires the services of others, which you pay for, to fulfill certain functions for your business. Among these services are resources such as the yellow pages, print and electronic media, advertising, public relations and graphics agencies, software providers, and your Internet provider. All of these can help you target your message to the right audience or assist in increasing your visibility in your market. Ask what such services can do for you to ensure that your target audience can find you. You may not have to buy that service, but if you do not ask, you will not know what that service can do for you.

As a business person you must not only engage in commerce with resources, you must also carefully consider the value of a resource. If you determine that resource has no value for you, do not use it. If the value does not appear worth the price, negotiate. The objective of messages to your resources is to generate maximum visibility and maximum efficacy for your messages and minimize the expense of your communication efforts.

Professional outreach opportunities abound; professional societies and professional groups exist formally as well as informally. You pay your dues to belong to these groups and expect something in return, but does simply adding a credential to your curriculum vitae have value? You also "pay your dues" when you purchase and administer specific pharmaceutical products, medical instruments, or brand-named services, but what do you get in return for your loyalty? Reach out: Ask what an organization has to offer to enhance your visibility as a provider. Take what they offer and use it, but do not expect that the relationship will be one-sided. Get involved: Offer your expertise by participating as a member with a voice, and as a volunteer with leadership.

Take the time to let your sales representatives know of your loyalty to their product and why. Share your experiences with their product. Then ask what they are willing to provide in return for your loyalty; ask how they can support you as the ultimate deciding factor in whether their product will be considered in fulfilling your patients' desires. If a representative is not willing to help you help your business grow, his or her product does not deserve your loyalty.

Source Purpose

Your communication with sources—those who lead potential clients or patients to you—requires messages that encourage them to refer individuals to you. Sources include referring physicians, patients, staff, even friends.

Communicating messages to sources must generate visibility among your established sources and create an ongoing opportunity for referral. You must generate direct channels of communication with your sources to maximize their confidence in referring patients to you; you must affirm your status as an expert in the specialized care you provide to validate that source's decision to refer to you.

GENERAL MESSAGES

General messages are those used in communicating with existing clients and patients. The primary purpose of using general messages is to maintain visibility for your practice among sources, whether the relationship is active or inactive, so they are regularly reminded of the services you provide. The second purpose, no less important than the first, is to create visibility and easy access for sources that have the greatest potential to refer to your practice. Your practice brochure, an article, or an update are valuable in sources' hands for generating referrals. Timely, relevant messages transmitted to a source, circulated among that source's staff, or passed along from an existing patient to an interested friend or relative create visibility and access to you, with or without direct referral from the source.

CONCISE MESSAGES

Concise messages are initially used to address a client's or patient's specific interests, such as sending a patient who has had a prior treatment an update on new protocols for that treatment, or a safety alert. However, concise messages can also be used to communicate treatments, procedures, or actions that can fulfill a potential referral's needs. Concise messages that are communicated to sources should include education about services and how you can provide these. In addition, concise messages to sources should engage the source to directly refer to you, providing information on how they can pass your message along to potential referrals. Your concise message should also show appreciation for the relationship. Patient education branded specifically to your practice and accompanied by a dialog gives the source the information and the means to recommend your practice to someone who expresses an interest or desire for an aesthetic treatment.

PROFESSIONAL OUTREACH MESSAGES

Messages of professional outreach maximize your status as a medical professional to tap sources for clients and patients. Communication with your peers conveys your value as a professional who can fulfill the desires of clients and patients the source may not be able to. When you confidently and professionally transmit concise and general messages to sources, they will respond by referring their clients and patients to you for the specialized services you can provide.

CLINICAL MESSAGES

Clinical messages provide information about your specialty or the particular services you offer. These messages update and support the current scope of your practice, the procedures and techniques you perform, and those you do not, and why. Although a physician or other professional source may not belong to the same specialty, he or she has an obligation to understand what you do and your ability to do it before referring someone to you. Examples of clinical messages include supplying published clinical updates, conducting informal or formal meetings to educate referring physicians, and speaking personally to referring physicians about a case they have referred to you.

❧ RELATIVE WISDOM: Just Ask

When a new restaurant opens in town, before you consider going there you do a little research on the menu and the atmosphere, and you read reviews or ask others if they have been there and for their opinion.

When you want to travel to a destination you ask a travel agent, visit a website, read reviews, or ask others if they have been there. You want a first-hand opinion. Before you arrive, you call the concierge and ask about tee times, restaurants, spa menus, and other attractions and activities. You want a trusted referral.

When you need a lawyer, a real estate agent, an accountant, a decorator, or a contractor, you ask those you know and trust—your banker, insurance agent, colleague, or even your neighbor for a referral. You select someone who you know has similar standards and expectations to yours and you ask someone who you know will be honest and sincere with you. But you don't just ask for a referral; you ask about the individual or the service to which you are being referred.

Your patients are researching you, and perhaps asking for a referral to you. To your prospective patients, aesthetic medicine is like a trip to somewhere unknown. Luckily for travelers, there is a travel agent or concierge who can provide the needed details. Unfortunately for your patients, there is no concierge, but there are those who can share first-hand experiences, such as patients, your staff, sales reps, and other physicians.

Everyone who encounters you, your practice, your staff, your patients, and even your professional connections may someday be asked about you. There is a significant opportunity for everyone you come in contact with, whether a mail carrier, patient, or sales rep, to refer others to you. But how do you know that they will? That they don't mind? It's an opportunity you should never overlook. Just ask.

Staff Purpose

As a proprietor of a medical practice, the purpose of communication with your staff involves more than transmitting the policies and procedures necessary for your practice to function. Communication with staff requires operational communications, quality expectations, and proprietary value.

OPERATIONAL COMMUNICATION

Operational communication must convey all the information necessary for your practice to function and to provide service consistent with your image, brand, and mission. This includes all procedures, policies, agendas necessary for operations, and standards of clinical care. It also must convey your views on operational proficiency, privacy, and an understanding of all the messages your practice extends to all the groups with whom you communicate. When these messages are clearly communicated and acknowledged by your staff, you may maximize the potential to extend those messages. Each member of your staff should be empowered to carry out his or her specifically defined duties and should be skilled in the communications attached to those duties. Every team member should also be aware of the communication attached to every aspect of your practice, internally and externally.

QUALITY EXPECTATION

Quality expectations are messages that define what you expect of your staff, and why you expect this. These messages include job descriptions and the goals associated with those descriptions. They include the expectations you have of your staff:

- Expectations to uphold image, brand, and mission

- Expectations to support, cooperate with, and maximize the potential of any practice segment

- Expectations to demonstrate respect for you, your practice, other members of your staff, and all of those you serve directly or indirectly

The success of your practice requires more than just the operational proficiency of your staff. They must consistently practice defined standards of quality and excellence. Define these formally in your employee manual and require employees to commit to them. Measure these standards regularly and recognize when they are met as well as when they are not met. Motivate your staff by example and reward them by sharing the credit for the fulfilled desires of your patients and practice goals attained.

MESSAGES OF PROPRIETARY VALUE

Messages of proprietary value are those that you, as a business owner, have a personal obligation to convey. They are important not only in avoiding risk and upholding quality care as you provide aesthetic medical treatments, but also in upholding the identity you have as a personal services business. They are messages specific to the operations of your practice, and to your quality expectations for operations. Messages to staff carry the following objectives:

- Create and support an aesthetic practice of clinical and personal excellence, efficiency, and consistency

- Create and maintain an environment in which staff are continuously informed of the messages your practice communicates and the manner in which you expect staff to communicate

- Create and maintain an environment in which staff can excel as individuals and as important contributors to the success of the practice

General Public Purpose

Any time you are a member of the general public can become a moment that has an impact on you as a professional. You may rarely be recognized as a provider and proprietor, but when you are recognized, your message should be consistent with all that you have built and founded your practice on. Staff members should understand that they too may be recognized as representatives of your practice. Although you do not have the right to restrict or scrutinize their private lives, you have the right to expect that your staff should practice public behavior that:

- Demonstrates respect for your specialty and those you serve

- Upholds the privacy of your practice and those you serve

- Is lawful and respectful of others

- Demonstrates your commitment as health care professionals to the welfare of others

In addition, when you or your staff have an opportunity to introduce yourselves as professionals in the business of aesthetic medicine, the foremost commitment must be to uphold your practice identity.

The purpose of all messages communicated by you, your practice, and your staff to the general public are very simple. You must communicate in a manner that consistently upholds your identity and your reputation, the excellence for which you are known.

🗡 IN PRACTICE: Damage Control

You might wish to remain anonymous in public, and you can, until you cross the line into what is legally defined as a *limited purpose public figure*. A limited purpose public figure is one who is thrust into the limelight, not by his or her own choosing (such as a celebrity or public figure), but by circumstance and personal action.

A case in point: A provider of aesthetic medicine was going through a nasty divorce. There was mud slinging; there were accusations; the physician even engaged in some very damaging public behavior. When he was arrested for this behavior, it received media attention. Thus a respected medical provider in the world of beauty was picked up for behaving in a very ugly way. What was his greatest worry? The damage this would do to his practice. And what did he try in response? Damage control.

However, when you get to the point that damage control is needed, no one can help you restore your reputation. Whether you are at fault or not, damage control is just that—trying to defend yourself against something you know has marred your image.

Although the example is extreme, the lesson is clear: Your actions as a private member of the general public must be scrupulous and dignified. Anyone may have personal difficulties, and we are all entitled to a private life, so keep yours just that—private. You cannot control what staff do or say when they are in public, but you should be careful in your selection of staff and emphasize to them that you have confidence that they will not behave in a manner that could damage your practice.

An example of the need for preemptive damage control: I stood at a department store cosmetic counter one day, and I did not have to eavesdrop to hear a woman talk about tooth whitening. She purported to work for a dentist who performed this service and her comments were very damaging. She was so vocal about the fact that the public were mere fools to be paying several hundred dollars for a treatment that uses only a few dollars' worth of product that other people around her began to engage her in conversation. So did I. I asked who she worked for and, incredibly, she told me. She publicly devalued not only her employer and the profession that she served, but she devalued herself as well.

Make certain this woman is not working in your practice. Also, ensure that those who do work for you understand the need to uphold the values of your practice and the very sensitive and private nature of the services you provide, even when they are in public.

CONNECTING WITH YOUR COMMUNITY

The purpose of messages communicated by you, your practice, and your staff throughout your community or among a close circle of friends does not alter the purpose of messages to the general public. The purpose is simply more pervasive.

How you behave in social interactions contributes directly to your success. If you find it does not, maybe you should reevaluate your social life. The best referrals come from those who know and trust you as a provider of aesthetic medicine. We have discussed these as patients and referring physicians, but referrals also come from your friends, neighbors, relatives, and acquaintances. They have the advantage of knowing not only that you are a credible professional, but they also know you personally. You should maximize this advantage, but do not exhaust it. There are three simple rules for communication with members of your professional and personal community:

- Ensure privacy and confidence all the time, in all matters. This demonstrates your character as someone to be trusted.

- Limit the discussion of matters relating to your practice to either general assessment or innovation, but only when others broach the subject first. Do not let yourself be pulled into a sideline consultation. The only exception to this is a formal presentation you are asked to deliver to your community.

- Choose to support only those community groups that have a personal connection to you or a relation to the service you provide. Otherwise, you may find yourself supporting nearly every group that approaches you so as not to offend.

These three very simple rules will allow communication with your local and personal communities to have professional value insofar as they align your private and professional lives as complementary.

TONE

The tone of a message can influence how the recipient interprets the message, and this can result in the recipient's responding by connecting, disconnecting, or simply feeling uncomfortable and awkward about the message. Definitions of the word *tone* include sound quality, voice inflection, attitude, elegance and status, color and shade, and muscle condition. When applied to communication in the practice of aesthetic medicine, tone has relevance as any one of these definitions. It is a significant factor in attracting those with whom you wish to communicate and in how you and your practice are perceived.

Your message's tone must be consistent with your image, brand, and mission. If the tone you set does not attract your target audience, your message is of no value to the success of your practice.

Sound Quality

What do others hear when you communicate? Are your messages clear, concise? Do they present you as articulate, yet not aloof? Does a message have little room for interpretation? Does it specifically address the needs of those you want to attract?

How your message sounds or reads or how it is perceived by others is an important component of tone. If you miss the mark with the tone of your communication, the objective of your message will be obscured.

Voice Inflection

Does your voice come across as high (anxious, urgent, stressed, and demanding)? Is it low (casual, relaxed, and informal)? Is it steady and confident, or does it waver and quaiver? Do those you communicate with want to listen, or are they distracted by an irritating tone?

The inflection, or pitch, of your message can vary greatly based on the purpose of the message, its urgency in relation to those you are communicating with, and the possible outcome of not acting on the message. It is a mistake to employ an exaggerated pitch. The most urgent message should not be so high that it creates alarm. A general informative message should not be so low that it does not garner a reply. Find a tone that fits the purpose and objective of your message while still maintaining a comfortable quality that is desirable to listen to and effective enough to generate a response.

Attitude

Is your message brash, attention-grabbing, and humorous, caring and empathetic, arrogant and detached, or confident and poised? Do those you communicate with find your messages to be consistent with your image, brand, and mission, or are they confused with who you are and the approach you take to presenting your identity?

Your attitude can make or break your connection with potential relationships. If your attitude is not well received, respected, and embraced, then quite simply you have an attitude problem. Others will not engage you to provide service, refer patients to you, or work with you if your attitude is not positive. If you are confident in your abilities, your attitude should clearly demonstrate that you put the needs of others first in fulfilling personal desire.

Elegance and Status

Is your practice a tony, boutique facility in an upscale world of glitz and glamour? Do you have an understated, sophisticated practice in an elegant, private community? Is your business a tranquil and holistic oasis, providing a world of serenity, peace, and natural beauty? Are your services high-tech and personalized? Or is your practice none of these things, but rather loud, bold, extremely trendy and cutting edge?

However you define your practice to be in terms of elegance or status, make certain of three things: (1) that your definition is congruent with the image, brand, and mission you convey; (2) that it is congruent with your practice philosophy; and (3) that yours is a definition you are willing to live with, even long after the message has stopped being disseminated. This is where you must carefully consider your target market to effectively attract them, persuade them to act, and retain them.

Color and Shade

Is your message soft and pastel, bold and primary, bright and neon, or glittery and metallic? Color and shade involve more than just the physical color of a printed message; they encompass the physical composition or design of a printed message as well as your persona in your communications.

Although all your messages need not be consistent in tone, they should be complementary and must be visually congruent with your image, brand, and mission at all times. Someone viewing your message should perceive a tone that is relative to your image, addresses your ability to fulfill the viewer's needs, and most of all, is attractive and inviting.

Muscle Condition

Does the power of your message punch, or stroke? Are you extending a firm, friendly handshake, or a half-hearted wave of outreach? Is your message from or to a chiseled hard-body, or a curvaceous and natural form?

The muscle condition of your message involves (1) the power your message has to carry out its objective and elicit others to act, and (2) the impact it has in defining your strength as a provider. Do not think of muscle as just your own personal tone; it applies to your practice and profession as well. Your credentials, accreditation, added qualifications, and professional recognition are all the muscle, or power, behind your validity and value as a provider of aesthetic medicine.

You must set the tone for your practice. Your strength as a professional is defined in a tone that effectively attracts those you wish to reach so they understand your message, process it, act on it, and respond in a positive manner. Once you have created the message and refined its tone to attract prospective patients, you must motivate those you have reached to respond through a call to action.

Tone Deaf

Tone is a factor in every message you send. It is real; it is perceived; and it is subliminal. It must attract attention in a positive manner as something by which others will define or judge you. Although tone must garner attention, it also must maintain attention and maintain the integrity of the practice or provider from where it originates. Every way in which you and your staff communicate—verbally and nonverbally, in print and in person, electronically and physically—carries a tone. Make certain the tone of the message your clients and patients, sources and resources hear and interpret reflects your image as a respected and capable medical provider.

IN PRACTICE: Two Tone

The physician's office was impeccably designed, polished, and well-equipped. His staff members, according to him, were stunning; but by all appearances they were not supermodels—they were "superdone." Their primary function seemed to be to communicate how fabulous the physician was, and how he could accomplish everything and anything. The physician projected an unmistakable tone: a sweep of shoulder-length hair, flashy clothing and jewelry. And to top it off, he parked his Ferrari right outside the office front window, for all to see that he had made it, that he was successful and rich.

But his patient base was in decline, because there were very few in his market who related to his tone. To most, what he expressed as wealth and success and extremes in personal appearance was interpreted much differently. His appearance and surroundings represented an excess that patients did not relate to—or want to pay for. His patients, naturally enough, preferred someone less narcissistic, who could focus on their desires, not on his own.

This provider scoffed when I told him to park the Ferrari in back of the building and to dress well, but conservatively. I explained that while it was nice that his staff members were attractive, it was also important for them to look like and relate to real people. A decor of leather and polished chrome furnishings is fine in its place but it is too hard and cold and uninviting for an aesthetic practice; it is not conducive to soothing patients who are already feeling vulnerable.

He didn't understand me; he believed his patients came to him because they expected his "greatness." So I asked him to allow me one afternoon of

Continued

🦋 IN PRACTICE: Two Tone—cont'd

experimentation to prove my point. The Ferrari was parked out back, jewelry put away, his hair bound in a neat ponytail, the bright lights turned down to allow natural light to emanate through the public areas, and soothing, fresh, light melodies replacing the jarring, synthesized music on the speakers. I put away some of the bolder accessories in the office. I asked the aesthetician to give the receptionist a very neutral, natural makeup application. I told the receptionist to put on a lab coat to cover her distracting cleavage, her black bra visible through a sheer blouse. I would serve as his patient coordinator for the afternoon, and to the staff's surprise, I refrained from singing the praises of the physician and concentrated on eliciting information from patients, focusing on their needs and addressing their questions.

Every patient that was seen that afternoon booked an appointment, and for the two patients receiving injectable fillers, I stood by their side and held their hand, something the physician had ridiculed as "too folksy." I left the office with a long list of little things this practice needed to do to change their tone so that it was more generally appealing and did not deter prospective clients.

The lesson here: Try to envision every message you project through the eyes of the receiver—this includes your actions, your appearance, and your words. While you may like your style, is it what your patients like and what they can relate to? Tone is highly personal, and while yours should match your comfort level, consider who you must connect with.

A CALL TO ACTION

You have defined and created a message with purpose. Your message is targeted to your intended audience. The tone of the message is appropriate and attractive; it is consistent with your image, brand, and mission; and it is designed to appeal to those you wish to communicate with and garner their attention. Now you need a call to action—a means or message to prompt your audience to respond or act.

In general, all groups you communicate with require a call to action. The defining factor to what the call to action will be is what that call to action must accomplish. A call to action is based on your objective when you communicate with specific groups; it is the response necessary to fulfill what is ultimately your goal. A common downfall in practice communications is not extending a call to action to your target audience. Your greatest opportunity to establish a reply to your communication efforts is a call to action.

Many practitioners feel that a call to action is distasteful self-promotion or could easily interpreted as pressure, and it can be. It can also be motivating for a reticent individual you hope to engage in a relationship, and it can be enlightening for an uninformed individual who may have the desire for your service or know someone else who does. Much like the practitioner who does not ask for referrals, the practitioner who does not extend a call to action is not likely to receive a reply.

Target Populations, Clients, and Patients

In your communications that generate interest, visibility, and acceptance, the objective is traffic, conversion, and retention. Your call to action may be as simple as letting people know where they can find you, or as direct as an invitation or query about an individual's specific desire for service. The caveat, as always, is that the call to action must fit your image, brand, and mission. In addition, that call to action must be clear, timely, and effective and must not overstep privacy or good judgment.

The best calls to action allow an individual to act on his or her own time, in his or her own way, with no deadline, money, or personal pressure attached. There can and should be time value, economic value, and personal value attached, but not pressure. Consumers today are savvy about their own desires and of your attempts to get them to reply. Use this to your advantage through a message that includes education and personal desire to create a call to action that fits your audience.

In external messages a call to action is usually found at the beginning, or introduction, of a piece and/or at the end in the form of logistical information that allows others to easily reply. Personally or verbally, one to one, a call to action typically occurs toward the conclusion of conversation, and directly asks the individual if he or she wishes to make an appointment, purchase a product, or book an appointment for treatment. When a call to action is in print, you do not have the opportunity to reply to hesitation; you need to be direct and accessible. However, if you are too direct, your call to action may be misinterpreted as pressure. With finesse you can be direct enough not to cause hesitation, but flexible enough not to appear as if you are arm-twisting. If the person hesitates, ask why. Is it personal uncertainty? Monetary concerns? A need for further education? A matter of simply needing more time to make a candid decision? The answers to these questions may provide insight into the strength or weakness of your communication methods and call to action.

"IN" ACTION

One mistake that practices of aesthetic medicine make when extending a call to action occurs either in tone or "in" action. Consider the message: "Call us now for your free consultation." Wherever an individual sees this, at whatever time of day or night it is, are you certain you will be there "now" to take that call?

"Fulfill your goals and dreams for a . . ." This is an implied warrantee that suggests that you, not knowing an individual's case, can assuredly meet expectations.

"Act now—this special offer is only available . . ." This is absolute. It is also marketing in the purest sense, making something attractive, and urgent, by price or special offer.

"Pain-free," "Incision-free," "No down time," and any other procedural qualifier designed to act as a call to action is absolute. Without knowing the individual's case or desires for service, do you want to risk making that claim and not being able to fulfill it?

Simply listing credentials, services, and practice contact information is also a mistake. Where is the call to action? What likelihood is there that this information alone will be attractive enough in tone to entice your audience to act? Not likely at all.

"Tired of . . ." "Looking for change . . ." "Improve your . . ." "The answer to your. . . ." What these call-to-action statements have in common is that they play on the audience's insecurities. Where is the ultimate result of your communication effort more successful: with insecure individuals or with confident individuals who seek enhancement and personal fulfillment?

Youth, beauty, vitality, restore, renew, radiance, self-image, body image, confidence, and personal fulfillment: certainly the personal desire to feel fulfilled or be defined as any one of these is a call to action, but these terms can also be stereotypical, generic, or offensive. Leave these terms as positives; do not make them the result of correcting negatives. Connect terms like these to what is unique about you and your practice. Your call to action will then certainly garner a reply.

Patients and Sources

Your call to action with patients and sources to generate added service or referral should be direct. The purpose of communication with sources requires that you ask for referrals, so the call to action in these cases requires that you support that purpose with the information and the incentive necessary for the patient/source to act. Ongoing patient education and outreach through newsletters, clinical updates, and special offers are tools that must include valuable information about what you want others to act on; the addition of an incentive is added motivation for the individual being referred.

Why not offer incentive for the source? Once you recognize the difference between incentive and gratitude, you will understand why incentive is unethical here, and why I stress the importance of gratitude. Quid pro quo (something for something, such as a gift or bonus for referral) to sources before their referral is totally unethical in the realm of medical treatment, much less elective medical treatment. Gratitude, not incentive, is essential when sources refer you. Gratitude acknowledges that you are aware of a source's effort on your behalf and, in turn, your gratitude fuels future referral. Gratitude can include a simple expression of thanks, or a token of thanks. Offering a gift of some kind is ethical when it is after the fact as a means of expressing your appreciation for the efforts of others, not when it is used as an enticement or trade-off for referral. In any respect, gratitude must exist. It is as much a call to action as providing the tools necessary for sources to refer you.

Incentive, part of your call to action, motivates an individual who is referred to you to act on that referral. When referral comes from other patients, incentive may include special pricing or an added service perk, or it may simply be the very powerful endorsement of personal service. There is no more powerful statement than, "Tell doctor you are a friend of mine. He/she promised me that he/she would treat any of my referrals with the very same attention I received." When referral comes from other physicians, your incentive can be special pricing, added service perks, priority scheduling, and a statement of cooperation in care with the referring physician. Incentive is any factor that motivates an individual who is referred to you to act based on confidence, convenience, or value. Your call to action in communication with referring patients and sources for referral must include incentive.

🖋 IN PRACTICE: In My House

Opportunities for referral exist in your "house"—within your practice, your existing patient base, your staff, and even yourself. Here you have every opportunity to be your own source, to build on the unknown or expressed interests of others and turn them into a referral. Without a call to action, however, you will not turn opportunity into referral; you will turn opportunity away. I have seen many practitioners, most with a practice mix of payor and nonpayor services, fail to act on opportunity.

Here is a classic case: A dermatologist was confused when the slick and dedicated retail function she added to her practice was not generating the volume she expected. She had a lovely storefront located next to a plastic surgeon in a convenient part of town. She was promoting externally in every positive way, but clinical skin care products were not moving.

On observation, her staff was excellent at discussing products with people who came by. However, people who came in for treatment with the dermatologist, the most likely group of consumers for the clinical skin care products, did not avail themselves of the retail function at all. I sat down with the practitioner and her staff to review how they communicated the value of clinical skin care to patients and how they communicated a patient's interests among themselves. Here is what we found.

The practitioner was not communicating the value of the retail clinical skin care; she expected that of her staff. Her focus was on prescriptive treatments. The staff felt it was her obligation to mention appropriate care to existing patients. This is why patients came to see her—for her expertise and advice. They felt that by making recommendations, they were not complementing her efforts but were possibly contradicting them, or stepping over the line.

To resolve this situation, because the provider was most familiar with writing prescriptions, we created a prescription pad with all of the retail clinical skin care products on it. The prescription pad stated that these were products available through the practice. This was the missing call to action to extend her services into retail. A successful retail function represents ongoing traffic for your practice. In addition, she was instructed that on using this prescription pad, before excusing herself from a patient, she was to say that her staff would assist in fulfilling the recommended products and could make any further recommendations for complementary products (thus building on the sale).

The staff, in turn, was instructed to take this prescription from the patient, indicate on it exactly what was purchased, sampled, or recommended, and return it to the file, so that on a follow-up visit, the physician could address how the products were performing for that patient, and also so the patient could not take this "prescription" home and order a similar product from some cut-rate Internet service. To make the purchase of skin care products even more attractive, the staff had coupons for first-time purchasers of product. When a patient was on the verge of purchasing something rather than sampling, the coupon prompted purchase.

Within 3 weeks, retail volume had nearly doubled. Within 2 months, it was more than triple what it had been in the past.

The physician was so delighted that we developed a call to action for walk-ins to the retail function that worked in reverse to the prescription pad. A skin care survey was designed to help any walk-in or potential patient define his or her concerns and goals with regard to skin health and appearance. Staff would walk a potential patient through this, provide patient education to address specific concerns, and make the appointment for a consultation. The information sheet gave patients incentive to express their concerns candidly and to have those concerns initially addressed by the retail staff without the investment of a physician visit. In addition, the information sheet became the basis for a patient file. To the practice, the benefit was that retail walk-ins now had a means and an incentive to convert into patients.

In addition, something new was born of both systems. The individuals who often accompanied others to the practice (such as a parent with a child who has acne or a friend shopping with another who stopped by to replenish a product) became the perfect additional subjects for both the "prescription" and the skin care survey. This in-house referral became a very productive tool.

Take advantage of every opportunity to educate and enlighten others in your house. This is only self-promotion when one has no familiarity or interest in your practice or services; when any interest or connection exists, it is an effective call to action.

Referral-ease

Your call to action with referral sources must not only be an incentive for the referred individual to contact you, it must extend that call to action and make it easy for a referral to come to you. You know that establishing relationships with referring physicians is essential to your success. You know that you need to make them a partner in patient care, keep them informed, and support and respect their status as a provider to that patient. However, you need to do more to make that referral source feel inclusive as a partner and to make referral easy.

When you establish relationships, also establish communication. Put your practice materials in the hands of those who refer patients to you. Tell them they are welcome to distribute these directly to patients, or to make them available in any way that fits their practice's means of communication. It is important to follow up to replenish or update materials. First, anytime you have new materials, distribute them to your referral sources. Second, have an administrative staff member establish a schedule and check in quarterly with referral sources to see if materials need to be replenished.

Let a provider know that his or her office is welcome to make appointments for referred patients directly, and offer a special physician-only extension to your telephone line to do so. Follow up with email or postal mail that confirms the patient has an appointment to see you. Include what you know the patient's interest to be, and affirm your gratitude. Immediately following the visit, update the physician on the outcome of that visit, and continue to communicate throughout the course of patient care. While this may seem cumbersome in administration, the outcome of not doing so may very well distance you from a source of referral. Keeping referral sources close keeps them active.

Don't overlook the staff of a referring physician's office. They can be an equally significant source of referrals. They are in contact with patients as much as the provider is.

Finally, although giving an incentive for referral is unethical, providing the opportunity to experience the services you provide so a source understands their value is perfectly acceptable and appropriate. Invite a provider and his or her staff for an afternoon or evening in your office. Give them a tour, demonstrate technology, discuss your mission, and offer them the opportunity to experience services that are appropriate. Extend a professional courtesy discount for certain services and extend the invitation to return. Build your relationship for referral through communication, calls to action, and practice referral-ease.

Resource Call to Action

If your objective for communication with resources is to generate and maximize commercial value in the opportunities they provide your practice, what should your call to action be? What is the motivating factor for them to engage you in a relationship?

If you answered "revenue," you are wrong. Revenue, for the resource, is the end result of a relationship with you. The motivation to establish that relationship is this: A resource wants to provide something of value to you that will help your practice communicate and operate so that you can continue to engage them. Your call to action defines how that resource can be of value to you. It is what you expect of the relationship and what you can offer.

Whether you are dealing with a commercial advertiser, a pharmaceutical vendor, or even the professional societies you belong to, you must state what your expectations are, why they have value to you, and how you intend to be of value in return. Your value in return is not just revenue; it is exposure, loyalty, and active participation in upholding industry standards and defining industry trends. Resources can earn revenue from countless businesses, but they cannot garner active, involved, and committed commercial relationships of value to their business unless you call them to action by stating your desire, expectations, and commitment.

HAND IN HAND

I have often listened to members of medical societies gripe about leadership always getting the media spotlight when it comes to society issues. Get involved, and you too might get that spotlight.

I have often had clients ask me how to get on a pharmaceutical or medical supplier's website of referring physicians. Simple: Ask your sales representative. He or she will tell you what the standards are.

I have had many practitioners of aesthetic medicine wonder how some practices can afford splashy advertising in certain publications, and why some publications always come to those providers as sources for articles. Negotiate your rates, commit to a publication, and appropriately establish yourself and remain active as a media source for material.

Your call to action is what motivates resources to help you maximize commercial value and opportunities for exposure. However, this will not happen if you are not willing to work hand in hand to help them in their objectives for a relationship with you. As much as you need to ask what they can do for you, know that they may be reticent to ask what you can do for them—so offer. Extend your hand in partnership; no exclusivity is necessary. If you are a medical professional who can offer your integrity and value, then they will take your call to action and work with you to achieve your success. When they have a vested interest, your success is their success.

🜂 IN PRACTICE: Simply the Best

I have seen providers, good and bad, some self-promoting and most reserved. The most successful practices not only communicate effectively, but they also have staff who are their greatest advocates and promoters.

Calling yourself the best is clearly unethical; being the best, especially in ethical self-promotion, is unbeatably powerful.

A provider of aesthetic medicine recognized the key to his success was his staff. They were the front line and direct link to all traffic, every potential client, and each patient. For a very busy practice, one with an immensely busy personal services and retail function, the practice was not heavily staffed. He choose his staff carefully; he empowered and trained them; he entrusted and allowed them to train him. Most of all, they were well rewarded.

He made certain staff had easy access to the services provided by the practice so they could understand the benefits and experience what patients would. Quarterly, he took one afternoon to review service and operations with staff, to listen to them, and to recognize their accomplishments. He never hesitated to consider paying for continuing education that had value to the practice. He treated his people well. They respected him and were devoted to him, but that alone did not nurture self-promotion.

The provider set high goals, and the rewards for meeting those goals had specific meaning attached to them. For example, if the practice met its revenue goals, the reward was stock (profit-sharing) in his practice. If retail goals were met, the reward was stock in the retail companies whose products he carried. After the staff meticulously prepared for accreditation review and passed, he rewarded them with cleaning services for their own homes. He had an appropriate and meaningful reward for every goal.

There were other perks. On surgery days, he always had breakfast or lunch delivered, so the staff went into surgery satisfied and energized and came out having something healthy to eat.

So how did this lead to self-promotion? It was the call to action for staff. Much like asking a source for referral and giving that source the tools and incentive to refer, this physician asked his staff to promote him. He gave them the tools and guidelines to do so ethically, and he extended respect and rewards that motivated the staff to be his greatest source of positive practice promotion and an immense source of practice growth.

If you have high staff turnover, explore why this is so. If your staff do not promote you, ask why. If you want success, do not let either of these things occur. Communicate with staff and call them to action.

RELATIVE WISDOM: At Work

We have a close family friend who is a therapist. Every time we are around him I feel as if he is analyzing me; I wonder what he might be thinking. I have asked him about this. His answer is simple. Like most people who are not thinking about or acting on their vocation at all times, he puts aside his role as a therapist when he is not actively at work.

Certainly as someone who is devoted professionally to enhancing appearance, you have had people outside your practice ask for your professional input on their desires. I hope you have never extended such input without an invitation. Much like my friend is not always in an active mode of providing therapy, you are not always in the role of aesthetic medicine provider.

How then do you handle situations outside your practice when you are called on as a physician? And how do you know if that interest is just a matter of conversation or genuine? You do not have to avoid such situations; you can turn these situations into opportunity by using a call to action:

- Offer a simple reply that lets the individual know that the present is not an appropriate time in which to go into detail.

- Indicate where the individual can get a complete and appropriate reply, whether it is directly from you at a later time or from an information source linked to you and your practice.

- Follow up with the individual privately, within a short time, if you feel the opportunity exists to translate the person's interest into service.

- Remain consistent with your image as a practitioner of aesthetic medicine in how you respond, because others may be listening as well.

It is that simple. You will preserve your image as a provider of aesthetic medicine, preserve your role as a private person outside the practice environment, adequately respond to the needs of others, and more importantly and appropriately, direct an interested person to a private and productive time and place where communication can focus solely on that individual's genuine interest.

Making a connection is the key to every successful relationship. Your success requires fulfilling relationships with those who wish to improve their appearance and their lives through the services you provide, so communication is vital. When communicating with various groups to acquire such patients, you must communicate:

- With purpose
- In a tone that will garner positive attention
- With a call to action that will direct others to respond

When communication is interpersonal, delivering and controlling your message is easy. When communication is not interpersonal, the vehicle you use to communicate has significant importance, because if the message is not received, it has no value.

CHAPTER 11

Connecting Outside Your Practice

> *When I started eBay, it was a hobby,*
> *an experiment to see if people could use*
> *the Internet to be empowered through access*
> *to an efficient market. I actually wasn't thinking*
> *about it in terms of a social impact. It was really*
> *about helping people connect around a sphere*
> *of interest so they could do business.*
> — PIERRE OMIDYAR, FOUNDER OF EBAY

Connecting with people you know, and those you don't, is a more complex process today than ever before. As author David Shenk noted in *Data Smog*, a marketing publication, the average American encountered 560 daily advertising messages in 1971, which rose to more than 3000 messages per day by 1997. Today various groups, from Nielsen to the Magazine Publishers of America, report that the average American may now be receiving as many as 6000 daily commercial messages—a truly overwhelming number. Add those commercial messages to the barrage of beauty, self-improvement, and medical information available on the Internet, in print publications, and on television as well as communications from friends, advisors, and family, and it becomes clear that a plethora of media outlets exist for delivering messages about your brand and your image to the public.

In the simplest terms, the targeted opportunities to connect with your market of current and prospective patients, referral sources, and personal acquaintances outside your practice include the following:

- *Advertising:* Paid messages created specifically to reach your target population of clients/patients and to provide visibility for your practice. These educate your clients and generate traffic. Examples include directories, magazine or other ads, your telephone message on your hold system, and even articles that you pay to have placed in a publication or online.

- *Outreach:* Unpaid messages that reach your target population of clients and patients that provide visibility and education and generate traffic. Examples include your website, social media and networking, or a seminar you plan or are invited to present. You may pay to have messages shaped, created, and managed, but you do not pay for message delivery to the intended audience.

- *Directories:* Whether paid (advertising) or unpaid (outreach), electronic or print, directory opportunities and options abound. Directories provide a structured platform for delivering basic information about your practice: brand (name), specialty, and contact information. In some cases they permit the inclusion of additional detail, such as your training, scope of practice, or service menu. Still others accept personal messages, before and after images, and even a direct link to contact your practice.

- *Media relations:* Media messages include credible, balanced, and attributed news (that is, the source of the news is cited) communicated via television, radio, print, or the Internet to inform and educate. Media relations are unpaid. You may hire someone to manage your media relations or to present your "pitch" to the media, but an editor has sole discretion for allocating time and space for your story.

These communication channels help you to:

- Create and maintain visibility

- Generate traffic

- Educate the public, your patients, and sources

- Keep relationships active

Your practice cannot function, much less succeed, without using one of these communication channels. These allow current and prospective patients to find and connect with you, to learn about your services, and to stay connected with your practice.

ADVERTISING

Many practices and providers of aesthetic medicine claim that advertising is unnecessary and distasteful. Others are zealous in their advertising efforts, placing numerous messages in multiple vehicles with high expectations for what advertising will produce.

Because it is impossible to be personally visible to all those who are potentially or fully interested in your services, you need paid vehicles for disseminating your message. Advertising is a form of communication that maintains your visibility to an outside audience; it is a controlled communication providing you with total command of the goals, message, purpose, tone, and call to action to be conveyed. In advertising, you control all the elements that make it an extension of you.

Advertising can be general, and serve the simplest and most far-reaching goal: visibility. It can also deliver a targeted message to an audience that you know is interested and will be responsive. Knowing your audience and its potential response is of primary importance when choosing the best method for delivering your message. This vehicle must be based on the demographic segment it reaches and the effectiveness of the message once conveyed. However, do not discount the value of a paid message that does not produce expected results from a specific audience based on the specific medium. First carefully reconsider your message to determine whether it was off course, or the medium was wrong for the message.

Advertising Essentials

Regardless of the moral issue, dishonesty in advertising has proved very unprofitable.
— LEO BURNETT, ADVERTISING EXECUTIVE

Advertising is not your only communication outlet; however, it is the one that most effectively characterizes you and your practice to the people with whom you have the least personal connection and wish to reach. However, when the truth is embellished or facts distorted, to compel others to respond, this is detrimental. For your message to produce results that promote trusting relationships on which your practice will thrive, the following elements are required:

- *Consistency:* For your brand and what your practice can deliver—every time, everywhere, outside or inside your practice

- *Compatibility:* Adapting your message to the audience or the situation without diverging from your brand

- *Precision:* Delivering your message with the right words, tone, vehicle, and timing

- *Truth:* If you cannot be sincere, be silent

Leo Burnett, the legendary advertising icon who created the Jolly Green Giant, the Pillsbury Doughboy, Tony the Tiger, and other indelible images, recognized that dishonesty in advertising will inevitably be unsuccessful. Any successful advertisement must:

- Have a goal—visibility, announcement, solicitation, education, news, novelty, or compliance. Pressure and price do not belong in ads for medical services, whether they are elective or essential. Define your goals so that you can measure the success of this connection.

- Call attention by making a visual and/or verbal connection to the audience (a headline). Whom does this message need to positively attract?

- Communicate clearly: describe your mission, announcing a new service; or introduce a new team member or product. The tone should be inviting, and familiar (words, images, and colors selected).

- Issue a call to action related to your purpose (how, where, and why others should reply). Determine how you want them to respond to this message.

- Tie all elements together concisely, clearly, and consistently; this may require a few square inches of space or a few seconds of time.

You can develop ads on your own, hire a professional agency, or use services offered by your medium of choice to help you create advertisements. Do not micromanage creation of the ad but do carefully control how you, your image, your brand, and your mission are represented. Two points require special emphasis:

1. Any paid message must be detailed and precise in its imagery and language, similar to the detail and precision you convey in your practice when meeting patient expectations. To someone who does not know you, this introduction should convey professionalism. To those who know you, it should be consistent with the professionalism they expect.

2. No provider of aesthetic medicine should ever allow any paid message to be disseminated without personally reviewing it first to ensure that it is representative of his or her image and practice. Trust your intuition and judgment if you do not feel comfortable with this message. Remember, you have worked hard to build your image, and it is crucial that the message be true to your mission.

The need for creating and delivering paid messages and for measuring their impact on your practice is fundamental. Every advertising plan should be monitored and evaluated continuously throughout its execution. Strategies that do not work can be modified. If you fail to reach your intended audience, reexamine their demographic viability and interest as well as the vehicles used. Messages that miss the mark must be redefined.

Paid messages today can be delivered through many channels, each with their own unique set of variables: print, electronic media, and hybrids (advertorials). Many of these advertising vehicles also have editorial content—true reporting of news and information. The hybrids attempt to blend advertising and content; these are touted for providing the greatest opportunities for disseminating your message, but they also have potential pitfalls.

BRANDING AND DESIGN CONSIDERATIONS FOR PROFESSIONAL SERVICES

Kevin McConkey, Grip Design

We define *brand*, as it relates to professional services, as an amalgam of experience, identity, and public perception. For some time now, the idea of a "brand" has been nearly inseparable from the visual execution of a practice; for instance, the development of a new logo is often referred to as a *rebranding*. We caution against the oversimplification of how a practice is perceived for many reasons, one of the most important being that patients are attracted by referral and reputation, two very important components of a brand that have nothing to do with the visual execution.

Visual identity reinforces the style and common traits of the target market and existing patient base. For example, an East Coast physician whose practice is defined by the latest technology, modern architecture, and the sparse, clean lines in the advertising and marketing has a different visual representation from that of a surgeon practicing in Santa Fe. Their differences are not based on variations in service quality, but rather on the common visual language of their constituency. Understanding your client/patient base is a key to practice growth. Appealing to their aesthetic sensibilities is the key to brand recognition.

Let's define a realistic expectation of what your identity can do for building a practice and why it is so important. Your identity will serve as a visual shortcut to how a patient feels about his or her experiences with your practice. What is perhaps more important for new patients is that it will provide a visual reference point that communicates the quality of your services. We have all been confronted with a choice between two unknown products; at the supermarket, the cosmetics counter, or when considering which hotel to choose, the visual component of a brand has the ability to increase consumer confidence. Consider the effect of a well-designed identity on the perceived value of services as a function of cost. Professional services need to be judged not by the amount of time required to perform a service, but by the value of that service to each client. Anyone can make an incision; patients hire their surgeon based on his or her ability to make *the right incision.* Visual elements that distract from conveying extreme competence should be eliminated.

The most important point to be made is that a modest investment in a professionally designed identity inspires trust among potential clients. The decision to undergo any cosmetic procedure is wrought with indecision and any element related to your practice that can engender trust is invaluable. While a healthy practice uses several channels to increase the customer base, the conversion ratio is most affected by conveying confidence, experience, and professionalism and by building trust.

Helpful to the process of beginning a redesign of your brand is to find a design partner with a process and personality you feel comfortable with, excellent typographic skills, standard operating procedures that guarantee deadlines, and a transparent billing process. You will need to share a great deal of how you see your practice evolving to get the most out of this process. The clients who gain the most and are billed the least tend to spend a great deal of time on the "front end" of a project, and once they feel an adequate direction has been determined, let their design firm guide the process. Just as your patients must trust you to make the correct decisions, so must you trust the partners involved in a redesign.

All of the visual elements involved in a redesign stem from a central triad: logo, type style, and color palette. Our mantra is to err on the side of simplicity. Be wary of any logo that attempts to define your practice with visual clichés or elements that may grow stale with time. A logo should be scalable (resizable) and have versions ready for any number of applications, such as a ball cap, a postcard, or a billboard. All of the logo usage guidelines, along with the type style for letterhead, correspondence, billing, and so on, should be contained in a brief "manual of style" created specifically for your practice. This document should also contain the color palette in each of the popular reproduction methods: Pantone Matching System spot colors, CMYK percentile breakdowns, and screen-based equivalents for television and monitor output. If this seems complicated, relax—the work to create this manual will be done by your design partner, and the intent is to create ease of use. Be clear at the outset of selecting a firm that the goal of this process is not just to create an enduring look and feel for your practice, but to do so in a manner that allows your administrative staff to replicate the professional design aesthetic on a daily basis.

Continued

BRANDING AND DESIGN CONSIDERATIONS FOR PROFESSIONAL SERVICES—cont'd

A successful visual identity overhaul is composed of the following steps:

1. Interview and identify a good design partner. The best partners will have a vested interest in doing research about your profession and be willing to show you up to three "comps" at the initial design presentation.

2. Invest time upfront to educate your team on your practice's messaging and style. Competent firms will work hard to define the appropriate look and feel for your business and should be well versed in your business plan for the next 5 years.

3. Hire or assign a "point person" to define and deliver your content. The single best practice to avoid investing more time and money than necessary is to have a single person funneling all content to your branding partners. Consolidated feedback focuses your design team on problem-solving and saves time and expense.

4. Create a competitive landscape to guarantee that your positioning and identity are unique. New practices are regularly carved out from existing physician groups. Understanding the landscape of your competitors or parent practices will allow you to craft a unique brand that reflects how and why you serve your patients.

5. Trust in the process and your design partner; let them exercise their abilities. A partner with years of training and experience can help guide your identity. Resist the temptation to become a closet art director. However, this does not preclude your providing feedback and direction. Great feedback does not address specifics, but rather thematic issues. Refrain from demanding a logo be larger and centered, but do ask how the brand can have a stronger presence on the page; you might be surprised at how many ways a problem can be solved.

6. Make timely, thoughtful, and final decisions. This falls under the rubric of progress and cost savings. Indecision and delays actually cost more than the time involved. The sooner you can produce your brand, the better.

7. Avoid designing by committee. Even in the most perfect of scenarios there may be some dissent about a final direction. Designing by committee destroys the possibility of unique positioning by averaging all work to the lowest common denominator. Consider the saying, "In all the world's parks, in all the world's cities, there will never be a statue dedicated to committees."

8. Establish planning guides that consider the entire year and marketing plan. This allows two very valuable effects: (1) it is easier to monitor and maintain the right amount of communication, particularly to augment slower cycles of the year, and (2) it facilitates efficiencies in production costs (printing multiple pieces at the same time greatly reduces the expense).

9. Set benchmarks in advertising and marketing and review progress quarterly. Establishing a creative brief at the outset of a redesign is one way of guaranteeing that year-long marketing and design efforts stay on-message and on-brand. Quarterly reviews can also provide a set method of reviewing and congratulating your team on projects that attained their goals.

10. Stick to your brand standards as defined by the manual of style. After all the time and effort spent to create a style and message, the manual will be your compass. Do not be afraid to police your brand and those who are responsible for its daily execution. We recommend annual checkups with your design partner to maintain consistency and effectiveness.

Certainly, at the end of this process you will have doubts about some of the decisions made along the way. It is human nature to reconsider our actions. But do not let eleventh-hour concerns delay production. As they say in sports, "If you don't shoot, you will never score."

Remember that your brand is composed of many elements working in concert. How a patient is greeted is just as valuable as how your logo is displayed at a charity function. The goal is to convey a sense of quality, build trust, reflect the values of your patient community, and inspire consumer confidence so every client/patient can serve as an evangelist for your services.

Just as relationships develop with patients, you will also develop a relationship with your branding and design team. Don't be afraid to have a good time! Building trust and experience among team members will benefit your practice over multiple projects and many years.

PRINT MEDIA

Advertising in a printed format is generally defined as a display ad, with artwork that conveys your message (as opposed to a classified ad, which consists of words used to classify a job or a product for sale). The current forms of display advertising and their format, range, focus, and audience include the following.

Billboards   Billboards, those prominent slabs of wood and steel scattered across farm fields and plastered on buildings, often hawk their wares in garish colors and outsized messages. A billboard's range is determined by the ability of passersby to see it as they speed by or stop for traffic. The focus has to be simple and clear, making a memorable impression in a few seconds when viewed from a distance. The audience is the public at large, and any targeting is related to the locale where the billboard is placed. Billboards can be expensive—tens of thousands of dollars, depending on location, lighting, size, and quality. Because of their varied dimensions and the requirement that they be visible from a distance, you will need to hire a professional to design a billboard. My view: Nothing as personal as aesthetic rejuvenation should be conveyed on something as impersonal and unattractive as a billboard.

Newspapers   In America, newspapers are dying. They are costly to produce and consume valuable resources (paper), but they are still favored by many traditionalists for their dose of national and local news. According to a 2006 study by the Newspaper Association of America, six of every ten respondents check the ads at least once a week for products to purchase. Newspapers can provide an accurate demographic of the audience they reach, whether a specific community or a large metropolitan region, or by the section of paper in which your ad is placed. Focus your ad to your demographic, but be careful: the low print resolution used for many newspapers can make images appear fuzzy and small text nearly impossible to read. In your market you need to measure who reads a newspaper as well as which potential clients have seen your newspaper ad. One of the advantages of a newspaper is that it affords you the opportunity to bundle your print ad with an online ad in the newspaper. Most newspapers have a short lead time; your ad may only require a submission lead time of 24 to 72 hours before it reaches your audience's hands. My view: Newspapers can be effective for seasonal messages, announcements, news, or novelty, depending on your targeted audience.

Magazines   Slick and gorgeous or cheap and cheesy, magazine formats run the gamut of quality, consumer interest, distribution, and ethics. They draw attention based on the focus of their content, from fashion and beauty to hobbies and sports, from travel to world news and business. According to a 2008 study by MediVest, magazines are used once a week or more by 47% of consumers in search of fashion and beauty information and by 37% of consumers seeking health and wellness information. Their range can be national or local. They are distributed by subscription or sold on newsstands, where their flashy covers compete with other similar magazines. Some magazines are unsolicited and distributed free of charge to specific addresses and demographic groups. National magazines often have regional advertising pages, or outside sales groups that resell a collection of national pages per region. Local magazines often feature societal or cultural activities in a community or metropolitan area. Like newspapers, magazines can bundle your ad to provide both print and online presence on the publication's website. My view: Good magazines with good ethical standards and quality content and production values can be effective for visibility, seasonal messages, announcements, or news. The caveat is knowing how frequently the publication is distributed and the lead time from ad placement to publication. This can be as little as 2 weeks or as much as 3 months.

Directories   Print directories are as staid and standard as the yellow pages or insurance, hospital, and community directories. Because their content changes frequently, and advertisers are diverse they are generally produced in inexpensive, disposable formats. Directories generally have a range defined by geography, with an opportunity for you to reach as narrowly or widely as you wish. They provide a basic compendium of contact information; their audience is looking for information about specific people, products, or services. My view: The only thing a directory is used for is to find contact information; therefore don't spend more than you must to list your contact information in the categories where directory users are likely to look for it. Each time the directory is published, read your entry to make certain the information is correct and current; it is damaging to your image if a potential client fails to contact your practice because of a changed number or a typographic error.

Programs   Whether for the opera or a local charity, a women's club fashion show or the local sports team, programs offer targeted opportunities to place display ads. They vary in format more than other forms of print media, and their range is defined by their purpose—the event or audience they serve. Unless your services have direct value to the audience, the only reason for advertising in programs is for visibility, name recognition and to inspire goodwill. My view: Programs are a great opportunity to share goodwill. Local athletic teams or charitable foundations may seek your support, and if you want to, give it, but don't place an ad if your message is not appropriate for this vehicle, offer your financial support instead.

Direct Delivery   Whether a postcard or a letter to your patients inviting them to try the latest and greatest in your practice, direct mail is a means for disseminating your message and making a connection. The format for direct mail varies, as does the source of the mailing and the opportunities to target or blanket an audience. Whether you are the source or you are using a direct marketing company, be certain that the quality of the material, the message conveyed, and the packaging are clearly defined. Direct mail has the greatest opportunity for flexibility: you can target a specific zip code or a specific subset of your patient population; you can produce variable data (whereby a specific field on the print piece is customized to the recipient) or send a generic mailer. But be careful: in sending any form of advertising or solicitation to your patient population, you must comply with HIPAA regulations; you must have your patient's permission to communicate in this manner. My view: Carefully define your audience, message, and the package you want delivered, then determine whether the effort to create and send your message is worth the time and money. Direct mass mailings require the support of automated systems, and the personal touch is lost. Direct mail to an individual requires careful targeting and careful messaging so that you are viewed as communicating a benefit, not pushing your services.

Co-op   Co-op is not a vehicle for advertising; it is an ad-sharing arrangement whereby a company with which you do business, such as the manufacturer of a cosmetic injectable, offers to pay for advertising promoting its brand in addition to listing your practice. This may be a print ad, an email, or another medium. The manufacturer may pay for all of the advertising, a portion of it, or for an aspect of the advertising process such as the printing costs for a direct delivery ad, while you are responsible for the postage. Coops can be great opportunities for companies to promote themselves and to show that the physicians who use their products report good outcomes and success. However, if the co-op doesn't reflect your practice brand and image appropriately, or if the ad looks like a co-op production that promotes other physicians along with you in your market, it's best to ask for the company's support in ways more consistent with your practice, image, and expectations.

Cost and Value

Before selecting a particular advertising vehicle, consider whether the format and content of that publication is consistent with your image. Evaluate the readership demographics to validate the publication's ability to reach the ideal audience for your message. You need to measure the cost in relation to the size of the audience reached, defined by most publications as cost per thousand (CPM). CPM does not refer to those who read your message; it indicates only those who receive the publication in which it is displayed. Any professional publication will have a rate card that breaks down advertising rates into your cost per thousand readers reached with any one ad insertion. You should require any sales representative to define this for you.

Also consider the publication's content when evaluating print media as a vehicle for advertising. Most publications provide an advance calendar highlighting special topics or articles to be featured in future issues. Paid advertising in an issue that includes content that parallels the service you provide or that is attractive to your target populations has greater value than unknown content. It is your relationship with the publication and its representatives that will inevitably result in an understanding of where your advertising should be positioned, or the assurance that your ad will not be positioned with content or other advertising that conflicts with or criticizes the services you provide.

If your evaluation of a publication's audience, cost, and content indicates that it would be a good place to advertise and you do so, you should validate your decision after publication by measuring the response that this publication has generated for your message. This can only be done internally by asking those who consult with you where they heard your message and what prompted them to act. With print advertising, validation can also be measured indirectly through the use of coupons or special offers, but you need to be certain that these are effective, tasteful, and congruent with your practice's image.

Print advertising can usually be created with images, is often less costly for display than electronic media, and is easily reformatted or revised to convey different messages at different times in different print formats. However, print advertisements can be easily overlooked, and many readers learn how to extract the content that appeals to them without direct attention to display ads. The flip side of this is that visually appealing display advertisements, much like appealing content, will garner attention.

What cost is involved in print advertising?

- *Creation of the artwork:* Some publications will resize or revise existing artwork at no cost to you just to induce you to advertise. Make certain that the revision is absolutely correct and meets your quality standards.

- *Cost of space:* This is usually referred to as an *insertion,* because an advertisement is priced by the amount of space it occupies and its particular placement in the publication. Newspapers measure advertisements in column widths by vertical inches; magazines and tabloids by page and fractional page sizes. Premiums are usually charged for color and with journals, magazines, and tabloids, for prime positioning (the front and back inside covers and the back outside cover). In addition, rates may be zoned—priced based on the audience size and demographics of a specific region to which an edition is targeted or delivered.

- *Cost of administration:* Whether you use an agent or a staff member to plan and negotiate your advertising efforts, there will be associated costs. Frequently, agencies charge you the full insertion rate and the medium you are advertising in will discount this cost by 15%. This is how agencies make their money. In other cases, the publication will provide a 15% discount if you pay in a timely fashion and commit in advance to a semiannual or annual advertising schedule.

Print advertising rates are usually negotiable, based on special promotions that ad representatives always have available to offer. However, if you call eager to advertise, why should an ad representative offer you a discount? You have tipped your hand, and there is little incentive to negotiate. The individual in your practice who manages and negotiates your advertising contracts must be aggressive and direct while maintaining a friendly relationship with your advertising representatives—even when you are not in an active cycle of advertising.

Direct Delivery

Direct delivery of printed messages or advertising, can be the best means of connecting with those you wish to receive your message, when a valid, targeted database is used, and when the message is targeted and attractive.

A great deal of junk mail is sent to businesses and residences on a regular basis, and no aesthetic medicine practice wants its message to be perceived as junk. If the message looks cheap, is confusing, or is delivered to an audience that is not interested in it, it is simply junk.

Direct delivery provides significant opportunities for creating added value for your practice. A single communication tool may have multiple uses for varying audiences, through different modes of delivery. For example, a newsletter may introduce your practice to potential clients/patients; it can serve as a visible link to your referral sources and keep your current client and patient population active, informed, and educated. Today's database management programs allow you to customize your direct delivery communications as well as your in-office communications. Your database can be sorted by topic, name, or another defined field; best of all, it can be used repeatedly, as long as it is kept current.

Is direct delivery negotiable? No, but it can be innovative and flexible. However, there are costs associated with direct delivery, and these need to be taken into consideration.

- *Creation of the message:* Your message must be developed. Because the message is so targeted, can you or, more important, should you trust an outside resource with this responsibility? On the other hand, because the message must be visually appealing and consistent with your image, can you afford *not* to have this professionally created?

- *Use of bulk mail:* Bulk mail is relatively inexpensive. Direct marketing companies and mail houses will print, sort, address, bundle, and deliver your direct delivery messages using various databases. There is a mail house charge, but postage rates are lower and the savings in time and effort to prepare the mailing are considerable. Even less expensive, but of much greater value, is hand-to-hand delivery through your referral sources, through your neighbors or other businesses with whom you develop partnerships, and certainly through your own office. Too many practices make the mistake of sending a bulk mailing but forget to print enough so that they have extras available to display in the waiting and examination rooms.

- *Administration:* Even if you outsource preparation of your direct delivery communications, this will still represent your highest cost of administration. The cost is in time invested because someone internally must define and develop your direct delivery or work closely with those who do. The value of direct delivery is its ability to target your audience and message, so no one other than you or your staff should be leading that charge.

Direct delivery is one of your best options for visibility, but may also be your greatest capital communication expense. It requires effective planning to identify your audience, define and develop your message, and select the most effective vehicle for each effort. If you are not committed to doing it right, do not do it at all.

RED FLAGS

Red flags set off warnings, and red flags in advertising can be costly.

Be careful about advertising your prices unless you can guarantee that the service or product at that cost is appropriate for anyone who responds. Be careful of advertising prices, unless you want to start price wars.

Absolutes are red flags: *best, most, complete, erase,* and *eliminate* are all words that convey absolutes. Unless you can prove those absolutes or achieve those absolutes 100% of the time, don't advertise that you can.

Descriptors such as *nonsurgical face lift, no down time, no risk,* and *no bruising* resemble absolutes. Unless you can absolutely guarantee that you can deliver on these promises, don't label your services this way.

These are not just my conservative views, they are the ethical standards that core specialty societies define in their membership guidelines. Before you advertise, be familiar with and respect:

- Professional society codes of ethics

- State or local regulation regarding medical advertising (pedigree laws and testimonials)

While only the ethical may be encumbered by ethics, it is also the ethical who are often the most successful.

Electronic Media

The words you write may sound perfect for conveying your message about aesthetic medicine, but when they are transmitted by electronic media, there is more to consider than just words. How are they presented? Does the program in which your commercial appears or the song that leads or follows set the right tone? How your message is delivered and in what venue—during a comedy, a drama, a news program, or a talk show—can influence your message. How your message will be interpreted is based on variables such as words, sounds, tone, volume, content, and images. Electronic media are more varied, unpredictable, and their success rate less documented than that of print media.

Similar to print media, electronic media can be used both for advertising and media relations. Electronic media must take into consideration the same basics as print: format, range, focus, and audience.

Electronic media also have "advertorial" value as "infomercials" or paid programming. No matter the name, if you pay for placement on radio, television, cable, satellite, digital or web channels, it is advertising. Before you place an ad on electronic media, you should determine what time of day and what day of the week are best. You also need details on the demographic market area (DMA) in which an ad will run. Electronic media are less targeted to the geographic location of the end user and more targeted to his or her interest.

Much like print media, your ability to evaluate the value of electronic media can be enhanced with media kits and rate cards published by the media provider. These provide specific demographic information about audience and reach. Factors to consider when evaluating electronic media vehicles include demographics, CPM, and content, just as with print. With electronic media, however, there are additional considerations. Print messages can be saved for later referral. Electronic messages, with the exception of Internet ads and interactive television, cannot be saved and referred to later. Thus all electronic applications have a shorter "shelf life" than print. Electronic media are also significantly more costly in retained value than print messages.

Outside of more traditional television and radio, the newest means of electronic delivery—Internet, intranet, podcast, email, and texting—are the fastest-growing communication vehicles today. These new methods are your closest link to interpersonal communication with current clients but offer the most remote possibility for reaching those unfamiliar to you. These wireless communications help you stay connected while allowing recipients to retrieve messages at their convenience. However, it is also highly disconnected because it allows individuals to boldly reject your message by either ignoring something sent directly to them (deleting it) or simply hanging up.

It is important to recognize the distinctions between print and electronic media to understand how the audience responds and to measure their response. Just as measuring response with print requires asking people where they encountered a message and what prompted them to act, this is also essential with electronic messages. Because these messages cannot always be saved or stored, how do you know that a message truly fulfilled its objective, especially if that objective is to draw potential clients/patients to your practice? Unless your audience already knows where to find you, electronic messages, to be effective, need to be reinforced with something concrete that can be retained. It is critical that you measure their exposure to messages as well as the defining catalyst that made them act, and how they found you.

Radio   Radio is a more targeted medium than ever as a result of subscription satellite services and Internet-based radio. You can listen to what you want when you want. Radio commercials (ads) have an unlimited range today; they may reach the listening demographic in a geographic area, or areas unknown. Radio is focused; formats include talk, news, and every variety of music. Radio commercials can be jingles, promotions, or sponsorships. If you wish, you can be the exclusive sponsor of the weather, sports, or beauty talk segment, or any programming the network or station offers. Your audience can be anyone or everyone in a geographic region who is interested in a certain format of music or talk show topic. My view: Unless your message or jingle is so memorable that the listener is both compelled to contact you and able to recall your specific name to use the radio website or another source to obtain your contact information, there is little efficacy in using radio.

Television   Television was once limited to a few stations, VHF, then UHF. Subscription services arrived, adding more channels and choices; then cable, satellite, Web TV, and now the digital revolution. For every VHF and UHF channel there can now be three digital channels. There was a time when we might have distinguished between broadcast, cable, and satellite, but the differences are no longer of consequence. With the advent of digital technology, broadcast television is now much more focused. Programming is designed not only to reach a certain geographic area but also to reach much more defined demographics. For example, among the four major networks, one digital channel can offer popular programming, one local news and weather alerts, and one topics targeted to specific demographics:

women, business, finance, or sports. Broadcast remains the most expensive way to advertise. Despite all the television channels and options, it still draws the largest audience (although that is dwindling). Cable and satellite offer very targeted channels and programming. Bravo, Discovery, and O! are among the favored women's demographic channels. CNN, MSNBC, and FOX provide news. ESPN has multiple channels; whatever your interest, there is a channel. Regardless of the television format, advertising can be national or local, and, as with print, there are opportunities to advertise on a station and its website. As on radio, you can run a commercial or sponsor a news segment or program. And if you feel your audience is awake at 3 AM, you might be able to purchase time for paid programming—which is advertising.

Telephone   The telephone is one of the oldest forms of personal electronic communication. Today telephones have more uses than ever. They have voice mail and accept text. Many are connected to fax machines, and, despite do-not-call lists, phones are used by countless solicitors to promote everything from mortgages to your vote on election day. Quite simply, telephone is your closest connection to the outside, offering the benefit of connecting in person. You can interpret voice and inflection and create a dialog customized to the individual. For this reason, it is my view that the telephone should never be used to advertise or solicit. It must only be used to communicate what has personal value, as though the individual were sitting before you.

Internet   The Internet offers advertising everywhere, in multiple formats. You can advertise through search engines like Yahoo! or Google media sites with sponsored links. You can advertise on specific sites with banners or click-through ads that are pay-per-click or bought at a defined advertising rate. You can run commercials that precede Internet TV clips for programs or news. The range is nearly endless; anyone can find anything on the Internet, but with so much available, the range is also limited to those who actually may find a needle in a haystack. The Internet can be diverse and dilute, or unbelievably focused and targeted; it depends on the actual site and format you choose for your advertising. The Internet carries a multiplicity of directories (advertising), some designed around your specialty, a special interest, a hospital or medical center, and some probably unknown to you on which you may be listed, without having paid a penny. Despite "cookies" and other means for tracking what websites a user has visited, the Internet is reasonably anonymous, which allows for imposter demographics (you may not be reaching who you believe you are). Does advertising on the Web work? My view is that carefully identifying your exposure on the Internet and maximizing the opportunities that bring those people who want to find you to your door (your site) is the only effective use of your resources: time and money.

Through the Internet you can video teleconference or videophone. In my view, this is as personal and distinct as a phone call or an in-person meeting. Use it for no other reason.

Intranet   Your hospital, health center, health club, car dealer, or maybe even your practice have an intranet, a mini-web of programming and information available only to those who subscribe or who are captive wherever the intranet is playing. The format of an intranet is anything the owner or creator wishes it to be. The range is limited to the audience who subscribe to it, are permitted on it, or are exposed to it. There may be very focused opportunities with an interested audience, but because intranets are private, it may be difficult unless you are in control to know what is being presented and when. My view: Intranets could prove to be a highly effective means for reaching a targeted audience; the variables of cost, control, and access must be carefully defined before choosing to advertise in this way.

Podcast   You can create your own podcast advertisement, or you can sponsor a podcast segment that is directed toward an audience that might be interested in your services. Podcasts must be downloaded by listeners; therefore they elect to view your commercial, or they encounter it when they download a clip or segment they want to watch. Podcasts are less effective for advertising than they are for media education.

Email   Some call them ads; some call them spam. If your emailed ad is unsolicited, meaning the user did not elect to receive your ad, it is spam. As a medical practitioner you must be very careful about email advertising; by reaching the user directly you must comply with HIPAA regulations. Don't send an email to anyone who has not indicated that he or she is willing to receive your message via email. This applies whether your ad originates in-house or through a third party.

Text Message   Text messages are short, to the point, must-act ads. I sometimes wonder how it is I receive them, since I never give my cell phone number out when I shop. But many consumers do give out their cell phone numbers, and get text message solicitations—ads. These bear the same characteristics and requirements as spam; you must be HIPAA compliant. Texting must be used for personal messages, such as confirming appointment times. It is not an appropriate vehicle for advertising.

Whether email, voice mail, or texting, the advantages to electronic delivery are substantial when you know an audience member will welcome your message. It is convenient, inexpensive, and easy to respond to. Because people can respond so readily, it also has advantages in measuring response. However, when used to disseminate messages to an unknown audience, electronic media can be highly disadvantageous. Consider all the junk email you receive and the annoyance of telemarketing. Although these would not exist if there were no individuals who respond to them, is the percentage of positive response worth the unfavorable impression unreceptive individuals will develop about you? Will you know how many simply ignore it or are infuriated by the intrusion? As the provider of something personal and private, is this important to your image?

These personal forms of electronic connection with your market have the most accurate means of measuring response of an unknown or highly targeted audience to your message, because the means of response is attached to the vehicle of communication itself. Those who respond are tracked directly through the technology, whether a telephone call or a mouse click that leads someone to your website. With electronic delivery, whether the reply is positive or negative, you can easily determine that the message was received, because the technology automatically tracks it. What you cannot measure in every instance, however, is much the same as with any form of communication: even though a message is delivered, is it seen, recognized, or processed in any way?

On the Air, In the Air

Electronic messages are great communication tools. Their greatest value to you, however, is not in paid messages such as advertising, but in patient education and outreach. When you consider the cost of paid electronic media messages and the fact that most people are engaged in some other activity while also using electronic media, assessing the effectiveness of this form of delivery requires some serious consideration. Electronic media should never represent the bulk of your communication budget.

A radio advertisement for plastic surgery, laser hair removal, or similar services is attention getting, but by itself it cannot achieve your traffic objectives. How many listeners will remember the telephone number to call, no matter how many times it is repeated? How many listeners will decide at the moment they hear your message that they are ready to act on a desire to enhance appearance? And if you wish to advertise your aesthetic services on television, you had better know your market well, because why would one use such a public medium to disseminate personal messages? How will your ad stand out from the assault of Internet messages? You must not only consistently present your brand and image, but also be the visible needle in the haystack while making certain the mix of messages is not counter to your own message, brand, image, or ethics.

Cost and Value

There are no generalities that can be cited about the visibility, attention given, or cost of creating and placing electronic ads. Television ads have three dimensions (audio, text, and video). Internet ads have connectivity (you can link from the ad to your website or even to a telephone call). Video can be inexpensively created with a digital camera or professionally produced by an ad agency. Internet ads can be compiled from simple art or be professionally designed for depth and effect. In all electronic vehicles there are multiple variables:

- You may spend as much to create an ad as you do on disseminating it. Use professional high production values for the best opportunity to capture your audience. There is no advantage to your business and image in paying a lot to distribute a cheap or amateurish ad.

- Unlike print ads, where you have a proof and know the date of publication, monitoring radio or television ads or even rotating Web banners is not so easy. You should request a full report from the medium on when and where your ad will run, and spot check it. If the message becomes corrupted and does not play, you should not pay.

- Make certain the receiver's primary take-away message is your brand and the audience knows how and where to connect with you. Be sure that not only the message but all surrounding programming or content complements your image, brand, and mission.

- Measure the response rate to your ads, not only in numbers, but in qualified leads. This means individuals who are appropriate candidates, interested in your services, and relative to the demographic you have targeted.

- Like print advertising, whether you use an agent or have a staff member plan and negotiate your advertising efforts, there is an associated cost. Agencies may be able to negotiate better rates.

Because radio and television messages cannot be captured or saved as readily as print media (a message heard on the radio while in the car, for example), the message must offer something easily remembered (thus the reason for the "jingle" on many commercials). What will electronic advertising cost you?

- *Creation of the message:* Many radio stations will have a voice-over specialist or announcer record your script as part of the cost of advertising. Television messages require professional development through a studio. Both can present your image well—or completely misrepresent you—especially if the tone of the message is off the mark. Oversee this creation carefully: it not only represents a significant capital expense, but it can also distort your image.

- *Cost of air time:* Air time is most commonly in 15-, 30-, or 60-second spots; 60 seconds is a lot of time. These spots are priced based on the time and the programming with which they run. They are also priced based on the market ratings of a particular medium in conjunction with its demographics.

- *Administration:* You will need an agency if you are going to use a major market network electronic medium to advertise. These organizations work only through agents, because this generally ensures that the advertising product will meet specific technical requirements. Smaller markets are certainly more flexible, as are some radio stations, even in larger markets.

Is the price of using electronic media negotiable? There is little room for negotiation in a thoughtful advertising plan with electronic media. The deals frequently occur only at the last minute, when air time has not been sold and is thus cut in price to sell quickly; there may be lower rates for off-peak times, when there are fewer viewers or listeners and advertising is difficult to sell. In my view, electronic media are not effective for advertising aesthetic medicine for an individual provider. The messages can be very attractive but are difficult to track and of little value unless the message is highly effective in conveying a call to action to connect with you. Who will respond to a repeated slogan of "Call 1-555-LIPO-NOW?" Pure marketing gimmickry works with electronic media, but providers with skill and integrity do not need to engage in this to succeed.

Just as every practice, every market, and every target is unique, so too must the vehicles you choose to disseminate your messages be individualized to these factors. There is a defined audience whom you know is interested and willing to take the next step to use additional resources to engage you.

CONVERGENCE MEDIA

Heather Frayn

Convergence media is the future for media and communications. It can be broadly defined as multimedia, or multiple types of media platforms converged into one. With newspapers beginning to fold all across the country, a new media form must replace them. People still need and want to receive news; they just want it in a more modern way. Convergence media is here to fill that void.

You have probably seen and used convergence media without even realizing it. Every time you go to a news website, such as *CNN.com* or *ESPN.com*, convergence media is dominant. When the Internet first began to burgeon, it was essentially limited to a display of text and photos. It has now evolved to offer so much more. In your practice, you can use this new technology as a way to connect with more patients and on a more intimate level.

- *Video:* Convergence video goes beyond the news story format that you might see on TV. It can be as simple as a brief clip from an event or as complex as a multisource, analytical, long-form story. This video transcends what we thought was possible until recently and has multiple applications. It can be a television station that only broadcasts online. For your practice, it can be a short clip of you demonstrating a procedure or a video montage of personal patient recommendations. Be creative in your use of this new tool.

- *Audio:* Convergence audio can also be used in a number of ways. It can accompany a photograph or a story to help the listener see an event in a different light. It can be a short sound bite from a press conference or a long string of multiple sound bites from an event. The important aspect of audio is to make certain the listener can still be in touch with all five senses. For your practice, audio can represent an anonymous way in which your patients can be heard.

- *Information graphics:* Convergence media includes many different ways to send and receive information, and graphics is a great attention grabber. Online information graphics usually consists of small visual pieces that enhance another form of media. It can be as simple as a bar graph showing the number of face lifts performed in the past year or may offer more visual and technologic interest, such as a map of the United States and when you roll the mouse over each state, it shows the number of practicing plastic surgeons in the state. The use of information graphics is an effective way to catch someone's attention because they are fun, quick, and easy to look at.

- *Interactive media:* One reason convergence media is so successful is because it is very interactive. From live online chats to opinion polls, interactive elements are important. Readers/viewers today don't want to just read a story, they want to read it, watch it, hear it, comment on it, and send it to a friend. For your practice, having a personal blog can make prospective clients feel closer to you. Or having an online forum for people to post questions on your website can make people more likely to choose your practice over a competitor's.

Convergence media will continue to evolve as the demand for new ways to receive information grows. It's important to keep up with the latest technologies, because chances are that your clients will be.

RELATIVE WISDOM: Look Like a Star

An acquaintance is a real estate agent who often puts television commercials together for her listings. It's a little unconventional to show a home in a 30-second spot during the evening news, but she does it frequently. What is interesting is that in these commercials, your attention focuses less on the homes and more on her rather flashy outfits and her behavior as she guides viewers through a mansion or condo, with extravagant adjectives and exasperating exclamations about feature properties. Anywhere you go in town, people love to talk about her over-the-top ads, but they never seem to talk about the homes; they always talk about her dress, her flamboyance, and her animated delivery style.

One day I ran into this agent at the grocery and we exchanged greetings. I decided to be bold and asked about her commercials. Were they helping her to sell more real estate? Were they worth the time and money invested?

"Oh, Marie, I am so happy you asked; you know everyone talks to each other about my commercials and how much they love them. Because they

Continued

RELATIVE WISDOM: Look Like a Star—cont'd

love my commercials, they list with me, and you know I take very good care of all my clients. Are you looking to sell?"

No, we weren't looking to sell. I just wanted to know if the commercials were worth the time, money, and effort. Did they give her clients whose homes were featured an advantage in selling faster, closer to the asking price, any advantage at all?

"Well Marie, of course there is an advantage! Everyone sees me and the home on television, and they just love the commercials, and I have the most listings of any agent in town. If you are not selling, why are you so interested?"

This woman could not get to the point, because she did not know the point—whether those commercials in fact made her business better. She simply loved being seen on TV, planning her wardrobe, and her well-scripted performances. She did not know whether the cost of her commercials afforded her clients a shorter listing period or a better selling price. She assumed that because of the chatter, her commercials were a success.

Because I was so interested, I asked a friend of ours who was a realtor to give me some numbers: what was the average time of her listings to date of closing, and how many of her listings sold for the original listing price. Guess what? Few of her listings actually sold within the contracted period, and many of her listings were relisted at lower prices or with other agents. Of those that did sell, most were within 3% of the listing price, but considering that she placed her commissions far higher than the industry average, her clients were losing as much as 10% or more off the listing price.

Relative wisdom: If you do choose to advertise electronically, or by any other means, define not only your goals, but also how you will measure the value of your advertising. It may result in your phone ringing all the time, but how many of those callers will elect to consult with you, how many will elect treatment, and how many are retained patients who are returning for treatment or are willing to recommend you? Because it is immediate, it is often that we limit our measure of value to the initial return: that phone call. But don't stop there; continue to measure the value of your methods through your patient's life cycle in your practice. And consider whether your ad is really effectively promoting your services, or is simply good entertainment.

Hybrids

Paid advertising today is often not limited to an ad; in many cases short articles, profiles, even full-length feature stories can be placed in publications or on radio or television. Meant to look like unbiased editorial content, these hybrid pay-for-play efforts are commonly referred to as *advertorials* (ad + editorial). These hybrids contain artwork and generated editorial content and are disseminated or published for a fee. An advertorial can be an opportunity limited to defined sections within a publication that are labeled as advertising, or an opportunity to support local publications with content.

Advertorial   Most ethical and credible publications will label advertorial ads that are meant to look like articles as advertisements. A quality publication will distinguish content that is researched, attributed, and vetted as factually correct and balanced from paid messages. Such a publication does not want to lose its credibility and reputation for objectivity or confuse and mislead its readers. They will not want to appear to be recommending, featuring, or presenting a product or service that has not been researched and reviewed through appropriate channels. My view: If you are not willing to have the advertisement labeled as such, then your intention is to deceive. If the publication allows an advertorial without labeling this as advertising, its policies and format should be clear to readers so they can easily distinguish between paid and unpaid content.

Special Advertising Section   Regional and metropolitan publications often include special advertising sections on a specific theme that allow a templated presentation of the advertisers (a photograph and a set number of words) or that allow a mix of advertising and content at special rates. Themes for such special advertising may be aesthetic surgeons, attorneys, beauty providers, bridal providers, and so on. Publications may invite firms or individuals to appear in these special sections, or they may simply invite anyone who fits the theme of the section. My view: If you know the context of the special section and all the other businesses, products, or providers featured, and you are comfortable being showcased among this group, a special advertising section can be a positive experience to reach a very focused audience. If the section is unlimited in how many providers like you are included, or undefined in the selection process of those features in the special advertising, it is best not to take the chance to be lost in a sea of unqualified providers or diverse and unrelated products and services.

Paid Programming   Whether on the radio or on television, paid programming seems to come and go in different formats and fashions. In the early days of satellite radio, some stations offered physicians the opportunity to be key experts on their own 30-minute talk show about aesthetic medicine in exchange for a predefined advertising contract on the station. This is pay-to-play and is deceptive to the audience, unless the programming in which the physician is featured is labeled "paid." Television has had a spate of programs that appeared and disappeared, for which a physician was contacted with an opportunity to be featured in a documentary, but expecting the physician to use his or her connections to secure $30,000 to $50,000 or more of sponsorship for the show. Then there are the less deceitful opportunities that simply entice physicians to star in their own television program for a fee, with additional fees charged for the program to air at 3 AM as paid programming on some little-known network or independent station. My view: What you spend on paid programming is better invested both in time and money on efforts to connect with serious prospective patients rather than those who randomly connect with your radio spot or television debut.

Pay-to-Play   Has a medium ever offered to mention you in an editorial context in exchange for your advertising? This is pay-to-play. Although publications and programs should support their advertisers (or they may find themselves without advertisers), they should never be so brazen as to offer pay-for-play, nor should you demand such a deceptive practice. If you have an established relationship with the medium, use it properly as a resource (see Media relations, p. 259), and their representatives will reach out to you with questions about your practice or upcoming story ideas. If you cannot support with your CV that you are a true expert on a topic or procedure, paying to be recognized as an expert in an article will not yield positive results.

Paid Features   An interesting phenomenon has emerged that combines either several articles or program segments featuring various topics or physicians to create a full publication or program. These paid features are just that: the opportunity to pay and have a well-trained editorial team shape an article or a segment about you or featuring you as the expert on a specific topic of interest, such as antiaging treatments. My view: Look carefully at the publication, the program, and all the other topics and providers featured. In most cases, no matter how straightforward the professional intent, these are easily read by your audience as paid efforts.

All hybrids, whether advertorials or paid programming, must be contracted as advertising, and you must carefully review the fine print. Consider carefully with paid programming precisely as you would with any form of advertising. Hybrids may not have the flexibility that your advertising might, but regardless, your logo, your image, and the quality you expect must be reflected. Accept hybrids for what they are, or choose not to accept them. If you consider a hybrid to be a fair way to make yourself look like more than the expert you are, you are acting deceptively. The key to building your practice is a strong foundation, with honest messages that build trust.

🦋 IN PRACTICE: The Best Advertising

A young physician in practice, a friend, called me, surprised and excited that she had been invited to be in a very well-known and well-circulated women's magazine, citing the very best aesthetic providers in her geographic region. She was thrilled.

I congratulated her, but asked, "Is there a cost in this?"

She replied that the representative from the magazine who contacted her was faxing over the required paperwork. I asked if she had this representative's name and number, that I would contact her as a favor to handle this. Surprisingly, the representative was not from the women's magazine; she was from a marketing company. To participate in this ad, which the magazine re-

Continued

🦋 IN PRACTICE: The Best Advertising—cont'd

quired be labeled "advertising," the physician would need to pay a $2200 "administrative fee" for any retouching of her photograph and for compiling her biographic information.

"So this is an advertising opportunity, not an independent study or poll of who the best doctors are?" I asked.

The representative replied that this was a showcase of the "best" doctors, and they were chosen by various factors, none of which she could seem to articulate.

The lesson here: There are a lot of "best doctor" opportunities being solicited every day. When you pay to be called the "best," it is not genuine; it is advertising, and according to the codes of ethics for most aesthetic core specialty societies, calling yourself the best or any other absolute is puffery and is unethical. If you are paying someone to label you the best, you are advertising that you are the best, and you may not only find yourself in the worst light among your peers, but your savvy patients and those in your market will see right through this and know that you have paid to call yourself the best.

AUDITED/NONAUDITED CIRCULATION

When you choose paid vehicles to advertise your practice, you may find the term *audited circulation* bandied about in rate cards and other material designed to help you make the choice of using that vehicle. In print media, audited circulation is certified by an independent publishing association called the Audit Bureau of Circulations (ABC). The ABC reviews subscription accounts and records, newsstand sales, and the like, and verifies that the distribution of a publication is within a certain standard of what it publicly publishes that circulation to be, and thus the number on which advertising rates or cost per thousand (CPM) is based. Most newspapers and magazines beyond those in small community segments will probably publish an ABC circulation statement on their rate card to assure you that your message is being circulated to the number of households or readers that you expect it to be. (Of course, this does not mean the readers pay attention to or act on the message; it just gets delivered.)

Electronic media have their own ways of auditing circulation. In radio, circulation is tied to Arbitron ratings. Arbitron is a company that monitors radio audiences, patterns, and habits on a regular basis to define the size of an audience for a given program or station at a given time of day. This gives the station a basis for advertising rates or CPM (in this case, cost per thousand listeners reached). Television works much the same as radio; however, Nielsen is the auditing group that measures viewership of programming, thus providing a basis for advertising rates based on CPM.

What does any of this mean to the success of your practice? Audited circulation is a tool that validates the distribution that any communication vehicle purports to have. Further, when circulation is audited by any one of the three most widely recognized groups—ABC, Arbitron, or Nielsen—it assures you of the validity of these claims. Your budget for communication may be small or large for paid communication vehicles, and you may have designated all, none, or some of those funds to print, radio, or television advertising. Shouldn't the decision you make to expend your communication resources be based on the vehicle with the greatest value for you?

AD(DED) VALUE

How do you determine whether an advertisement has value to your practice? By measured response. But exactly what measure of response makes an ad valuable? At a minimum, one that pays for the ad, and beyond.

Suppose that over a 3-month period a practice spends $4000 on display advertising. Through that advertising, it generates five people who were prompted to contact the practice for service specifically as a result of that advertising effort, and another nine who recall exposure to the effort. Half of these 14 individuals (seven) translate to patients. Just to recover advertising costs, each patient would have to spend roughly $1140 on services: $4000 ÷ 7 × 200% (which is considered a fair markup of services based on the actual cost of providing those services). Is the ad effort of sufficient value to be pursued?

Suppose further that the practice's ad offered an incentive, such as added personal services or extending service. I do not like using discounts on services, because this demonstrates to others that at certain times one is willing to devalue what the practice provides. So if the incentive has a listed value of

Continued

AD(DED) VALUE—cont'd

$200, each individual who engages the practice from this effort must now spend $1540 to make the effort of value (recall the 200% markup). This is the return on investment (ROI), the amount of revenue that can be attributed directly to the marketing effort.

ROI is just one measure of value. Consider where the practice's time and money may have been better spent to attract those 14 people. Consider the immediate and long-term value of those 14 people—whether they elect treatment today, will return tomorrow, and will refer other patients to the practice. Of those who don't elect treatment, what was the reason? Did the ad reach the wrong demographic? Was it confusing or misleading? What would the practice traffic be without those 14 people, of whom seven are newly satisfied additions to the patient base? This practitioner must assess whether there were other means by which to attract those 14 people and the seven who became patients.

The ROI in the business of aesthetic medicine, or any brand-based, loyalty-based business, is more than simply a matter of dollars. It is also a matter of image, loyalty, and future opportunities.

IN PRACTICE: Ad Slam

A good advertisement can be a slam dunk, a point in your favor, traffic at your door, added service, added revenue, and practice growth. A mistake in an ad can be a slam to you, your image, and your practice. You must never allow a paid message (much less any message) to be disseminated until you or someone you unquestionably trust reviews that message in every detail. Ideally, more than one person should review the ad scrupulously. Do not trust a spell-check system; do not trust the graphics people you hire, and do not trust chance.

A reputable, well-known plastic surgeon had a beautiful ad professionally created to generate identity in the yellow pages, an upscale regional magazine, and a women's magazine. It was to reflect the core of his visual brand. The ad was one of general interest and identity and contained a short list of the types of procedures in which this plastic surgeon specialized.

Unfortunately, this tasteful ad received an unscheduled appearance on a late night talk show. Why? Because not even spell-check identified an error in typography that proclaimed this skilled, reputable surgeon as one experienced in "beast surgery." This tiny error—one mere letter of the alphabet—in a costly, professionally designed campaign became a huge slam to the reputation of this skilled surgeon—made him the butt of a cheap joke. You might think such a small error is something most people would understand, but do you ever want to be the victim of such an error?

When you cannot personally extend your message and a communication is made on your behalf, you must make certain that the communication is wholly what you expect it to be; that it correctly, succinctly, tastefully, and consistently conveys the message and reflects a skilled medical provider. If you overlook detail in your communication, what might others think you overlook in providing care?

OUTREACH

Advertising is a fee-based message to reach your target population; outreach includes all nonfee messages to reach these audiences and carries the same functions: visibility, education, and generating traffic. Outreach messages have a cost to you in time, effort, and productivity, but they are not a paid means of delivering your message.

Outreach is any event or opportunity that allows you or a representative of your practice to deliver a message of purpose, with a relative tone and a call to action (subtle or direct) to those you wish to engage. This includes one-on-one and group communication inside and outside your office, such as patient education and audience communication, seminars, special events, public education, professional philanthropic contributions, community education, professional education, and the contribution of your expertise to any of these efforts. Nonpaid directories, those of your hospital, for example, also provide outreach. Electronic outreach may include online referrals and consultations as well as the questions and dialog that your own website may elicit.

In the business of aesthetic medicine, outreach creates visibility for you and your practice at a defined time when you or a representative of your practice can personally extend your message. Through outreach, much like advertising, your practice must directly convey your brand, image, and mission to a target audience. Unlike advertising, where a message is concise and controlled, in outreach, your audience and the vehicle or partner you rely on may take control of the effort. It is important to look at outreach in distinct categories:

- Outreach efforts that originate from your practice, such as patient and public education and networking, are most commonly focused on the individual, either in person or through methods through which your practice normally communicates.

- Outreach efforts individualized to your practice that are focused on a targeted audience, such as seminars or distribution of practice publications, or participation in blogs or online communities.

- Outreach efforts shared or driven by another group with which you have a professional affiliation, such as seminars in which you participate, or educational efforts to which you contribute.

Outreach in the form of patient and public education that is focused on the individual is essential to your practice. It includes all of the things you need to provide for a client/patient to make an informed decision to engage your practice and to keep your practice visible and attractive. In the most basic sense of one-to-one patient education, outreach is critical to your ability to practice aesthetic medicine. To contribute to the success of your practice, not just your ability to practice, outreach must extend beyond individual patient education to focus on a specific audience, keeping your patients and interested public continuously aware of the services you provide as well as the innovations and opportunities attached to those services.

The use of outreach individualized to your practice and focused on a specific audience is much too commonly overlooked, despite the immense value it has to your practice. Consider the discussion of patient retention and the value ongoing communication has with inactive patients in the form of added service, referral, or simply maintaining visibility. You need to reach out beyond the confines of your practice to keep people coming in. Who better to reach out to than those who already have an established relationship of trust with you?

Some outreach efforts, such as seminars and special events, can be golden opportunities to put you in the spotlight for those truly interested in you but who are not yet ready to make an appointment for a consultation. However, this type of outreach can also tarnish your image: If you do not have the finesse or patience to manage the unpredictability of an audience, even in carefully planned outreach efforts, you can find yourself in an awkward or uncomfortable situation.

Do not participate passively in an outreach effort that is shared with or driven by another group. Make certain your image and message can be delivered in a predictable manner with a set agenda. Participate in planning and carrying out these forms of outreach and make certain that you know the other participants and their expectations and contributions as well as your audience's expectations.

What are the connectors, the vehicles or strategies of outreach? There are traditional means, and then there are the widely growing means of *social media*.

Networking   Whether you are at the hospital visiting with other physicians or playing squash with physicians, network. Talk business—ask them what is new in their specialty and discuss what is new in yours. Don't be afraid to ask if a colleague will accept your referrals, and don't be shy about saying you would sincerely appreciate and accept their referrals. Don't stop there: referrals and networking are a constant, not just the initial connection. Offer in-service sessions for your colleague's staff on the procedures you provide; invite them into your practice to experience what your patients might. Offer to take your colleague's practice materials and keep them on hand so that you may provide them when you make a referral, and ask if you may give your colleague your business cards, service menu, or any other items that are clearly branded and unique to you. Further, you must keep this valuable connection going. On a consistent basis that is appropriate to your relationship, whether once per month or once every few months, contact that referral source, ask how things are, ask if there are questions, and ask if materials remain in good supply. Whether another physician, a spa, salon, concierge, personal shopper, image consultant, or your very best referring patient, networking is an active role. Keep it active.

Events   Events may be in-house gatherings or at another location, small and intimate, or large and staged. Some may take the tone of an intimate afternoon tea; others may be the size and tone of a three-ring circus. Events that provide outreach opportunities include:

Seminars/Lectures   Whether for one individual or a ballroom filled with varying demographics, seminars and lectures must be of interest to the audience. Individuals must walk away having learned something to benefit them personally or professionally. You may conduct a seminar or lecture before invited guests, or you may be invited by a specific group. Whether educating referral sources, a women's club, or your own patients or staff, make certain you have a clearly defined agenda and goals for your seminar, and deliver on them.

Treatment Events   Treatment events may be as small and private as a pre-bridal party preparation, or an event that draws complete strangers to experience what is new. Seminars are often combined with treatment events. Be certain that the participants are willing and that all appropriate procedures are followed, including screening of candidates, patient education, and informed consent. Before anyone is treated, confirm that you have consent to treat, whatever the procedure, and that the individual is at ease accepting treatment in the group. I personally don't like treatment events that go beyond aesthetician services, skin care, and cosmetics. Anything more is a truly personal endeavor and should be provided in private.

Expos and Trade Shows   Employers, hospitals, media companies, hotels, health clubs—trade shows and expositions can be hosted by any number of businesses, or they can be a collaboration by a large marketing company to bring together similar businesses. Expos and trade shows take time and preparation, take the right staff to interact with and educate visitors, and can be unpredictable. You may find yourselves standing idle, or busy and exhausted. The most important thing is to know who is hosting, know the audience, ask about prior history for the event, and gauge your time and investment wisely. Do not hand out samples of products unless you anticipate you'll have enough and they will be appreciated; bring ample and quality branded information about your practice and try to make beneficial connections. Offering things such as complementary skin analysis will draw the hordes who ordinarily would not partake of your services—and you should understand that it is unlikely you will ever see that person again.

Social Occasions   Whether you are the host or a guest, social occasions offer a great opportunity to network. Don't arrive at you neighbor's cocktail party and hand out business cards, but don't be shy in asking people about what they do, so you can share what you do. Even among those you do know, social occasions are an important time to network. Put others at ease in your company so that when they need your services or want to refer someone to you, they will not hesitate.

Philanthropic Events   Charity gatherings can be as diverse as the local women's club fashion show to fund the arts, a free skin cancer screening, gang tattoo removal, or a retreat for cancer survivors. Philanthropic events are an important way for a physician to give back to the community and to create goodwill. You may find the audience is not of the demographic you would ordinarily attract, but giving of your skill and time is recognized and appreciated. Make the most of it, using these occasions for media relations, announcements, and demonstrating for your existing patients and referral sources that you selflessly give to others.

Aside from philanthropic events, there are many ways to give of your time and resources that effectively reflect on your practice and reach out to others who may be your patients and referral sources, or your prospective patients. You should engage in philanthropy because you want to give back, not because you expect to get back. But the things you do to give back should not go unrecognized or undocumented. Philanthropy can be as simple as participating in a cancer screening, donating to a silent auction, or sponsoring a local sports team. Be careful how you represent yourself and how the audience may view your efforts.

PHILANTHROPY AND THE AESTHETIC SURGEON

Steven L. Ringler, MD, FACS

I recall, when I was a third-year medical student, sitting in the darkened auditorium at Butterworth Hospital in Grand Rapids, Michigan, where I was doing my surgical rotation, and watching as Dr. Ralph Blocksma, a pioneer in the field of cleft lip and palate surgery and an internationally renowned plastic surgeon and humanitarian, presented a case of a woman who had a severe hemifacial atrophy. He had used injectable silicone to help fill the deformity. The result and subsequently his ability to transform her life were so dramatic; it was at that moment I decided that I wanted to become a plastic surgeon.

It was also well known to the medical students and residents that Dr. Blocksma had done a lot of mission work and had not even billed a patient until he was more than 40 years old. He had dedicated his life and his practice to helping people who couldn't afford medical care. He was my first mentor in medicine, and I still recall with great admiration his quiet confidence and the joy he possessed. It was his inspiration that led me to consider volunteering once I completed my training.

People go into the medical profession for myriad reasons. I believe that most idealistic medical students choose medicine because they want to help people and that they are caring and compassionate human beings. Although we help our patients every day through our aesthetic practices, in a competitive marketplace and busy world, it is easy to lose track of the reasons we chose the profession to begin with. Sometimes our bottom line takes precedence over our commitment to care for other people.

Over the past 20 years I have volunteered my time to Operation Smile, the not-for-profit, volunteer medical organization that provides plastic surgery for children with facial deformities. Operation Smile was started by Dr. Bill Magee and his wife, Kathy, more than 25 years ago. Since it began, Operation Smile has operated in over 42 countries and treated more than 120,000 children. Bill and Kathy Magee created an unbelievably successful organization by simply saying "Yes" where they saw a need. They have created a legacy that will continue to inspire us for years to come.

Anyone fortunate enough to go on a mission with Operation Smile, or any other medical mission where you have the ability to share your talent and your good fortune with others, will benefit enormously from the experience. There is simply no greater reward in medicine than handing a child back to his parents after surgery and to see the tears in their eyes and the shared joy of knowing that the child, their family, and their village have benefited by your effort.

There are countless stories that will touch your heart from the experiences of medical volunteers. Some examples: a 19-year-old male with an unrepaired cleft, living in a cardboard box in Nairobi because he couldn't get a job with his facial appearance. Or a female infant actually discarded in a trash dump in China simply because of her cleft lip deformity. Three generations, mother, daughter, and grandmother, all with unrepaired clefts because treatment was never available to them. Then there are the families who travel 8 to 10 hours by bus, donkey, or on foot, ready to hand their child over to a total stranger in the hope that they can be helped.

The experiences one has when volunteering in different parts of the world also help put your own circumstances into perspective. There are so many people in the world who struggle to get by with so little in the way of material goods, and who often face enormous challenges just to get through the day. Yet the joy, appreciation, and their sense of family and community are not diminished in the slightest.

My decision to do volunteer work has been rewarding in so many ways. Beyond the grateful families, the gratitude prevails both at home and abroad. Whether it's the volunteers in a country halfway around the world welcoming my return to treat their people, or my patients who have commended me on my efforts and taken pride that I am their physician. I often have patients say that one of the reasons they came to my office was because of my volunteerism. This becomes a reflection of you as a caring and compassionate physician they can trust.

You might ask if I am continuing these efforts just to market my practice. Certainly this is good PR, but it's not the primary motivator. I do not look for anything in return from these trips other than a safe flight home, where I can share my experiences with family, friends, and patients. I didn't go into medicine to win awards or accolades. I went into medicine to help people!

So when I ask myself again next year if I can afford to take a week off from my busy cosmetic surgery practice to travel to some far-off country to help a child or 100 children in need of surgery, the answer is simple. If my participation can improve the life of one child, then the effort will have been worthwhile. I have made a commitment to donate my time and expertise both at home and abroad to serve those who need help. The personal rewards far outweigh any sacrifice.

Besides, I like being a hero and inspiration to my own children.

Viral Marketing   Although it may originate as advertising, viral marketing is a ploy designed to be so intriguing, so infectious that people share it. It's "the buzz," such as the Super Bowl commercial that never made it on the air because it was far too risque for the public airwaves, but became the greatest hit ever on YouTube. It's the trend of slogans that are so bizarre, they become part of public vernacular to mean "Take it easy, brother." Viral marketing is what you do to get everyone talking, sharing, forwarding, listening, and engaged in your message for reasons that sometimes have little to do with you. Does viral marketing have a place in aesthetic medicine? If it follows the rules of defining a goal, having a purpose, sharing the right tone, and calling for the right response, all within ethics and good taste—maybe. To think that something so personal as improving one's appearance could become an infectious phenomenon—unlikely.

Social Media   The term *social media* refers to a means of connection with others in a virtual or online world. The trend is growing quickly and is actively used by younger populations. It is a free means to convey your message and to connect with others. However, you must consider the time and regular participation required for social media to be effective, and the anonymity of participants can result in outreach to poor candidates or individuals who are not honest about their intentions.

There are five key facets of social media that are used by those who elect aesthetic procedures or that may be useful for you to connect with your referral sources and patients:

- *Networks:* Social networks range from Facebook and MySpace to LinkedIn and Yelp. There are general social networks for making friends, and specific social networks for everything from business to travel; mothers; specific ethnic, religious, or interest groups; and college students. The premise is that you establish yourself with a profile (information about you), then you network with others on the site through blogs and chat rooms and interact via email and through instant messaging. These virtual communities have rules, but that does not prevent people from acting dishonestly or maliciously. Networks may remind you when a member's birthday comes up, or may post general topics and conversations you can engage in. Social networks are the place for social discussion and connection; they are not a place to give advice or solicit patients. Even if you don't engage in social networks, you should know what they are and monitor them, because your patients may just be talking about you.

- *Sharing:* Whether YouTube or Flikr or a multitude of other sites, sharing is a means to share videos, images, and stories. The reality is that these sites are free and accessible to host your video or pictures, but they are like needles in a haystack and are not an effective means for sharing with a prospective patient or a wider audience. Sites like these are generally unmonitored and somewhat unrestricted, and you may find your well-intended message has been morphed into something damaging to your image.

- *Blogs:* A *blog* (the term is derived from Web + log) is an online conversation. People share experiences, ask questions, and engage in conversations through blogs. Blogs are often read by those who don't participate. Like social networks, blogs have rules, but sometimes it is unclear who is monitoring to ensure that participants follow the rules. Some physicians choose to start their own blogs on their website or intranet for patients to ask questions and discuss topics of interest. This may be beneficial to your audience, but more important than starting a blog is the need to keep it fresh and moving. Much like social media, while you might not want to spend the time on blogs, you should know what they are and monitor them carefully as you may be the subject.

- *Reviews:* Like vacation spots, restaurants, movies, and plays, reviews of physicians, medical procedures, and beauty products are now available online. You may be the subject of a review but not know it; multiple sites crop up that offer patients the opportunity to anonymously review your practice and your services. The best means to know where you are reviewed or discussed is to regularly search for your name and brand through a search engine and see what listings come up. Contact the webmaster of any site that has incorrect information about you. They will likely try to sell you enhanced profiles; however, they must either correct erroneous information at no charge or remove your information from their site.

- *Wikis:* Wikis (the term is derived from the Hawaiian word for "hurry quick") are sites with collections of Internet content that are interlinked and can be accessed by anyone to add content. If you post to a wiki, you do not post about yourself, but for public education purposes.

Many practices are hesitant to engage in live or social outreach beyond individual patient education for two common reasons: the potential for unexpected outcomes, and lost time away from productive practice. However, the most successful practitioners of aesthetic medicine realize that if you do not reach out to those with interest in your field of expertise and those in your geographic or professional community, you cannot expect that others will reach in.

You may scoff at the potential value of these new channels of communication as too faddish and gimmicky, but multiple forms of online networking are here to stay, their use is burgeoning, and the current modes will inevitably be superseded by still more innovative methods. The generation who will be your target population in a few short years are extremely Internet savvy, and you must be too.

Cost and Value

Outreach has immense value because it is immensely personal. Although outreach itself may not directly expend capital resources, outreach efforts can still be costly. However, the rewards of that cost may not be found in any other communication efforts.

- Outreach is visible. It puts you in front of an individual audience that is interested in you and your services.

- Outreach is essential to patient and public education.

- Outreach can be altruistic. When attached to philanthropy, it elevates your image to one of generosity in human spirit; when attached to community support, it elevates your image.

- Outreach can be unpredictable, especially when you are not familiar with the expectations of your audience; likewise, they may not know what to expect of you.

Outreach can be delightful, or disillusioning and exhausting. Some practitioners find the time invested is far too great for the exposure they receive. For patient education efforts, your patient coordinator must be your empowered partner if you feel you cannot fully invest the time your patients require.

What will outreach cost? That depends on your level of effort and participation.

RELATIVE WISDOM: Fishing With Pirates

My boys love to fish and every vacation we take as a family must include some form of fly, deep sea, back bay, or other fishing adventure. I often seem to be the one who takes charge of investigating the right fishing guide or charter to keep us safe and happy fishermen (and fishermom). On a recent excursion to Mexico, I did all the homework necessary, contacted the concierge for the recommended deep sea charter, looked at the company's website, and perused travel sites online. All seemed to be in order; however, there were no reviews about one particular fishing charter company. But their boats looked the newest, cleanest, and largest, the video on their site was impressive, and the price was right. So we chose them.

Our fishing day began with ours being the only boat leaving the harbor. Cabo San Lucas was very quiet that morning. As we set out on the Pacific there were 30-foot swells tossing the boat everywhere. The day before there had been an earthquake in southern California, and the Pacific Baha coast was feeling the aftereffects. When we left the resort, no one told us of the sea conditions, but then, we didn't ask. When we boarded the boat, we were so excited to head out that we failed to ask about conditions. But when the conditions hit, we were hit hard. Our full day of fishing ended in less than 45 minutes, with a Coast Guard helicopter coming to the rescue and a hospital trip in Mexico.

When all were safe and well, I called the charter demanding my money back; they had nearly killed us. The company stood behind their contract policy and would not refund our money. So I did the very next best thing: I went on every social networking site I could find, rated the company, shared

Continued

RELATIVE WISDOM: Fishing With Pirates—cont'd

our story, and flooded the Internet with this one experience. Suddenly I had people responding to me online—others who had taken this charter and told of personal belongings stolen, trips cut short, and dangerously unprepared and unqualified boat captains. Other people thanked me for alerting them to this very dangerous business.

But I had more. In short order I had webmasters contacting me asking me to prove my story, because the charter company had complained that my postings were false and biased. Thankfully, I had the Coast Guard record and hospital bills to prove the event, and my blog posts remained. In no time, the company contacted me with the offer to take us out fishing at no charge the next time we were in town. No more pirates for us—I demanded and got my money back.

Relative wisdom: Social media can make or break your business with the extremes of stories told. But credible sites with strict rules will in fact investigate to prove if claims are real or not and will remove those that are not. If users cannot trust what they read on the site, the credibility and the usefulness of the site is lost. Don't flood social media with extraordinary, glowing accolades and reviews of yourself as a doctor, or ask your patients to do so. You'll be caught out. And if you are the victim of unfair slam on a blog, contact the webmaster and ask for investigation of the validity of the claims. The burden of proof lies with the source of the information, not you.

DIRECTORIES

Print directories are a thing of the past, right? Who really needs a telephone book, a hospital directory of staff providers, or any other printed medium that lists contacts in alphabetical order, or by service specialty, geographic location, or any other specific category? Given the cost of dialing telephone information and the easy access to the Internet, does anyone still need print directories?

Electronic directories are easier to search and keep current, occupy less space, are less costly to maintain, and can be targeted specifically to the user's interests than telephone directories can. These indexes have not made print or telephone directories and referral services obsolete, but they offer by far the greatest advantage of any form of directory.

Directories come in print, electronic, and Internet-based formats, and there are still telephone information services. Your car GPS may have a directory on it, as well as your PDA and the applications you choose. Directories can be very narrow (all the physicians on staff at your local hospital) or broad (the national directory of all members in your specialty society). Directories can be individual (a patient or personal contact database) or mass (online). The focus of directories may be broad (the yellow pages of your metropolitan region) or narrow (a listing of providers in a specific state who perform a specific procedure with a specific device).

The advantages to directories are many:

- When they are free of charge as part of a membership or professional service for a group to which you belong, you should take full advantage of such directories.

- Although many other forms of communication will include information on where to find you, a directory offers the easiest and most readily accessible means to obtain your contact information with no need for technologic devices.

- Although someone may not directly be seeking your practice, in searching a directory he or she may come across your listing, credentials, and practice information— anything that may create interest and prompt that individual to make the connection.

The disadvantages to directories are also many:

- The value of the information degrades over time, because it quickly becomes obsolete and is rarely reviewed for updates and revisions. Print directories become obsolete more quickly than any other directory, because they are printed far in advance of distribution. With telephone directories, there are so many offered, by so many known and unknown companies, that not only are you confused by which directory you should be listed in, but directory users are confused by which directory is the most comprehensive and current.

- The cost of listing your practice in some directories can be prohibitive, and some directories may require specific actions by the participants, such as offering free consultations or accepting a set fee schedule for any procedures performed on patients who find you through the directory.

- Unpaid directory listings often have the disadvantage of lying latent. You do not know they are there for you to take advantage of unless you search for them. These are usually directories of the medical instruments and pharmaceutical companies whose products you use, of the professional groups to which you belong, and of other general information guides (most commonly on the Internet) addressing consumer interest in a subject on which you are an authority.

Measuring response from directories is much the same as with any other communication vehicle. First, the question is one of exposure; then it is a question of which directory prompted an individual to act and contact you. With electronic directories, the added advantage is that there can be built-in tracking mechanisms. However, such systems measure numbers, not the quality of connections. The most reliable form of measuring response to the success of communication vehicles you choose to use is by simply asking these questions:

- Who or what referred you to our practice?

- Where were you exposed to a message from or about our practice?

- Where did you obtain the contact information you used to contact us?

Cost and Value

Directories can be targeted geographically, demographically, to a resource or professional affiliation, or to target interests. Consider the yellow pages, a preferred service provider directory published by a media or marketing company, or a hospital or professional society directory. Also consider the online services to which you can subscribe to be listed as a provider of aesthetic medicine for a specific type of service.

When your participation in a directory requires certain commercial activities on your part, such as providing free consultations or agreeing to a set fee schedule, the cost of these losses of revenue must be considered part of the cost of participating in that directory.

Directories can be interactive and link a target directly to you, or can be static, requiring additional efforts by the target audience to reach you. Some telephone services will make the appointment for a consumer who contacts them or forward the interested consumer right to your phone line. The same holds true with some Internet-based directories. They can provide links directly to your website. Other directories require the consumer to retain your contact information to manually and directly contact you.

What do directory listings costs? Again this is the most variable category in cost and value.

- Creation of the listing can carry no direct capital expense if you simply input the information electronically. It can also be included in the cost of your subscription to the service, or it can cost you the physical creation of materials when it appears in print or as a banner or page on an Internet directory.

- Subscription to directories can carry no direct capital expense if they are part of a professional affiliation such as the hospital where you are on staff; your national, regional or local medical society; or a pharmaceutical or medical instruments company for which you are a preferred provider. Subscription can also carry huge direct capital costs, such as with the yellow pages and electronic subscription directories. There exists little, if any, value in paying a high price for directory listings when less expensive resources of equal or greater value exist. Your capital resources are much better spent in more active communication efforts to build traffic.

- Administration of directories can rarely be left to outside resources. This is something that must remain in-house and should be on a regular maintenance schedule. Rarely do directory services remind you to update; they only initiate enrollment. Make certain someone in your office is empowered to keep all directory listings, especially electronic listings, as current as possible.

So how do you plan your directory listings? Take advantage of all noncapital opportunities and invest in administration to keep these current. Include yourself in other paid directories, but when the subscription fee is variable based on content, make certain that content is concise, simply listing who you are and what you do. Do not pay a high price for large displays and directory visibility for something as personal as aesthetic medicine. Anyone who identifies or contacts you through a yellow pages listing most certainly has heard of you elsewhere and did not choose to contact you by the design, size, or flash of your listing.

IN PRACTICE: All Things to All People

I love to scan the yellow pages and websites devoted to aesthetic medicine. It amazes me how many of these try to be all things to all people, and in the end probably contribute very little to the success of a practice of aesthetic medicine.

Consider a yellow pages ad featuring a sunbathing twenty-something blond beauty in a listing for a practice offering everything from facial rejuvenation and body contouring to male breast reduction and hair removal. Consider the advertisement of a well-groomed, reasonably attractive plastic surgeon stating that he or she is there to "make your dreams come true." (I cannot believe someone would choose a surgeon based on the surgeon's appearance—disqualify them, maybe, but choose them, doubtful.)

Then there are practice websites where the physician puts countless before and after photos of patients, illustrating every possible procedure with little explanation of exactly what techniques were used and what adjunctive therapies were included.

I received a call from a surgeon who was frantic because the money he had spent on directories was not generating the traffic he had hoped for. I asked him how most of his patients came to him. Referral was the greatest, and surprisingly, the website was his second greatest source of referral. You would guess the website was in itself a success, correct? No. The website referrals were quite significantly tipped in the direction of breast augmentation and reconstruction patients who arrived at this surgeon's website from the breast implant manufacturer's site, where he was listed as a resource. Is it surprising to know that the yellow pages were merely a means for people who already had a basis to want to contact him to do so?

The lesson here: Few individuals will choose a provider to fulfill something as important as their personal desire for appearance enhancement by searching the yellow pages or a website. They use these merely as a locating reference, but their initial awareness of the provider has come from someone or something else. Although listing your practice in directories is essential, how elaborate or comprehensive your listing must be in a vehicle that has not proved its ability to garner new traffic is questionable.

MEDIA RELATIONS

Media relations—involving interviews, press releases, story placement (in short, publicity)—is not for everyone. Coming from a media background, I can tell you that there are individuals who should not appear on camera or speak to a group over the air, or in interviews with reporters. However, there are many appropriate opportunities for media efforts.

Through media relations you and your practice can be a source for public information about your profession and practice. Journalistic integrity requires unbiased, authoritative, balanced reporting that does not include any compensation from or to sources of information. Those engaged in media relations who do not adhere to these principles lack integrity, and I would not trust them to accurately convey your message to the public. Certainly, the rules are often bent, and gray areas do exist. This mostly exists with frequent media spokespersons and media "darlings." However, unless you are a spokesperson or darling (and even if you are one), stick to the rules.

There are two ways to go about national and major market media efforts to garner publicity:

- If you are a strong enough presence and personality who has significantly greater value or standing than the peers in your profession, you can drive your own media relations efforts.

- If you are a strong, dedicated, and articulate personality who is active in research or teaching in your specialty; in the local, regional, national and international professional organizations you belong to; and with companies who manufacture or supply the treatments you administer, prescribe, or sell, you will have value to a media outlet.

- You can garner media relations through your contribution to these groups, either by driving your own media relations efforts, by partnering, or by acting as a spokesperson for the group you represent.

You must accept how media relations efforts are driven and realize that if you want reputable media coverage through channels that have value to your target populations, you must adhere to the principles of ethical media, and to your own principles.

- Make certain a media outlet or organization has integrity and that it will fairly and accurately transmit your message.

- Prepare for any meeting or interview. Ask for the specific focus and your expected contribution to any comment or interview as well as an agenda so you may prepare accordingly. Practice the dialog you expect to undertake with any journalist. When this conversation does take place, have any information readily at hand that you may wish to provide to support your points.

- Ask for the opportunity to review any portion of your contribution to a media effort for clinical accuracy. This is fact-checking. (The caution here is to check facts and make certain you are not misquoted. Do not make the mistake of trying to direct a journalist how to present his or her story, or you will never again be a source for a media story.)

- Be conscientious about patient privacy when media are present on your premises or when speaking with media. Certainly the best story is a personal story; involve your patients in a general way when you can and be candid about the effort. If a patient agrees to be part of your media relations efforts, it cannot be a quid pro quo arrangement (in exchange for free service) unless that service is nominal and unattached to the effort at hand, and you *must* obtain a specific release from the patient for his or her participation whether this is to be in person or through photographs, even if the patient is not readily identifiable in the photographs.

- Communicate well and consistently with any media organization. Provide supporting data, follow up all questions with supplemental information, and make certain you know when your contributions will be broadcast or printed so you can make certain your office staff are ready to field the attention and phone calls.

- Maintain the media relationships you develop with verbal and written appreciation. Don't do this for the attention, but for the professionalism, much as you would maintain a relationship with patients through correspondence related to patient care and innovation.

Once you understand the principles of media relations, you must determine how you wish to communicate with the media. Determine whether you want to drive your own efforts or engage in efforts of partnership, and establish the results you expect. Know who to contact, and regularly update your contacts. Reaching the wrong editor or reporter at an organization rarely results in your message finding its way into the right hands. For your message to be effective, you must put it directly in the hands of the journalist who can most effectively use it to address the interests of his or her viewers, listeners, or readers. Ask about and continuously follow the rules.

Be realistic about subject matter. Unless it is truly news, something of interest to the audience of the targeted media that is not self-promoting, it will not have any value in garnering media attention. Don't think that you can slide unproven methods, innovation, self-named procedures, self-serving inventions, or theories and non–American Board of Medical Specialties (ABMS)–certified credentials by any journalist. Every day there is a plethora of self-serving releases put out on the wires, and any reasonably skilled journalist will see right through the fluff.

Even the smallest organizations have strict standards when it comes to reporting on medical issues. They will check the validity of your credentials and your reputation as well as your ability to speak on the subject. Your story will be thoroughly vetted, unless the organization already has a relationship with you, unless the effort is one driven by a credible affiliation with a research or professional organization, and unless the effort is of exceptional news value and is presented accordingly.

Publicity Value

Media relations have immense value to you when properly undertaken. They are a drain on time and practice communication resources, and statistics show that in practice, fewer than 3% of perfectly executed medical media relations efforts result in coverage. This is not measured by the occasion or the effort, but by all media targets in your efforts. Thus if you were to send out 100 perfectly targeted, content-appropriate, accurately delivered releases throughout the year, your practice would receive coverage from fewer than three of those releases. Although the value of this in improving your public image and elevating your status as a noted spokesperson in your specialty is immense, using media relations is an individual decision, the caveat being whether you have the resources to expend on media relations, and whether you wish to be thrust into the spotlight when the opportunity arises.

Media Relations Cost and Value

Your communication efforts may be very strategic, and media relations may be unnecessary. On the other hand, by virtue of your professional affiliations, you may find yourself thrust into the role of spokesperson, and media relations may be one of your outreach efforts. Technically, media relations should cost nothing and offer excellent inherent value, which includes reaching an audience, disseminating a valid message, and enhancing your image and visibility. The media offer current dissemination of information and are strategic to your public and patient education efforts. Media reports can reach those you never thought you could—but they take a lot of effort for results to be achieved, although those results may be well worth the effort. Media relations must not to be engaged in by trial and error; you have to know what you are doing or hire someone who does.

Creation of media campaigns can involve nothing more than the cost of delivering a press release on letterhead, or can be as costly as a video press release with full professional agency efforts to present and place your message.

Administration cost is low when outsourced, high when kept in-house. Someone in your office must be empowered to effectively follow up and maintain relationships.

How aggressively you wish to engage in media relations depends on the value it will bring to your practice and the cost of your time and efforts.

🐝 IN PRACTICE: On the Spot

Media relations is a tough business; I have worked both sides as an agent and as a journalist. What I will tell you is that regardless of journalistic integrity and standards, there is a lot of patronage among medical reporters and agencies, just as there is among sports reporters and the hometown teams they cover. Few are as slick and alarming as this case, however.

The thriving practice of a personable provider was approached by a media relations agent who had been referred through a pharmaceutical company, who offered to pursue on behalf of the practice a media effort "guaranteed" to produce exposure on a top local network newscast. The focus was breaking news, a new treatment from the pharmaceutical company. As a member of that company's "preferred and referred providers," he was to act as a spokesperson.

The provider, never having engaged in media relations before, was persuaded to accept the opportunity.

A few very significant things went wrong that illustrate exactly why media relations require not only careful planning, but also a thorough understanding of the process.

A local media reporter called the provider's office one day to tape a news byte with barely an hour's notice. The physician was performing surgeries that day. Not to miss the opportunity, he finished the procedure he was in and cancelled the next procedure. The surgery he was completing ran a bit long. The news crew had to wait 20 minutes, and although they were graciously accommodated by the practice staff, the crew grew irritable. They were not concerned for the safety or the satisfaction of the patient in surgery, as was the provider. They wanted their news byte.

Once he was able to meet them, the reporter began to direct questions to the provider that were completely unanticipated. The event unfolded so quickly there was no chance to prepare in any way. The provider had never been before the cameras, and his first experience was not only unplanned,

Continued

![icon] IN PRACTICE: On the Spot—cont'd

but unnerving. A man who was generally soft spoken and quite articulate was suddenly stuttering, rambling, nearly incoherent.

The media organization presented all of three bytes of the provider speaking that totaled 26 seconds. The editing distorted his statements significantly, and he looked terribly unprofessional in the segment.

Two weeks later, the practice received a bill from the media relations agent for $7200. The provider had never agreed to contract this man, nor did he expect that the services would be paid for by him. They were presented as being initiated by the pharmaceutical company. When the provider questioned the bill, the agent said that by accepting participation in the media effort (even though he had not formally engaged the agent's services), he was expressing his agreement to engage the media agent's expertise in obtaining media placement for him.

This is completely unethical, but it would have been difficult to dispute in court whether an oral agreement existed for services, because the effort did result in media coverage for the practice.

For the fee, the practitioner received little from the agent: no preparation, no participation, no respect for the practice or its patients and privacy, no management or control of the effort, and certainly no sense of principles. Not knowing what to expect resulted in quite the opposite of the positive visibility for which the physician had hoped.

There are multiple lessons here, but the most important is this: You must make certain any opportunity for visibility in media is planned, timed, prepared, and that you know the source. What happened in this case is that the media agent caught an assignment producer on a slow news day. Crews were paid to sit around with nothing to report on, so the producer took advantage and sent the crew to the provider's office, whether in patronage to the media agent or to get him to stop pestering with his effort of placement.

The provider and the public were the victims in this case. What might have been a valuable news story presenting a prepared and articulate expert in aesthetic medicine was an ill-conceived story that offered the audience little valuable information on an innovation that may very well have been of interest to them.

CHAPTER 12

Connecting Inside Your Practice

You can close more business in two months
by becoming interested in other people
than you can in two years by trying to get
people interested in you.

— DALE CARNEGIE

Outside your practice, you attempt to attract individuals who might be interested in your services, to make a connection. Inside your office, you have already made the connection of interest; now you must convert that interest into services; then the services and connection translate to loyalty.

COMMUNICATION

Communication consists of interest, education, and comprehension. One of the keys to effective communication is its availability on demand, or as close to on demand as possible. It is a vital component of any successful practice.

You are involved at every level of your practice, as you strive to attract potential clients/patients with your services, image, brand, and mission. Your target audience must be educated about the clinical care you recommend to meet their personal expectations. You must also make judgments as to whether an individual client fully comprehends a recommended treatment, and its potential outcomes and risks.

Despite your involvement in your practice, you cannot be the key contact at every stage every time. You must empower your staff; at each level of contact you require a core communicator—a familiar, trusted resource for clients and patients—who can address every detail except the core clinical function of the practice.

No staff member should ever suspend clinical care in progress to attend to on-demand communication of a client/patient, unless it is clearly of clinical urgency. No one other than the physician should ever recommend, direct, or provide clinical care to any client or patient. But core communicators provide a link between a client's or patient's need for information and your availability to provide it. Furthermore, without a core communicator, a potential or existing client may not be able to get timely answers to their questions from a trusted and familiar contact in your office, which risks the possibility of that client looking elsewhere for an immediate response. Although communication must always be secondary to quality care and skill in fulfilling needs, it is nevertheless essential for converting interested clients to patients and to ensuring patient satisfaction.

Communications within your practice or emanating from it must be personal. But the one thing it must not be is a paid endeavor—an advertisement. It must have a goal, purpose, tone, and call to action.

Within the office, you will communicate with prospective and existing patients, staff, visitors, and outside service providers who help your office operate effectively, such as the cleaning crew, an accreditation inspector, your publicists, and industry sales representatives. The connections you make or break in your office can have positive or negative consequences.

THE FUNDAMENTALS OF IN-OFFICE ENCOUNTERS

Five basic components are integral to nearly every encounter in your office, no matter who the subject may be; these include the environment, greeting, function, administration, and closure.

Environment

Your office environment, from the upholstery on the chairs to the color of the walls, from the music to the flowers to the lighting, conveys something about your office. In a business focused on fulfilling the personal needs of patients, this environment must focus on the individual. The surroundings may reflect your tastes, but they must also invite and welcome the individual and offer individualized attention.

- Leave personal and political messages outside the office environment. Pictures of your children and spouse are appropriate in your office, but not throughout the facility. This is as much for their safety and privacy as it is for those in your office to focus on their tasks, not on your private life. Your passion for hunting, golf, or motorcycles may not be shared by others. It is perfectly acceptable to personalize your office, but remember that it is in your patients' interests that the office exists.

- Consider comfort and function, not simply design. An environment that is too formal may be intimidating; too casual may seem unprofessional. Floor-to-ceiling windows may be stunning, but for the patient in a state of undress, they can be horrifying. A high examination table may be perfect for you to reach your patient, but awkward to climb up on. The general lighting should be soft, flattering, and natural.

- Temperature and volume play a big role in client/patient comfort and confidence in your environment. A warm, draft-free temperature, quiet ventilation, and soft voices that don't carry from one room to another are essential. The ability to change the level of sound, such as background music, in individual rooms can be important for putting an individual at ease or for ensuring his or her undivided attention. Adjustments should be made for the season with appropriate temperatures maintained for unclothed patients, not for your personal thermostat.

- Choose bold, bright colors or soft, muted shades to convey different messages. For walls, clothing, and brochures, select colors that attract, not tones that distract or overpower.

- Be aware of the scents that permeate your office environment. An overcooked lunch in the microwave, the smell of alcohol or disinfecting agents in an examination room, and the smell of burnt hair in a laser room are offensive. Recognize that these scents may be unpleasant to those who have come to you for a pleasurable experience.

- Lose the clutter: minimize posters, pamphlets, artwork, files, piles of old magazines, overstuffed binders with photographs, displays of skin care products, necessary medical instruments or supplies. Keep accents to a minimum and organize the mainstay items so they are easily accessible, not randomly scattered.

- Keep things soft. Anything that touches the body should be soft, warm, and discreet, even if it must be disposable. If you would not be comfortable in a paper gown, don't expect your patient to be.

- Maintain a comfortable pace. If you are hurried or dragging, flustered or inattentive, it will be reflected in your environment and will affect your patient's comfort and mood. Keep things well paced and call attention to matters that require handling when and where necessary. A sense of urgency should be reserved for truly urgent matters.

- Listen to what you say, to whom, and how and where you say it. When scheduling goes out of sync or a nuisance occurs, it's easy to slip into a terse, irritable tone. A quick change in tone can change the air around you, altering the environment altogether—and it can take time for staff members to rebound. Before you snap, consider who will hear you, whom it will affect, and how it may be perpetuated.

These subtle elements and so many more contribute to creating an environment in which you will make multiple connections with multiple individuals. Take control of the environment in your office.

Greeting

When someone enters your office, there must be an initial greeting to acknowledge the person. This welcome must be immediate; although it may not be possible to attend instantly to the individual's needs, it is important to say, "Hello, nice to see you. Can you give me just one moment and I'll be right with you?" Do not allow an individual to stand in the doorway waiting to be acknowledged. The same holds true for telephone, email, or text messages. These should be answered as promptly as possible, and if necessary, the individual should be told when a response will be possible.

Whether on the phone, in person, or by any other means of connection, there are three ways to route one's actions after a greeting. Immediately ask who the caller or visitor is and the individual's purpose: "Hello, welcome to Doctor's office. How can I help you today?" Then depending on who you are dealing with, the caller or visitor is routed in one of the following ways:

- *A patient or prospective patient:* Do not delay; learn the purpose for the connection and the appropriate response. Never keep a patient or prospective patient waiting unless he or she is waiting to speak to someone more appropriate than the initial greeter.

- *A visitor:* A sales rep, the friend of a patient, another physician, or someone stopping by. Perform triage: Respond immediately to those you must, and have others wait until you are able to respond.

- *A delivery man, an essential service to your practice, the lab driver, or a supplier:* Teach these individuals your operating procedures and protocols from day one. Don't overlook a greeting, but do what you can to automate these visitors or callers.

Begin a greeting in a warm, focused manner and you will get compliance. If you offer an insincere or unfocused greeting, you'll create doubt or discomfort. Never overlook the power of the greeting—the tone you set will leave an indelible impression.

Function

Whether for a consultation, treatment, or follow-up, to deliver the mail or check the smoke alarms, any individual who comes into your office has a reason to be there. Knowing that reason and responding appropriately are essential.

Patients come first. Whether their arrival is expected or unexpected, for an emergency or simply to replenish their supply of a skin care product, patients are your priority. Some will drop in unexpectedly because of a miscommunication about appointment times, or on purpose. If you are not aware of the patient's reason to be there, with no opportunity to prepare (for a consultation, preoperative or postoperative visit, photographs, payment, a treatment, or follow-up), the first thing you must determine when that person arrives is his or her purpose for being there, and attend to it appropriately with minimal disruption of the schedule of other patients.

Visitors who accompany patients can be helpful or a distraction to effective communication with the patient. No office should provide a babysitting service, and appointments must not be social occasions for your patients and their friends. Set policies on the level of the visitors' participation in your patient's experience and make these guidelines clear to everyone. Such a policy protects the interests of all of your patients and should therefore be welcomed.

Visitors who are not accompanying patients may have an obvious function such as sales, service, or delivery. Where you can, set policy as to where these visitors should enter, with whom they should connect, and where they may and may not leave deliveries. Set a policy so that all sales calls require appointments, and limit those appointments to the days and times when they will not disrupt serving your patients.

All other visitors must be greeted and immediately asked the purpose of their visit. Strangers should be addressed without delay because, quite simply, the safety of all persons in your office may be at stake. There is no need to panic or get defensive about unknown visitors, but staff must be trained to follow proper procedures to greet and inquire about this person's reason for being in your office and to act accordingly.

Although maintaining a visitor's log may seem like an unwarranted burden, it is an important means of protecting the safety and privacy of everyone in your office and it is important that you keep one. Patient appointments can be tracked, as well as all other people who enter and exit your office each day. This may serve you well historically and will be of benefit if any incident arises that requires recall of everyone on the premises.

Administration

The administrative function in your practice involves scheduling appointments, taking messages, signing for deliveries, or providing forms that a prospective patient is asked to complete. Administrative staff are connectors, communicating what is needed and why and making the process simple for everyone without losing the personal character of your practice. Administration is a nonclinical area where process and procedure are most important, and where the personal touch can readily be lost. Some important ways for administrative staff to make a positive connection include the following:

- *Making eye contact:* Whether handing over a form, directing a patient to an examination room, or jotting down a signature or a message, before and after this act, make eye contact. Let the individual know that although the brief exchange may seem impersonal, you are in fact connecting personally.

- *Affirming:* Any detail or instruction that is important or may be unclear should be confirmed before you administer.

- *Personalizing:* Use the individual's name when you know it, or ask if you do not and it is appropriate. Be personal and personable.

- *Remaining private:* Whether collecting personal or basic information in person or on the phone, keep conversations private for those you are speaking with and for the comfort of those around you. If necessary, allow patients or staff a private place to carry out administrative functions. I once sat in a plastic surgeon's waiting room as his receptionist was calling a referring physician for records on a mastectomy patient. Right in front of me, and within earshot of the entire waiting room, this poor woman's name, address, social security number, and condition were broadcast. This is not only a violation of HIPAA, it is simply terribly inappropriate.

- *Investing the connection with personality as well as process:* Yes, they need to sign your privacy policy or photo consent. Yes, you expect the housekeeper to review her task list and its completion with you, or the laboratory to review the orders communicated. Although this may be process, it does not have to be impersonal. Say "please" and "thank you." Demonstrate that the person you are connecting with is more important than the task at hand.

Administrative functions can be like the automated, robotic, impersonal phone calls we make to get customer service—or they can be like your own personal shopper, butler, concierge, or confidant. In a personal services industry, strive to leave the impression of the latter.

Closure

A simple matter of tone to the word "goodbye" can close a meeting or phone conversation and express "until we meet again," "I hope we'll meet again," "get lost," or "get out." For reasons of interpretation, every connection in your office must end with some form of closure, and the tone of your closure message must indicate the direction you hope your future relationship will take.

Early in my career I worked with a director of communications whose method of closure for any phone conversation was to abruptly hang up. He did not seek closure, he did not say "thank you" or "goodbye"; he just hung up. He didn't last very long in that job, which was no surprise: he did not know how to communicate, but he certainly did know how to disconnect. On the phone, closure is essential, but more important is the timing for closure. Closure requires recognizing when the other party has completed his or her part of the conversation. You should acknowledge that the other party accepts this, and leave the door open for the future. It is much more than "goodbye"; it must be "until we meet again, soon," and it must be sincere.

In person, closure requires something equally sincere: a handshake or a gentle touch of the shoulder, and a smile. If possible, it means escorting the other party to the door, or if necessary, providing the privacy and time for the person to leave when ready, such as when freshened, dressed and composed after a treatment.

The nature of electronic response is brief, such as voice mail, text messages, or email from your office, but it should not be impersonal or terse. Closure follows an opening, an invitation, and the distinct call to action that ensures the recipient will respond and provides the details to make that method of response as easy and accessible as possible.

VEHICLES OF COMMUNICATION

Today we communicate almost as frequently with those inside the office with one-on-one meetings as we do with other external communications. The vehicle you use is not as important as how you use it: setting a positive environment, offering a proper and prompt greeting, realizing the function of the interaction, carefully managing administration, always offering a sincere and inviting closure, and most of all, even if the communication is not in person, keeping it personal.

Interpersonal Communication

Interpersonal communication within your practice is within your control. You are not only the basis of knowledge; you set the standard. With interpersonal communication, you can define the practice's purpose and objectives, set the tone, and convey a call to action that garners an immediate response. When you and your staff are the communication vehicle of choice:

- You know your own function and your audience. You are face to face with them.

- The alternative is input from someone outside your practice, one you do not want to have influence.

- Caution lies in all things defined earlier as red flags (see Chapter 8). It is your obligation to communicate appropriate, candid, and sincere messages.

- Active obligations are the standards you set and demonstrate consistently for interpersonal communication within your practice. If communications are inconsistent, you risk confusion and alienation.

- The physical and financial cost of interpersonal communication is reflected in how the value of your time spent in interactions translates effectively to providing service (thus generating revenue). The physical and financial cost of interpersonal communication is vital to your practice.

Interpersonal communication delivers your message directly to an individual and allows him or her to respond directly. Without interpersonal communication, no practice can survive. However, your practice cannot survive, much less succeed, without other means of disseminating your messages. Even a consummate expert at interpersonal communication will require additional vehicles of communication, some of which work in concert with interpersonal communication, and others that work either together or alone to present your message outside your practice.

We often hear the term *bedside manner*. Some medical providers are wonderful in one-to-one communication, whereas others have surgical skills that far exceed their people skills. In aesthetic medicine and in fulfilling the needs of others, poor personal communication can be an Achilles' heel. You cannot possibly succeed in fulfilling the personal desires of others unless you can communicate with those you serve about their desires.

You must frankly evaluate your own communication habits, skills, and patterns. It is difficult to recognize your shortcomings in this regard and to make accommodations accordingly. If you tend to be succinct, brief, and businesslike in your connections, this may be interpreted by patients as brusqueness or lack of attention to their concerns. If this is the case, empower a patient coordinator or nurse who is an effective listener to handle a significant portion of patient communication. If you are warm and tend to converse at length with patients, taking joy in learning about them and their desires, have the patient coordinator or nurse keep you on track. If you and a patient do not seem to be communicating well together, draw in your patient coordinator or nurse as a participant in the discussion so he or she can buffer or translate. If your patient coordinator or nurse has difficulty with certain patients who want to speak with you and only you, make yourself available and stress to that patient that you and your staff practice interpersonal communication within the office that is a team effort. Empower the members of your team to optimize their communication strengths.

Although interpersonal communication within your practice is person to person, it need not be solely to one person. So long as the lines and responsibilities of communication are clear, make your interpersonal communication a team effort. A team that works together is always more likely to succeed than is a team member who functions solely on his or her own.

IN PRACTICE: Well Scripted

So many practitioners know they need to communicate better and up-sell or cross-sell the value of the services they provide, but few are truly successful at this. Up-selling is adding more to the patient's desired services, cross-selling is adding valuable complementary services or products. The more I observe practitioners and staff in situations that can easily grow into service or added services, the more I realize that often it is not an individual employee's lack of effort or desire to communicate; it is a lack of confidence that keeps growth or added service from materializing.

In any office of varying demographics, practice mix, missions, and images, you must take the time to ensure that staff members understand your standards and objectives for interpersonal communication. Interpersonal communication is the single greatest communication tool available to the success of your practice. Your messages must be consistent, positive, effective, and influential. How do you accomplish this? With scripting.

From how the telephone is answered to how patients are greeted, from how messages are delivered, from informed consent to up-selling and cross-selling—all the very simple phrases and actions that lead to retention and referral must have scripted guidelines. These will give practitioners and staff the material to customize their messages to meet their objectives. Scripts are not verbatim recitations; they are a means of defining and organizing the thoughts or points to communicate.

Case in point: A practitioner was sending countless patients to purchase products from his retail function, but his associates sent few. I spent time with them all, discussing all the opportunities to enhance service by directing patients to the retail function. After a very short time, the problem was clear.

Continued

⚘ IN PRACTICE: Well Scripted—cont'd

One practitioner was an adept communicator who controlled and steered conversations with patients. He had no difficulty finding a way not only to suggest, but to invite others to consider added services or retail options. His associates, on the other hand, were so focused on the one issue a patient presented with that they overlooked the opportunity to extend the conversation beyond the patient's immediate need.

After creating one very general but thought-provoking script, after several sessions of role-playing, and after setting goals for invitations to added service, we reassessed the volume of the retail function. Not only was it experiencing enormous growth, but personal services were too. The benefit to the practice was not just in volume and revenue; satisfaction surveys illustrated that patients were so pleased at the practitioners' thorough discussion and candid recommendations that they consistently rated their experience as exceptional and noted the experience afforded greater value than they had expected from a particular visit or treatment.

Although you do not have a choice of vehicle in your interpersonal communication efforts because it is you and/or your staff, you do have a choice of vehicles for messages that you and your staff do not directly and personally deliver. Making the right choice on which vehicles to use requires:

- *A basis of knowledge:* How a vehicle delivers your message, to whom it is delivered, and the specific characteristics of that vehicle

- *Evaluation of options:* An analysis and comparison of cost, opportunity, and audience demographics in relation to your ideal target audience

- *An ongoing review of results:* Your most vital, and often the most overlooked, component of choosing a vehicle; if you do not measure how successful a vehicle is in eliciting direct response, you do not know whether to continue using that vehicle

Telephone

Next to interpersonal, in-person communications, your office will communicate most frequently with prospective patients, current patients, and anyone else by telephone. For this reason, the telephone should be used for the most personal communications, not for telemarketing. Your telephone conveys your image:

- How many rings before someone answers?

- Who is the voice on the phone, or is it a machine that answers?

- Is the caller given the opportunity to state his or her reason for calling, or simply put on hold the moment the call is answered?

- How many prompts or transfers until the individual calling connects with the person he or she is trying to reach?

- What is the background noise, the volume? How many times is the person who answers the phone distracted, distant, or simply seems uninterested?

- Does every caller receive the necessary answers or information on that first call? Does your office track the number of messages that need to be taken and the time it takes to respond?

I do not believe in receptionists or telephone operators; I do believe every individual in the office must be trained and ready to answer the phone at any time. There is no reason a phone should ring more than three times. There is no reason for music on hold unless you feel your callers expect to be entertained, or for messages on hold, unless you plan on having people on hold so long they hear the whole message.

Call where you have permission to call. Consider the environment your telephone creates not just for those calling in, but also when calls are made out. In addition to greeting the recipient of your call, ask if the individual is free to speak at the moment, and if the time is convenient to carry out the function or agenda for which you called. Be prepared for the call with all notes, comments, questions, and information necessary. Carry out your function and then determine whether the recipient of your call has questions, concerns, or comments. Look for closure with the recipient of your call, even though you are the one who made the call. Closure must, as always, be personal and inviting. Even if the call is simply an appointment reminder, make certain the patient knows where to arrive, what to expect, and that you are looking forward to welcoming him or her. Automated appointment reminders may save you time and money, but they are impersonal and sound uncongenial.

TAKE A MESSAGE

There are times when it is acceptable to take a message, so long as someone responds to the message in a timely, sincere manner. Today medical advancement occurs regularly and rapidly. Media reports on legitimate and questionable medical innovations are pervasive, particularly in aesthetic medicine. Why? Because our society is focused on youth and beauty, a fact the media use to attract an audience.

When someone from that audience is curious enough to seek more information and calls on your practice, you do not want any of your staff to say, "I have never heard of that." The reality, however, is that not everyone can answer every question, all the time. Therefore, if for some reason a staff member is not familiar with the subject of the patient's query, make certain he or she is astute enough to know when and to whom to refer a call. Otherwise, you will lose a potential client, and may lose credibility. This too is an area in which scripting is invaluable.

Email

Email is a wonderful communication tool when it is welcomed, informative, and personal. Email that is overused or generic will be ignored. If your office emails people for multiple purposes, be certain you have a distinct sending address for personal patient email: one for general messages and one for business. Appoint one person to check personal patient email consistently, all day, because you never know when the message from a patient may be urgent.

Email carries all the same requirements as any other form of communication: environment, greeting, function, administration, and closure. Yes, email may be quick, but it need not be impersonal, and it must not be impolite. Email that includes sensitive information or information specific to an individual's course of treatment is better left to telephone. Why? The tone of text can be easily misinterpreted and leaves no room for personal discussion or clarity.

Today email is best used for administration: collecting or sharing information or documents that will be used, discussed, returned, or reviewed during a personal visit. Email is great for reminders about personal appointments and specific instructions. I know a physician who emails his smoking patients daily before procedures to remind them not to smoke. He requires that they reply to him every day. Not everyone needs this type of regimen, but for his practice, it works.

Email is an excellent means for narrowly targeting general messages from your practice, such as an invitation to a special event, a new product in stock, or simply to fill appointment slots that are open. For example, if you notice that hair removal appointments for next week are slow, email all those who have not been in during the prior 4 weeks but have been to the office in the prior 4 months for hair removal and remind them to schedule to achieve or maintain results.

Voice Mail

If you must leave a message, ask that the intended recipient return your call; never offer details, because you cannot know who will listen to the message. If you must use voice mail, do so only when absolutely necessary and to the advantage of the caller. Define a policy for the office's voice mail; require that it be checked regularly and that no call go unanswered for the day.

If you and a patient get into an exchange of voice mail questions and answers, stop the cycle. Set up a convenient phone conversation or an in-person appointment. If it becomes too difficult for patients to connect with you, they might just disconnect the relationship.

Texting and Instant Messaging

Text messaging has become popular, and many use it in the same manner as email. You should not, however, see texting as an equivalent to email. Even if your patients or those you are communicating with accept text messaging, keep messages as simple as possible, such as appointment reminders, and only if the person has indicated that this is an appropriate way to be reached.

Print

Despite the immediacy and many other advantages of electronic communication, printed materials are still essential. A printed piece can be transferred electronically, or hand to hand. A printed document may be easier to view in total. Moreover, a handwritten note, when appropriate, sincere, and legible, is still the most gracious way to say "thank you." Some communications, such as congratulating a patient on an exciting life event or achievement, or expressing sympathy at a loss, should only be sent as a written personal note. Such courtesies and civilities should not be lost in the rush of daily communications, and the personal touch will have deep meaning for the recipient. This is part of building and maintaining an ongoing relationship with a valued patient.

Unfortunately, too often today, handwritten notes seem to be limited to phone messages and Post-its. Formal letters are still the standard when a signature is required. Even if your office is completely paperless, don't overlook that some documents, such as preoperative and postoperative instructions, medication instructions, and informed consents, should also come in a printed format.

Computer

Some practitioners use PowerPoint, computer animation programs, and other automated functions to educate and communicate with patients. These may support or enhance interpersonal communication and education, but they do not replace it, nor must they be the primary means of communicating. You are in a personal services industry; keep it personal.

Multimedia

Whether used similar to a computer message or to play video messages of interest in your office, don't allow multimedia to dominate the environment or replace the personal connection, or you will simply lose your connection.

Display

Skin care samples, tabletop posters, even the syringe tray setup on the examination room counter are all displays that communicate within your office to your patients. If you clutter your office with diverse or unrelated display messages, you will distract your patient's attention. If you clutter tables with skin care samples, you'll have a breeding ground for organisms and the potential for a sloppy mess. Leave needles or instruments on the counter, and you'll invite patient stress.

Make certain your displays are inviting, informative, and most of all, consistent with your image and brand. Do not use space in your office to advertise a company's product unless that display also promotes you.

> *Climbed a mountain and I turned around*
> *I saw my reflection in the snow-covered hills*
> *till the landslide brought me down*
> — FLEETWOOD MAC, "LANDSLIDE"

EMOTIONS

You can control the process and vehicles you use for connecting and communicating in the office to make solid, enduring connections. The one variable you have very little control over, however, which can make or break your connection, is emotion. Emotions can get the best of anyone, patients, staff, or visitors, particularly when emotions are permitted to get out of control.

The strongest of men and women have their emotional moments. Those who have come to you to improve or enhance their appearance are already in a confident or vulnerable state, or perhaps something in between. Some people embrace their challenges, succeed, and suddenly feel they have fal-tered. Whatever the reason, the most conflicting, intense, and unexpected emotions are those that bring the person you are connecting with crashing down—like a landslide.

No communicator in your office must be so arrogant as to think he or she can manage every type of emotion with one course of action, one means of communication. Even for an effective, seasoned communicator, the greatest variable to deal with is emotion.

Excitement is a positive emotion, as long as it is realistic and doesn't over-look the reality of what is to come. A patient who is extremely excited antic-ipating the outcome of a procedure must be made aware of the realities of the experience it will take to achieve that outcome, and must accept them realistically, or after a procedure that excitement may turn to a landslide of disappointment.

Anxiety is most often a little worry that can sometimes go haywire. It is a natural emotion in the course of treatment. What is most important is to al-low those you are communicating with the opportunity to share their anxi-ety. Listen, ask questions, and then provide the data, evidence, and com-passion to allay their anxiety. If anxiety is so severe it stands in the way of someone's trust and comfort, take a step back and start the education process again. Medicating anxiety is easy, but mitigating it yields the most productive outcome for you and the other party.

Fear in moderation helps people to accept reality and to control their own behavior, because they fear the outcome if they do not comply. But when fear turns to panic or to mistrust, you have reached a disconnect. To recon-nect, identify the source of the fear, respond to it sincerely and logically, and allow some time and distance at hand to permit fear to either resolve, be-come manageable, or become so obvious it is a risk to all those involved.

Reluctance is not the emotion that you must change; it is the condition that causes reluctance that you must address. Like anxiety or fear, there is a reason for reluctance. Seek that, then use facts and reality to make the connection.

Curiosity is a good thing, but when people ask too many questions, you must take control. I believe in transparency and educating others fully, but sometimes there are things better left unknown or unspoken. For example, you don't need to let a patient watch his or her own surgical procedure. Instead, offer the opportunity to watch a clinical video on the subject, after the fact.

Melancholy can result from something as insignificant as a change in the weather, or it can be pervasive, and hide some far deeper unhappiness. When dealing with someone whose emotions are difficult to read or who seems sad, take the time to give this person your support, but keep it professional. Taking a personal interest in the sadness of a patient or any other person in your office can be misinterpreted as taking an intimate interest. Do not allow yourself to be vulnerable when a compassionate gesture can be misconstrued.

Demanding people want it all. Give it to them and they will expect more. Don't give it to them and they may turn against you. Demanding people need boundaries; they need to be allowed control of themselves—not of the entire office or situation. I am a demanding person—control everything but me, and you'll make a connection.

Educated individuals can be an asset—or a liability if they believe they know more than you, and can dictate to you. The best way to deal with overeducated or wrongly educated individuals is to let them have their say, then to clearly state your point of view and document with evidence and examples why you are the expert.

Comparative people like to measure you, your office, your recommendations, or your actions against those of others. If you respond to such comparisons, you will find yourself negotiating, for example, on price. Clearly and firmly define who you are, set that tone with your communication, and if others must compare, allow them to. Don't respond with your terms; respond in your terms.

Hostile individuals may be antagonistic for the moment, or it may be part of their nature. The key to understanding whether you can have a successful relationship with someone who is hostile or whether you can make a successful connection is to assess the source, the validity, and both sides of the hostility. Hostility that is focused on one occurrence or incident may be resolved. Overwhelming, continuous animosity or hostility that is unfounded is trouble waiting to happen. This is the one situation where making a polite disconnect from this person is your very best strategy.

Most humans inherently read emotions well, but we sometimes simply do not understand them. Some have a gift for interpreting and dealing with emotions, and others don't. For this reason, interpersonal communications in your office rely on a team approach—you must not do it alone. Discuss your observations about patients' emotional responses honestly with your staff to seek solutions. There are books and training on how to handle conflict, difficult people, and how to take control of situations. These are all helpful, but remember, your practice inherently presents unique situations where individuals are self-focused for a service they hope will fulfill a very personal desire. It's not a contractual negotiation or a political debate with which you are involved; you are dealing with a human being with vulnerabilities and expectations.

RELATIVE WISDOM: Remain Calm

Have you ever called 911? One of the first things the operator says is "remain calm." But when there is an accident, a fire, an intruder, a real reason to call 911, remaining calm seems almost impossible. Even those who are normally rational can panic in an emergency situation and behave in ways they would not under other circumstances.

We were at the riding stables ready to enjoy a lovely summer afternoon on the trails. It was the type of day when parents brought their young children for a pony ride around the ring. It was such a beautiful day that Ivan, the crazy stallion, was let out of his stall and into a corral to enjoy a little of this beautiful day. Then the beautiful day turned ugly. A pretty painted pony was quietly being walked outside the corrals by a guide with a small boy on top, his mom videotaping his first ride. Within a few seconds Ivan threw himself over the rails at the pony, the pony reared, the boy fell, and the next instant there was screaming and blood. My first instinct was to get off my horse and get my husband to call 911. My next was to attend to the child and his mother, who was hysterical.

We were dealing with a lot of emotions, and all I could remember is what a 911 operator will tell you at every turn: "remain calm." The boy was bleeding from his mouth, clearly frightened and crying. His mother was fearful for her son; she could not stop screaming. I wiped the blood with my sleeve and found the boy had bit his lip. "Remain calm," I told her. "He only bit his lip."

My then 5-year-old was curious, "What happened? Why is he bleeding? Is he going to die? Did he break his back? Is the horse going to get punished?" Remain calm, I told him.

When the stable manager ran out, he demanded, "Who led a pony past Ivan?" Remain calm, I told him. This is not the time for fault-finding; this is the time to care for this child and keep all others safe. The stable hand arrived and was hostile; letting Ivan out was not his problem. The pony guide was reluctant to step forward and become involved in what had happened. Then another mother who had her children riding ponies decided to get involved; she knew the answer to everything, insisting we sit the child up so his lip would stop bleeding, or pick him up off the ground and carry him to the shade. I asked her, too, to remain calm; until we knew the extent of this child's injury, no one but a professional was going to move him. The whole situation provoked a maelstrom of emotions from a simple unexpected event that went wrong.

No matter how large or small the emotion, or the number of emotions that may be culminating in any one given moment, calm is the solution to bring a resolution. There is nothing wrong with telling patients to remain calm, to reassure them. There is nothing wrong with telling staff to be calm, whether during a patient emergency or a dispute. There is no wrong time to suggest and ask for calm; only wrong tones to take and methods for delivery. Even if it is not an emergency, remember what they always say when you call for help: "Remain calm."

PATIENTS

The patients you serve are the reason for every connection you will make in your practice, whether the connection is with those patients, your staff, or any other resources or services to your practice. You will communicate with others for the benefit of your practice and your patients for innumerable reasons, but there are some very specific reasons for which you will only connect with your patients. Inside your practice most of those reasons are specific to the service you provide and treatment that is either sought or necessary.

Patients may come to you for necessary treatment: to treat illness or a traumatic injury or to improve function, or for elective reasons: to improve appearance for personal desire. Regardless of the reason patients come to you, there are specific actions you must take:

- *Consult:* Review the patient's goals or needs for seeking your service. All the subsequent actions generally take place in the consultation environment, whether these are carried out by the provider or a core communicator.

- *Examine:* The physician will perform a physical examination of the patient and assess his or her condition, as well as health factors that may influence the course of treatment. If the physical examination requires a state of undress whether the patient is male or female, ask if the patient would prefer a chaperone, or you may elect to always have an assistant in the room.

- *Diagnose:* The physician will identify the condition the patient has. In elective cases, it is inappropriate to communicate such things as "unsatisfactory appearance" as the diagnosis to your patient. If you must use such phrasing, keep it in your record; there is no need to share such descriptors with the patient.

- *Prescribe:* The physician will define the course of treatment, whether drug therapy, treatment with a device, surgery, or a combination of procedures to best achieve the patient's goals.

- *Discuss alternatives:* The physician will offer alternative courses of treatment that may or may not achieve similar results, or offer what will likely occur if no treatment is rendered.

- *Inform:* The physician or a core communicator will inform the patient of the specifics of the proposed procedure, the potential risks and outcomes, the recovery, and the patient's responsibilities.

- *Take photographs:* The physician or a core communicator will take photographs and secure appropriate consents for those photographs. This is a very vulnerable and intimidating time for some patients, and it is essential to be discreet and sensitive to that and provide privacy.

- *Measure:* The physician or a core communicator may take measurements related to treatment or other vital anatomic information.

- *Instruct:* Pretreatment, treatment, and posttreatment instructions must be detailed by the physician or a core communicator and documented. It must be clear that the patient understands and accepts these as his or her obligations.

- *Obtain consent:* Consent requires securing a signature from the patient confirming that he or she accepts a course of treatment and acknowledges awareness of the potential risks and outcomes. This is the ultimate connection to your patient and his or her choice for treatment. As a practitioner and proprietor, you know and accept the importance of informed consent. It is essential to risk management. Informed consent is so varied and comprehensive, based on the individual procedures and clinical preferences of practitioners that it must be individualized. As a legal tool, thorough informed consent must contain:

  - A clinical definition of the procedure

  - A definition of the condition for which the procedure is being performed

  - Alternatives to the procedure (where they exist)

  - Defined benefits or outcomes of the procedure

  - Definitions of risks associated with the procedure

  - Definitions of any possible uncertainties

  - Verification of patient's competence in voluntarily accepting treatment

  - Verification of patient's state of health relative to treatment

As a vital measure and contributor to the success of your aesthetic practice, informed consent must be more than a legal tool to define clinical risk. It must be a document that verifies by patient signature that he or she willingly accepts treatment and understands all clinical implications and potential risk. Trust between provider and patient, specifically defining that a patient:

– Has personally chosen this provider based on confidence

– Willing and unwaveringly wants to undergo treatment

– Is not being pushed or influenced by anything or anyone other than personal desire to undergo treatment

– Understands and has honestly communicated expectations for outcomes

– Understands and has honestly communicated any question of the processes necessary to achieve those outcomes and all the associated risk

– Will actively and accurately follow all preoperative and postoperative instructions

- *Treat:* Until you reach the point at which your potential patient actually converts, accepting treatment, you have made countless connections for multiple reasons, all culminating in this one point: treatment. Whether the process takes a few moments, several visits, several weeks, or even months of consideration and time, this is the point you strive for; it is where you make your livelihood, providing treatment. All of the basics for connecting in your practice—environment, greeting, function, administration, and closure—must be conveyed with the same care, delivery, tone, and manner throughout your patient's experience. Your goal is not to make the connection for this treatment alone; you are striving to fully satisfy the patient's desires and make the entire experience satisfactory, from accepting treatment, to receiving treatment, and beyond.

- *Follow up:* After treatment, three things seem to happen: (1) patients follow procedures for a necessary visit such as suture removal, or (2) they return when something just isn't right, and (3) sometimes they revisit the practice when they want additional treatment. Some practices suggest when to follow up; they don't insist on it or schedule the appointment—they wait to hear from patients and believe that no news is good news. In rare and truly appropriate and exceptional cases, proactive practices will use one of the many communication vehicles available to stay in contact with patients and will reach out and follow up a day, a week, a month, and even a year later. However you maintain contact, follow-up must not simply be a function of posttreatment necessity or to address a complication. Follow-up must be de rigueur—it's not a written rule; it is simply a matter of good practice.

Satisfaction and loyalty are not the result of a single connection you make; they result from the numerous connections you will make inside your office to achieve a satisfied and loyal patient. Satisfaction and loyalty are critical to your success; they are not where you connect—they are why you connect, and why you are in practice.

☘ IN PRACTICE: Just Procedure

It is sometimes difficult to see things from the inside out. Role-playing has great value in allowing a practice to do this, and I encourage practices to do this often as a learning and improvement exercise. As an outsider, I often have a provider take me through the patient process, sometimes without letting the staff know that we are role-playing. Poor informed consent practice, not in a risk-management sense but as an operational tool and one of patient satisfaction, is among the most common scenarios I identify. It happens with new practices as well as with established practices who are hoping to improve and polish their methods.

Continued

IN PRACTICE: Just Procedure—cont'd

Here is what happens: The consultation goes well, acceptance is communicated, and informed consent begins. The practitioner zips through documents, stating what they are and that they were discussed during consultation, then asks hurriedly if there are any questions and hands things off to a patient coordinator. The coordinator indicates what and where to sign, shuffles documents, gives the patient a loose stack of copies of what is required, asks again if there are questions, schedules the treatment, then collects any payment required at that time. This is unfortunate. Hurrying through informed consent risks two things:

- Something will be misunderstood.

- You will be perceived as someone who hurries through other areas of the patient experience.

Shuffled, loose, nonpersonalized, disorganized documents, either in the patient file or in the patient's hands, create the following risks:

- Something will be lost, misplaced, or misunderstood.

- The origin of the document (your practice) will be unknown.

- You will be perceived as disorganized.

- Informed consent will be perceived as merely an administrative protocol, not as a component of patient care and satisfaction.

The message here is about more than just informed consent; it is about every aspect of the client/patient experience. Take the time to make informed consent valuable without impeding productivity or validity. Show the client/patient that you take care in every detail of the process because he or she needs the assurance that you are consistent with your attention to detail in clinical care, operations, or administration. Be visible; be consistent. Demonstrate to each patient that there is nothing to hide and nothing to gloss over. Make certain nothing is perceived to be trivial or minimal. Through a consistent, individualized, quality experience, you and your patient are better assured that acceptance will lead to satisfaction.

RELATIVE WISDOM: Service Mapping

My dear friend Mary Lind Jewell is the practice manager for Dr. Mark Jewell in Eugene, Oregon. Eugene is not a big city where you would expect ground-breaking theories to be born, but Mary has taken one of the best business principles and applied it to the practice of aesthetic medicine.

Service mapping, also called *experience mapping*, is all about the journey needed to get an individual from point *A*, some unknown place outside your practice, to point *B*, where he or she is within your practice and is completely fulfilled. It requires taking every point along that journey, every contact, every communication, every variable in which your practice connects with the individual and placing that point on the map.

Pull your staff together one day and select one procedure—just one that you offer and service map it. Identify every potential point where you may connect, or fail to connect, with an individual you wish to serve and fully satisfy. Who is involved, what is involved? How much duplication of effort is there? Is something missing? Are messages and image consistent? Where do we most commonly fail to connect or lose someone? Use this exercise to improve on your means for making consistent and valid connections.

STAFF

You cannot run your business alone. You have staff—a team, who together act as your connectors to others, including the most visible and consistent communicators with your patients and prospective patients, and who you must connect with individually on so many levels. In any situation in your practice, you set the tone. If you are stressed, you will stress others. If you are secretive, you will raise suspicion. If you are fair, consistent, and polite, your staff members will trust you. If you are communicative, they will communicate with you. As with any daily connection, connecting with staff requires a greeting: a friendly "Hello, Mary" or "Good morning, Zack," acknowledging these people by name who are an integral part of your team. Don't ask "How are you?" if you don't want to hear the answer. Your communication with staff must have a function:

- *Patients:* Discuss patients in the most candid and professional manner. First, you must rely on staff and their assessment of individuals based on the time they spend communicating. Your impression and a staff member's impression may be entirely different, or you both may have the same doubts about or assessment of a particular patient. Next, you must be discreet and respectful. It is inappropriate to gossip about patients and comment about matters that do not relate to the patient's goals and role in your practice. These actions convey that you feel comfortable gossiping about anyone, perhaps even your staff.

- *Business:* Matters of business are entrusted to your staff, but also are *your* matters of business. You have the right and reason to ask questions, have discussions, give directions, and expect certain actions and information in return. But realize this person is not only your confidant; he or she is an employee who can come and go at will, and when that individual goes, your confidential business matters may travel as well. Be careful, be confident, and build trust over time. Most of all, communicate to your staff precisely what you entrust these individuals with, and formalize this with job descriptions, regular tasks, performance goals, and appropriate performance reviews.

- *Other staff:* In groups that work, play, or live together, confidence, cliques, partnerships, teamwork, and conflict can arise. Egos can clash or co-workers can support one another. There are leaders, there are team members, and there can be weak links. If you must discuss a staff member with another employee, speak briefly, professionally, and constructively; it must be about how this affects your ability to practice and do business, not about gossip or trivial disputes. It is better not to get involved in office infighting, and you must make it perfectly clear that you do not intend to be the arbiter of petty grievances. Taking sides is not your role; evidence, performance, and accountability are the measures by which you review and resolve disputes, if and when you must get involved.

- *Personal matters:* When you consider that for many work is 30% or more of one's daily life, an employee's personal life can have an impact on his or her professional life. Where personal matters are clearly affecting a staff member's work, you have the right to call attention to this and ask for your employee's attention. When personal matters affect other's safety or emotional or physical health, you have the right to direct that person to the right place to get help. This should be done discreetly and with compassion. I discourage physicians from getting involved in staff members' personal matters, unless they are willing to accept the consequences of those personal matters. Never lend money to staff members unless you know they will be there to pay you back, and unless you can lend it to everyone. Don't get involved in divorces or disputes, and don't offer personal advice unless you want to be the prop your staff can lean on. When it comes to staff relying on one another, make it a policy to keep personal matters outside the office. And what happens outside the office must stay outside the office.

In a well-run practice, your staff members are professionals whom you trust, empower, and rely on. They are an essential part of the success of your practice, and it is important to acknowledge this. Why you connect is as important as how you connect:

- *Individually:* Connect individually and privately when matters are individual and private or pertinent to the staff member or the practice. Praise in public, and praise in private. Corrections and concerns, cautions and discipline must be conducted in private. Where messages may be uncomfortable, confrontational, conflicting, or unwelcome, always deliver your message individually and privately, and with a witness who is entrusted to the intimate details of the human resources function of your practice.

- *Teams/pairs:* Whether with your clinical team, administrative team, aesthetics team, or a pair of staff members, make certain messages that must remain confidential are not shared in teams and those messages which are clearly indicated to be passed on do get passed on. In conversations with one or more staff members, make eye contact and acknowledge each individual in the conversation, even if the conversation is relative to only one. No one wants to feel ignored, even if the message or the connection was not immediately directed at the other individual.

- *As a group:* You will have formal meetings, and informal meet-ings, emails, messages, memos, and more that are addressed to the entire group. If a message is intended for the group, but cannot be delivered at once to the group, make certain there is a response mechanism to ensure that the message was delivered and received. A sign-off on a group memo, a reply receipt on an email, whatever policy you establish, make it clear that you are reaching the group for a reason: you want each member to connect and to respond.

Staff members are your extra hands in creating, supporting, and maintaining a practice environment of personal excellence, efficiency, and consistency. None of your efforts has value if your communication objectives with staff are not met. Those objectives require staff to support you and operational excel-lence, and must support staff excellence, both individually and as important contributors to the success of the practice. What is your call to action? What motivates staff to want to meet these objectives? Today's employees are no longer motivated only by money. Human resources research shows that vested interest, empowerment and professional development, flexibility, and respect are among the most highly regarded benefits that individuals look for in employment. Your call to action for staff should include:

- Establishing systems that compensate staff for their devotion to and efforts toward your success

- Empowering staff and imposing responsibility so that indi-viduals are recognized as essential contributors to the prac-tice's success

- Offering a work environment that, within guidelines, respects and accommodates personal needs

- Displaying your respect and the value you derive from those who work for you

If you expect staff members to embrace and support your goals as a provider of aesthetic medical service and as a personal services proprietor, your call to action must motivate them to want to be a part of your success.

FULLY STAFFED

Would your practice exist without staff? In a world where good, supportive, and loyal individuals are slow to come and quick to leave, is your greatest investment your staff? Does it make more sense to have a revolving door or a closely held team? Must you effectively communicate with staff to operate productively, safely, and successfully? Should your purpose in communication emphasize what you expect of staff and what they can expect in return for helping you to succeed?

Here are some examples of messages that many practices overlook with staff:

- *An employee or operations manual* (as required by many accrediting organizations): As much as this needs to succinctly define policy and procedure, it should also define your image, brand, and mission as well as how you expect your staff to uphold it and how you as a proprietor apply this in respect to the contribution the staff makes to your practice.

- *A formal system of review:* This is not so much for salary increases, or even for identifying areas of improvement, but moreover to demonstrate to your staff that you are attentive to their contributions. Review and recognize, individually and in defined cycles, that staff is fulfilling potential and maximizing skill. Further, if you make a commitment to them, they will make one to you.

- *Continuing education:* This is a message that clearly states you believe in your staff, you want them to grow, and you want them to grow with you. Nurture learning, nurture training, and set a good example yourself. Education need not always be formal. In-house clinical updates and training from your hands sends the message that you do not stand alone nor practice alone. You need staff to understand what you do and how you do it, so that they may play a continuing valuable role in assisting you.

- *Informal recognition:* Praise is an immensely powerful communication tool and is more important for reinforcing behavior patterns than is correcting someone's poor performance or error. One should use praise to acknowledge the staff's conscious efforts to help your practice succeed.

Continued

FULLY STAFFED—cont'd

- *Incentive:* This is a compelling communication tool that must be carefully thought out and administered. While attaching sales goals or commissions to aesthetic medical service is flirting with the bounds of ethics, attaching incentive to meeting overall practice goals, not just in productivity or revenue but also in satisfaction, is not. The incentive need not be cash, but it should be something your staff finds of value.

- *Integrated communication and cross-function:* All of the staff within your practice need to understand the expectations and the contributions of others as well as the vital role that each staff member plays in the overall operation of your practice. This accomplishes two things: the ability for those performing different functions to work together cohesively as well as developing the knowledge and cross-training necessary to fulfill the role of another staff member during a planned or unplanned absence. As a business owner, it is compelling to your success to have staff work cohesively and to simply be able to work when one team member is unable to participate.

- *Collective input:* Few practices find the time to regularly meet and share experiences based on each others integrated roles, needs and agendas. At a minimum, physician and staff should meet together on a monthly basis to review innovations, changes, specific cases, observations and opportunities for the practice, for patients and for quality improvement.

There is a purpose to all of these communications and connections: your team has value, and can be invaluable to you if you send the right messages.

🦋 IN PRACTICE: I Am the Boss

I was visiting an efficient, strong practice with loyal patients, but a high turnover in employees. The physician was well liked by his patients. He was busy and successful; he was often the recipient of referrals. But though he could attract and keep his patients, he could not keep his staff. The pay scales were reasonable, the office hours and environment were lovely. There was structure in the job descriptions and the employee manual, and there were excellent perks, including free treatments for staff.

But it took little time for me to realize just why the staff would not stay. The physician's behavior was a case of Dr. Jekyll and Mr. Hyde. In "Dr. Jekyll" mode, he was warm and spent quality time with his patients. He was compassionate; he put people at ease. "Mr. Hyde" berated his staff. He barked orders, snapped and threw his hands in the air when things didn't go his way. He cursed around his staff, and often at them. The most unbelievable action I witnessed was when he called his receptionist into a consultation and ordered her to remove her blouse and allow the patient to see and feel her breasts. I was dumbfounded.

That afternoon I brought the practitioner and the staff together for a group meeting. I went around the room and asked each member to tell me what they liked about where they worked. Then everyone shared what they did not like. The short outcome of this exercise was that the physician felt he was not only entitled to act the way he did, he felt it was necessary to motivate his staff—he stated that they lacked initiative and never acted unless directed. The staff felt they were belittled; they were afraid to act without direction because the doctor's expectations varied so greatly. I gave both the physician and staff homework. He was to refrain from cursing and berating staff in front of patients, and they were to communicate more, not less with him. They were to take initiative and be prepared.

Two months later, I revisited the practice. Things were improving but not great. Our next step was to pull together a staff mission they could all refer to and reflect on in their expectations of one another. I asked the physician to define goals for his staff, and the staff to define requests of him. We set up regular staff meetings to discuss office policy, progress, and advancement. Part of every meeting was an agenda item specific to team building.

The lesson here: The reality is that different personalities will have differences. Finding good people, training them, and keeping them is as much an effort as it is finding a good employer, learning the ropes, and growing in one's role and aspirations. Never overlook the value, feelings, and trust you have in your staff, and the respect and trust they should have for you.

REFERRAL SOURCES

Within your practice you will encounter and connect with the people who are your sources for referral, those who help you to grow your practice. Patients who refer others to you will come back as patients again, or will accompany friends. You may see them on social occasions hosted by your practice, or you may reach out to them regularly to show your gratitude, support, and personal acknowledgment of them as an important source for your practice.

Professionals, whether other physicians, other service providers, or even your direct peers who may refer to you may connect with your office to refer, to confer, to learn, or to observe. Invite them in, keep them connected, and in turn they will continue to connect others to you. No matter the source, there are important means for connecting and staying connected inside your practice:

- *Remain personally connected:* Remind others that they are in your thoughts, that they are welcome, and that you appreciate them as individuals, not just referral sources; they are important to you. Birthday greetings, annual follow-up calls, and/or a personal note any time that is appropriate is always welcomed.

- *Remain clinically connected:* Keep your sources abreast of what is new in your practice and in your specialty and what is relevant to them or to the patients they refer to you. Rather than simply putting this in writing, invite them in for a luncheon, a seminar, a treatment, or to observe. Keep them educated, and they will keep others educated about you.

- *Show gratitude:* The most common reason for a disconnect with your sources, next to arrogance, is failure to show your appreciation. If you cannot say thank you, don't expect to get that referral again in the future.

Sources grow your practice from the inside out, so keep them inside in as many nonintrusive, personal, and appropriate ways that you can.

RESOURCES

Inside your practice you will need to connect with sales, service, and patient resources—those whose efforts support your practice or who want your support in their endeavors. Resources can be the most overlooked connections inside the office, simply because they are more often viewed as "selling" rather than "servicing." When connecting with resources, you certainly don't want to tax your valuable time, yet you don't want to miss out on good opportunities:

- *Screen and team:* Screen all visits and functions for resources carefully before any meeting; make certain the time is time well spent for both sides. Assign a team member to manage the relationship, review new products, data, research, procedures, or services and bring you the most pertinent information so that you can make a valid overall decision.

- *Pay attention:* If you only have 10 minutes, give that resource your attention during that time. If you are not willing to give that time, have a team member screen and report back to you; be sure that team member follows up with the resource, because you never know when you might need the one person you have avoided for the past 2 years.

- *Ask for data and analysis:* Resources often come to you with an opportunity. Expect and ask for data and analysis that show whether that opportunity would be attractive to your practice. In doing so, your resource has the opportunity and the tools to connect, and you have the opportunity and the information to make a value judgment.

SECTION IV
When

CHAPTER 13

When Do You Seek Opportunity?

> *No one gets an ironclad guarantee of success.*
> *Certainly, factors like opportunity, luck and timing*
> *are important. But the backbone of success is usually*
> *found in old-fashioned, basic concepts like hard work,*
> *determination, good planning, and perseverance.*
>
> — MIA HAMM,
> AMERICAN GOLD MEDAL OLYMPIAN IN WOMEN'S SOCCER

Timing isn't everything, but good timing, or the lack of it, can certainly make or break nearly any enterprise. No matter what we do in life, there are good times and bad for even the most well-intended actions and well-thought-out plans. Although you can plan to achieve success, attaining it requires that you recognize and act on opportunity—when the time is right.

In large measure, you control your success as a provider of aesthetic medicine. Timing is a critical factor in the success of anything you do. However, you have little control over timing unless you identify key factors to synchronize your practice operations and the opportunities essential to your success. The key factors that influence well-timed decisions include the following:

- Opportunities to fulfill patients' appearance enhancement desires.

- Cycles or trends that recur, and the cycle of your patients' experience in your practice that may be seasonal, clinical, or individual.

- Privacy is not a question of timing; it is an absolute. Privacy is relevant to the way you practice every day, with every patient.

All of these factors influence your ability to succeed, even if you have a firm grasp on the things you can control. No matter how carefully you carry out measures that are within your power, unless you do so when others are receptive to what you offer, your efforts will not achieve their goals.

When opportunity knocks, open the door. However, the wait
for such an opportunity may be long—a never-ending phase.
True success lies in the hands of those who seek, create,
and seize opportunity realistically and passionately.

Which Bus Do I Get On? And Who Do I Let Ride With Me?

John E. Gross, MD, FACS

Don't let the pursuit of perfection or the worry about not making the "right" choice get in the way of your pursuit of excellence and expanding your horizons. Opportunities require decision-making, but don't let the process of decision-making get in the way.

We all develop strategies for making difficult decisions or choosing a path. We balance the upsides and downsides of every choice. We look at the risk-benefit ratio of outcomes for our patients, our practices, our profession, and our families. Even with these tools and careful assessment, the "best choice" still may not be clear.

A few years ago I heard a story told by Coach K (Mike Krzyzewski) at a Duke basketball camp I was attending with my son. He told a story relating life's journey to that of being a passenger on a bus or being the driver of the bus, and the importance of "getting on the right bus." From that story I realized the bus I was on: I no longer trusted the driver, and I made the decision to get off.

Relate some of the decisions you make to that of being on a bus. There may be busses that we are passengers on, or we may be the driver. When thinking of getting on a bus, one needs to consider who is the driver, and where is this bus headed? We are essentially putting our lives in the driver's care. Do we trust the driver to get us to the destination safely? Do we trust his or her judgment to make a great decision in case of an emergency or a detour? Do we believe that the driver will not just worry about maintaining a schedule, but will be able to balance the needs of the passengers? Are we comfortable with the route and destination? Is it a reputable bus company with a respected name, or an unknown that may not have good business practices? When seeking excellence, professionalism, and safety, do we really want to get on that bus? And once on the bus, will we know when to get off? Do we still trust the driver with our lives and livelihood? Did the driver change the route or destination? Does the driver still care about the passengers' interest?

Who do we want on our bus? If we invite someone along, will they get along with others on the bus? Are they interested in getting to the same destination using the route you plan? If there is a detour, can they accept that? If there were a flat tire, would they pitch in and help? Will they be respectful of others on the trip? When thinking of bringing on an associate or a new employee, consider do you want that person on your bus?

Sensible diversification is important. Embrace opportunities and be willing to take a ride.

Although you are a skilled medical professional, you must create and seize opportunities to make your practice visible and achieve your goals. You may have impeccable credentials, an appropriate image, a well-developed plan, a sufficient number of interested clients, and an effective staff, but these will not in themselves bring success to your door. You must search continuously for the opportunity to extend your services to those who have a valid reason to respond to you. This includes the following:

- *Public opportunities:* What you extend outside your practice to your target audience, patients, and the public

- *Professional opportunities:* What you extend of yourself and of your practice to other medical professionals and members of your professional community

- *Private opportunities:* What you extend of yourself to other individuals

In a world in which consumer demand for aesthetic medicine is high and the competition among providers is fierce, you will not succeed if you focus primarily on capitalizing on that demand. You must focus on satisfying consumer demand first, and the capital returns will follow.

PUBLIC OPPORTUNITY

Some practitioners do not feel the need to publicize their practices. Why is it important? Because public opportunity involves bringing your practice to the attention of the public through advertising, media relations, and other channels. However, to a provider of something as intimate as aesthetic medicine, the idea of publicity can cause true discomfort and hesitation.

If you ignore opportunities to bring your practice to the public's attention, how will you generate the interest and traffic you need to sustain your practice? It is difficult to meet your productivity goals by pursuing opportunities only among your professional affiliations and existing patients.

Other providers hesitate to publicize their practices because they question whether the return of value will justify the time and expense. Still others worry that public notice will open the practice to public scrutiny. But if you have skillfully shaped and maintained all the elements you can control—credibility, image, goals, and communication—why hesitate to present yourself to the public? If you control these variables and have planned appropriately, the return on pursuing public opportunity should be relatively predictable and the value easy to confirm.

If you are hesitant to publicize your practice, your reasons are likely one of three things: (1) You are unprepared or have failed to plan, a poor situation for any proprietor; (2) you are unwilling to have someone try to copy what you have worked to create; or (3) you are fearful you might open yourself up to competition, scrutiny, or ridicule.

"I don't need to" is not a credible reason. Even if you feel you don't need advertising and publicity for your practice, you undoubtedly engage in public opportunity in some way. Why not identify that effort and maximize it through control, planning, and timing?

As a physician, you are trained to prepare for anything and everything. As a proprietor, you know that planning is essential to effective operations and to attaining your goals. If you are unprepared for public opportunity, there may be a weakness in your control of the variables on which your success and survival rest. You will need to reevaluate all of the variables in your control within your practice. Define these as individual components as they relate to your goals; then evaluate the value these have to your practice. Prepare and plan, then reap your return.

If you are wary of imitation or competition, perhaps you are not fully confident of what you have built. Physicians who have developed a sound, thriving practice can withstand competition and imitators. Imitation is not a threat when it cannot improve on a solidly built original. If you are concerned that publicity will reveal the secrets of your success, then your success is not solidly founded; it is not built on your skills and accomplishments as a provider and your savvy as a proprietor.

If you avoid publicity for fear of ridicule or a lack of return on investment, you demonstrate a lack of faith in your methods and your practice. Solid credentials will stand on their own. An appropriately targeted image, brand, and mission cannot be gainsaid. If you are the center of your practice around which everything revolves, and all the things you have control over are well managed, let the world know about it.

There is no secret formula to the success of any aesthetic medicine practice. It is one that maintains high standards, integrity, careful planning, and appropriate procedures. Planning includes advertising, outreach, and media relations. Timing these efforts effectively is as essential to planning as is your budget.

✎ IN PRACTICE: Hidden Treasure

In the late 1990s the medical spa concept was born. Such a facility encompasses what I consider the right combination of personal services and retail. The medical spa concept takes services that are not necessarily administered by a physician and offers them in the comfort and tranquility of a spa setting. The advantage is that the minor discomfort or inconvenience associated with the treatment is now made attractive through the pampering, amenities, and relaxation that a spa atmosphere provides, inviting repeat service and building loyal patrons.

A provider in a metropolitan area that was on the cusp of innovation built a beautiful spa. He spared no expense in the surroundings or in the staff to provide a full range of added personal services, from skin care to holistic health care and nutritional counseling, as well as services that were designed purely for personal indulgence. His theory: His upscale patrons would quickly become devoted spa clients, and word of mouth would quickly generate additional traffic.

However, 6 months into his endeavor, traffic was building, but slowly. His patient base continued to be strong, and although he did everything right internally to motivate patients to try the personal services, the daily patient traffic of that one provider was not enough to sustain all of the services offered in his new facility.

When we met, I was impressed by the detail and procedures of his operation. The physician was very private and soft spoken but very confident, and certainly someone in control of all his practice variables. However, although his plans were meticulous, his goals were unrealistic. His process for generating the traffic necessary to sustain the new business extension did not reach beyond those already in his practice. The only time people were exposed to messages about his new concept was when they were on the premises.

I asked him why no announcement had been made to publicize his new spa, expecting his answer would be that he did not want other providers in his market to begin competing on this level as well. His answer, however, although very impressive, was ultimately short sighted. He did not want his loyal patients to feel that their secret to aesthetic rejuvenation and tranquility was public domain. He believed that any publicity would diminish the valued privacy and exclusivity of his practice.

But how could he sustain this expanded and expensive enterprise if only his existing patients, who visited only a few times per year, were aware of the services available? Clearly, he could not, but he felt the need to remain focused on his existing patient base. He also thought that any attempt to promote to them would diminish his image of discretion and control.

This was what we had to work with to get the spa to start living up to its goals of reaching beyond the practice while maintaining this very private image among those who trusted and valued that image.

Careful planning was the key. This involved maximizing the practice's existing database information to target personalized messages to different categories of patients based on demographics and prior services. Keeping close to the image of privacy and strict control, both in service and operations, messages were delivered through channels the staff could identify that patients were comfortable with, such as mailings and personal calls. Some providers of personal services in the spa called patients directly who were identified as likely candidates for their services and invited them to come in for a visit. For example, patients who had previously booked appointments with the physician for noninvasive facial treatments more than 6 months in advance because he was so in demand could now obtain the same service on much shorter notice at the hands of someone chosen and trained by the physician. The invitations came directly from that trusted, hand-picked, personally trained staff member.

Others patients received a personal letter from the physician recommending that as an enhancement to his services, they make an appointment for a specific service now offered by someone chosen and personally trained by him. Still other patients who were young and more adventurous in their tastes received invitations to experience some of the new and trendy services the spa offered, with incentive packages that were complementary in service and price. His most devoted patients, and those who clearly hit the appropriate demographic for his spa, were all given a private tour of the facility when they arrived for appointments with the provider. The tour was one of the most strategic of hands-on methods to make his patients aware of the possibilities the spa offered.

Did this work? Over time, it did. Time was a factor in planning, not only to get the message out but also when to send it out. They wisely did not contact all patients in the database at one time. Sometimes patients know one another, and if they shared this news it would nullify the concept of an individualized personal message. To call dozens of patients at once and invite them in would have bordered on telemarketing. However, a patient's history and patterns could be reviewed so an approach could be targeted directly to them. This required planning these efforts directly around opportunity: favorable circumstances that in this case took a very private practice and enabled it to reach out publicly, yet in an individualized manner to draw people to the practice and the provider's very controlled image, brand, and mission.

SPIES AMONG US

When you advertise, you know your competition may see the ads. When you reach out, you know they have the opportunity to reach in; when you speak out, you know they have the opportunity to listen. When you address an interested audience or open the practice's doors to the public for a special event, you must be aware that the staff and friends of competitors and perhaps even the competitors themselves may be among those watching and listening.

There is nothing wrong with paying attention to what other practices are offering and advertising, and there is nothing wrong with responding, so long as you keep in mind that spies who get caught are generally inept or insecure. I hope you are neither. A negative response has negative value, so do not denigrate your competitor's practice. Doing so cannot enhance the integrity of your image, brand, and mission, because nothing negative should be associated with you or your practice. A direct response, such as lowering your pricing or attacking the credentials of another, is simply begging to get into a battle.

Pay attention to what others are saying and doing simply so you can do it better. Don't become anxious when others pay attention to you; if you are providing excellent care and producing satisfying results in your practice, no one can take away your patients, your image, or your success.

Timing Public Opportunity

Should you act publicly when opportunity arises? Too late. If you wait for opportunity and then act, you will miss your mark with a poorly planned reply that cannot possibly maximize its potential. Although you can anticipate opportunity, the best approach is to seek it out.

Favorable conditions for targeted public efforts in advertising, media relations, or outreach are generally:

- *Time sensitive:* When innovation, change, or accomplishment occurs

- *Target sensitive:* Reaching those you identify as your intended audience

- *Theory sensitive:* Responding to a new theory, treatment or other innovation in aesthetic medicine

Cycles that are seasonal, clinical, or individual also present public opportunities to accelerate or build on the success of your practice (see Chapter 14).

Time-Sensitive Public Opportunity

Time-sensitive public opportunity requires real-time reactions. This can be either your easiest opportunity to prepare for, or your most difficult. It is easy when you have advance knowledge of an impending opportunity; you can then plan your response in detail so you will be prepared to seize opportunity when it occurs. This clearly has value across advertising, outreach, and media relations.

Consider an innovation in treatment; for example, injection therapy of fillers for wrinkle reduction. This treatment was used off-label for years, and practices were very quiet about offering injections so as not to cross the bounds of regulations or professional ethics. The day that the FDA made its announcement that it had approved injection therapy for use as an antiaging treatment, physicians scrambled to make it known that they provided this treatment. The glut of advertisements and direct mail as well as media coverage lagged by several weeks, because most practices waited for that approval before they acted on the opportunity. However, FDA approval was confidently anticipated, so any practice might have scored a coup by having the ads, mailings, and press releases ready the moment approval was official.

Time-sensitive changes include the addition of a new service or provider to your practice, a change in location or affiliation, or even the addition of new forms of outreach, such as a website. Why wait until this transpires to announce it and fuel your growth? Why not plan the announcement before the change is in place and thus build anticipation of your expansion among your target audience?

The time-sensitive opportunities you can least plan for are those linked to accomplishment, endorsement, or accreditation, because you cannot verify or announce these in advance. It is absolutely unethical to advertise that you are board eligible, or that you have a credential you do not. The awarding of a credential cannot be verified until it actually happens, nor may it be communicated until it is a reality. However, the tools necessary to make this news a public opportunity can be ready in anticipation of this. Recognition by a third party of your services, innovations, research, or outreach is difficult to predict; your advance notice may range from a few weeks to no time at all. However, if you are prepared for such eventualities and have an ongoing relationship with the outlets you need to act on this public opportunity, you can make the announcement promptly.

Target-Sensitive Public Opportunity

Certain clearly defined groups are favorable targets for your efforts. Consider the value of an opportunity to distribute practice information and extend an invitation for quality care to new homeowners of appropriate demographics in the area. Consider the value of presenting a seminar on breast surgery to breast cancer survivors, or on body contouring to those in clinical weight-loss programs. Consider the value of advertising in a special edition of a local magazine with a defined editorial stance on "living young," or in the fashion guides of media that reach your target demographics. (If you do not believe an interest in fashion has a direct correlation with an interest in aesthetic medicine, you are in the wrong business.)

Target-sensitive public opportunities abound. To take full advantage and maximize your efforts, you must evaluate such opportunities carefully. Do the demographics of that target audience relate to your practice demographics? Can you or do you want to serve the interests of a new demographic group without alienating your current client and patient groups?

The most likely opportunities involve advertising and outreach. Attempts at publicity through the media will probably yield little return, because sources for information on media coverage that are target sensitive will probably be pursued by the media themselves. The exception is providers who have established themselves as trusted sources with reliable media outlets. This requires very savvy and appropriately managed media relations. However, very few providers in aesthetic medicine can do this without their efforts being attached to research or being designated spokespersons. Be realistic in your assessment and strategic in your approach, and targeted opportunity will help to build your success.

Theory-Sensitive Public Opportunity

Unless you are a noted researcher with institutional or other backing to support your theory or innovation, your options for using theory-sensitive public opportunity are limited to disputing unfounded theories and unsubstantiated aesthetic medical treatments. A credible researcher's public efforts will be somewhat restricted until research outcomes are fully accepted and applied in practice. A researcher who lacks credibility will quickly fail in media relations, because any media organization today will verify not only your credentials, but also your credibility in the research you are conducting. Although you can advertise ongoing research, it is only effective to enroll participants for your research program. Few individuals will risk their appearance to unproven methods; therefore this is not something a credible individual practitioner or practice should do.

If you are not an active researcher, the only theory-sensitive public opportunity available to you lies in disputing theory, but this requires caution and strategy. Take, for example, the glut of organic or therapeutic breast enhancements that have been advertised. Use this to your advantage with media relations, outreach, or advertising. Affirm that the surgical methods in which you are trained and skilled are the only proven means to enhance the size, shape, or appearance of the breast. But do not dispute another's claims. If you approach opportunity by attacking someone's theories and their validity directly, you risk two things. First, if the method is later proven and accepted, you have marked yourself as a disbeliever. Second, a negative approach is unnecessary to reap positive results. Your image, brand, and mission should never be associated with something negative, nor should your messages. Instead, focus on positive, proven methods to achieve your goals.

PUBLIC THEORY

Some physicians are meeting the rise in consumer demand for aesthetic treatments by brazenly taking what is a generally accepted treatment or procedure, attaching a catchy name to it, and touting this to consumers as something innovative, improved, and exclusive to them. You know who they are. They are certainly not appropriately trained or credentialed practitioners of aesthetic medical service, or are they?

Surprisingly, as educated as consumers are today, and with public education tools so readily available through medical societies, boards, and the media, some consumers still fall prey to such tactics. Before you employ similar tactics, consider carefully whether the value of such a public opportunity is worth the damage that can be done to your reputation.

If you engage in accredited research to advance care through innovations in treatment and procedure, successful outcomes will redound to your benefit. If you engage in research simply to elevate your public name or garner a few extra dollars direct from the consumer, your theory will not only eventually discredit you but will also discredit all you have planned for and built.

PROFESSIONAL OPPORTUNITY

To succeed, you must take advantage of favorable professional circumstances or situations; in fact, you should actively seek them. You must not only engage professional opportunity; you must initiate it.

Professional opportunity contributes to your success when you reach out to other medical professionals and to members of your professional community as a source, a resource, a partner, and a peer. Outreach approaches may be as narrow as establishing relationships with referring physicians or as broad as participating in the professional societies of your specialty. Professional opportunity requires that you seek opportunities rather than wait for them to find you. You must search for opportunity:

- Outside your specialty, with other medical professionals
- Inside your specialty, with your peers

- With those who support your specialty, the businesses that are your resources, your professional service support, and your suppliers

Much like public opportunity, there are time, target, and theory considerations to professional opportunity. Most professional opportunities fall into specific targeted categories defined by specialty, by professional or personal relationship, and by geographic proximity. These can be individual targets or groups and can benefit your practice through referral, peer and resource support, or education—yours or theirs. Maximizing your effort requires defining who your targets are among medical professionals and engaging them individually or in targeted groups, as well as determining the timing of your actions.

For your professional relationships to present favorable conditions that will benefit the growth and success of your practice, others must first understand your principles and guiding actions, and you must understand and respect theirs. This is necessary for relationships that generate referrals or that provide general professional support. You cannot build a mutually fulfilling relationship if others do not understand your principles of practice.

Timing Outside Your Specialty

Professional opportunity outside your specialty requires prior planning to maximize its value. To gain the relationships that will benefit your practice through professional opportunities, you must first lay a foundation.

If another provider needs to refer a patient to you quickly, will he or she know where and how to reach you? Know whether you are willing or able to address such a case? Will he or she have materials available to educate that referred patient about your practice?

Professional opportunity to enhance the growth of your practice through clinical service is time sensitive. If you have not established relationships that invite professional opportunity from outside your specialty, professional opportunity cannot exist.

🖉 IN PRACTICE: ER (Emergency Refused)

Despite the prevalence of ambulatory surgical facilities, it is likely that you are still on staff at one hospital at least, and that you may be required as a staff member to be on rotating call. Few providers like to be on call, and many refuse to take it. Before you refuse, be cautious of when and how you do.

An established provider of aesthetic medicine was called to the emergency room late one night by the attending physician. A child was in need of immediate attention and the mother was adamant that a specialist be called. He asked the attending about the case, and then refused to take the call. The attending never shared the patient's name, nor did the specialist ask for it.

The next day, the provider's practice received a call from a patient who was scheduled to undergo extensive aesthetic treatment. The treatment was cancelled. Why? Because this patient was the adamant mother from the night before, and when this provider failed to treat her son when called on by the hospital, she felt she could not engage him to treat her. He was furious that the hospital never released the patient's name to him because that would have resolved everything—or would it?

The lesson is not the lost patient, but rather, had the specialist taken the time to establish a relationship with the emergency department, his expectation of them and the information important to him when deciding to take a call might have resulted in a far better outcome.

OUT OF SIGHT, OUT OF. . .

There is no greater importance in timing than to make certain you are visible among professionals with whom time-sensitive opportunity exists. You may not often have the occasion to encounter them, but you should make the effort to maintain contacts and keep their interest fresh. This includes taking the time to engage them, refresh and update referral and patient education materials, and even to follow up on past cases.

Maintaining your own visibility and that of your practice increases the likelihood that you will be the provider that comes to mind when a colleague wants to make a referral. Remain visible by inviting professionals to your practice to learn more—not to teach them how to treat others, but to learn more. Pick up the phone and follow up with a referring physician on a patient from several months past.

If you remain visible, you remain memorable. If you drop out of sight, you will drop out of mind.

Timing Inside Your Specialty

You cannot expect the professional groups to which you belong to support you as a member if you do not support the group in theory and practice. In addition, you cannot expect that if and when you do have a practical theory of medicine or theory in practice to share, others will find this an opportunity of value, much less pay attention, unless you have established relationships that are mutually fulfilling.

Specialists sometimes question the value of building relationships with their peers, because they view them as competitors. But given the demand for aesthetic medical service these days, the benefit of peer support far outweighs the influence of competition. Your competitors are probably located geographically close to you, have a similar practice model, and target the same demographic group your practice targets. Combine these variables, and your competition among your peers is a very narrow group. Do professionals within your specialty present greater opportunity as peers to engage, or is your best opportunity to view them as competitors to monitor and avoid?

You and your peers probably face the same or similar clinical and operational issues. It is likely that you have similar educational needs to keep your skills and knowledge current. You also have similar proprietary issues. So why not learn from one another? Who better to support you, in theory, than members of your specialty who face the same issues you do as a provider and proprietor?

Should you engage your competitors? Does professional opportunity exist? Indeed, it does. Among the many potential patients who seek your services, there is no possible way that you can fulfill the needs of every individual to the best of your ability and the best of their satisfaction and comfort. Some individuals will come to your practice but you will choose not to extend service to them, for clinical or personal reasons, and there are some individuals who will not choose you. Which is the better scenario: to know your competitors well and defer to them when appropriate, thus maintaining with the trust of the individual you cannot serve, or to simply turn that individual away, severing any present or future link, and allowing them to leave your practice with an unfulfilled experience?

Remaining a contributing member of your professional society presents an ongoing opportunity to remain networked and visible. This connection can be as basic as reading your society's newsletter and casting your vote for society officers, extending your expertise in an instructional course or to a society committee, or even remaining close to your competitors and peers.

There is another constant professional opportunity: your dedication to your specialty and to upholding the ethics and standards it imposes. You represent not just your practice, but your specialty. If you fall short of upholding the image of that specialty, you not only tarnish yourself, but also the image of that specialty group. If you think you can succeed without your credentials and your professional affiliations, I dare you to try. If you think you can be a success without upholding all of the ethical and clinical standards of your profession, give up your credentials. Do not tarnish the efforts of a group through your own reckless arrogance. One bad apple cannot spoil the bushel, but it can make the bushel unattractive.

A LACK OF ATTENTION

Practitioners complain about the lack of attention they receive from the professional groups within their specialty. They argue that unless you are in a research-based practice or training program, you have no opportunity to serve in leadership. Wrong. They argue that unless you are in a research-based practice or training program, you will not be asked to serve as a media spokesperson. Wrong again. They argue that participation on committees is just a waste of time; it contributes to a bureaucracy that favors the elite (the research, training, and high-visibility practices). Wrong one more time.

Would your professional society exist without the individual members who are in private practice? Is the value of research-based practices and training programs essential in the growth, innovation, and advancement of your specialty? Do you as peers have a common ground? Then why not participate?

I have seen society leaders and presidents come from private practice. To know these men and women is to understand their passion and devotion not just for their practices, but for their specialty as well. Passion and devotion alone present the opportunity for you to succeed, so exercise this in all you do. You will reap the rewards.

SUPPORT AND PROFESSIONAL OPPORTUNITY:
Learn by Teaching

Mary P. Lupo, MD, FAAD

As a second-year dermatology resident at Tulane in 1983, I asked my program director, Dr. Larry Millikan, if I could start a cosmetic clinic for our residents to "learn by doing" bovine collagen injections, chemical peels, and sclerotherapy. It was easy to do this because we already had a clinic to perform dermabrasion and hair transplants under the supervision of Dr. John Yarborough. I recruited patients from my local health club, because there are always people who wish to have, but think they cannot afford, cosmetic procedures. The "see one, do one, teach one" motto of Charity Hospital was never so true. By my last year of residency, I was instructing my first- and second-year residents in the nuances of cosmetic procedures.

When I left to begin my practice, I continued to staff that clinic, and I do so to this day. In addition to training at Tulane, I welcome my aesthetic peers in dermatology, plastic surgery, and other core specialties into my office to share my treatment pearls and practice methods, perform live injection sessions at AAD and ASDS meetings, and began The Cosmetic Boot Camp in 2005 with Dr. Ken Beer. To keep the meetings at the highest level of learning, we allow only board-certified dermatologists, plastic surgeons, facial plastic, oculoplastic, ENT, and ophthalmology MDs to attend.

As a result of this constant interaction with my fellow aesthetic specialists, I continue to hone my skills. My patients benefit, because I have found you learn just as much as the person you are teaching. You see things through different eyes, and as you explain while you are doing, it advances the imprint on your brain of the skill you are demonstrating. By teaching my fellow core aesthetic physicians, I am advancing and strengthening our specialty. But at the heart of it all, I feel that I am helping patients by taking physicians who have the "core" training in aesthetics from their residency training and helping them reach their full potential to effectively and responsibly make their patients look better.

Like many of you, I have been to industry-sponsored seminars where nonaesthetic physicians and nonphysicians are signed up to jump on the economic bandwagon of nonsurgical rejuvenation. Frankly, I have found many of the questions asked at these seminars scary, to think how little some of these individuals understand about wound healing, laser physics, and the basic aesthetic principles that we know from our residency training. It disturbs me to think that they are physicians, yet they have allowed economic

Continued

SUPPORT AND PROFESSIONAL OPPORTUNITY:
Learn by Teaching—cont'd

pressures to compromise the basic tenet of our physician responsibility: to do right by the patient.

Physicians should always refer to another physician who has the advanced training in the procedure the patient needs, rather than to perform it themselves just for the revenue. When one's bank account is more important than patient welfare, you are no longer a responsible physician. I now regularly see patients who have untoward complications as a result of weekend-trained noncore physicians who have gone beyond their training. The ASDS has documented an alarming increase in the trend of nonphysician practice of medicine and its sometime serious sequelae. By helping each other within the core aesthetic specialties, we can strengthen our position with the public and ensure that we remain the experts for patient care. That will result in both our economic success and the improved safety and success of these cosmetic procedures for patients.

PRIVATE OPPORTUNITY

Private opportunity—the one-on-one communication between you and another—is critical to the success of your practice; it is the most universal yet least visible form of opportunity. It occurs most commonly within your practice as well as outside. It is linked directly to who you are as a practitioner and proprietor. It is the catalyst that brings a client or patient to accept your service or not, based on what you extend of yourself as an individual and a professional.

- What do you extend of yourself to your patients and those close to them?

- What do you extend of yourself to your staff and to those who support your ability to treat patients?

- What do you extend of yourself to your peers and the professional relationships that support or provide your ability to treat patients?

These are all your private opportunities: those that lead an individual to make a confident decision to choose you as a provider and to be satisfied by that choice.

The greatest occasion of private opportunity is in consultation with a potential patient. However, the consultation is rarely the deciding factor when a potential patient accepts treatment and becomes your patient. This conversion is not your ultimate goal; the goal is forming an enduring relationship built on trust.

Private opportunity is targeted directly to the other person in an encounter. It carries the likelihood that the individual will share his or her private experience with you with other potential patients. Even when you discover that conditions are not favorable to your success in this instance (such as with a patient who is not a good candidate), you still must make that encounter into a positive and appropriately timed experience.

Timing Private Opportunity

Public and professional opportunities are planned for and sought out. Private opportunity is the basis of your practice. Your career is founded on privately fulfilling another person's desires for appearance enhancement. If this to you is not inherently private and restricted to the individual who is engaging you, and if you do not see your ability to make every personal encounter a private opportunity, you are in the wrong business. Every personal encounter you have should be one that:

- Affirms you are a caring and skilled provider

- Affirms you can fulfill the desires of the individual you are engaging

- Affirms you can fulfill the expectations of someone who refers a patient to you

- Demonstrates your compassion, skill, and devotion as a provider who not only can provide treatment, but also understands the individual's desire for aesthetic medical treatment

- Demonstrates your dedication to your practice and patients

The timing of private opportunity is not strategic, planned, or sought. It must sincerely exist at all times. Even one instance when you do not fully embrace a private opportunity to enhance the success of your practice can result in diminishing your value as a provider of aesthetic medicine.

🦋 IN PRACTICE: Not Me

A woman scheduled a consultation for a procedure that was purely aesthetic in nature but essential to her self-confidence and her ability to feel fulfilled as a woman. She entered the office of an aesthetic provider, clearly anxious, accompanied by her husband.

The patient coordinator addressed them and did her best to allay their anxiety. She took them to wait in a private room, carefully reviewed all the elements of the case, and then the physician came in. His exit was as abrupt as was that of the patient and her husband.

Our provider could not meet this woman's expectations, and he openly stated so from the very beginning. Rather than work with her to educate her and help her understand why her expectations would be difficult to fulfill, he let her go. His answers, although private to her, very publicly exclaimed, "Not me."

Moreover, when the woman left, she did not feel that someone had listened, showed compassion, and addressed the issues candidly; rather, she felt as though something so deeply important to her was either unimportant to this provider or simply a lost cause. Was she angry? You bet. Was she hurt? You know it. How did her husband react? He left calling the practitioner names, because he thought that they had found someone with compassion who could fulfill her desire. Instead they experienced even more frustration and disappointment than for the condition for which they came.

What is the lesson here? Although this was not an opportunity that would have resulted in immediate patient satisfaction and the continued contributions of such satisfaction to the success of this practice, it was still a missed private opportunity. Although the provider could not achieve what the woman wanted, he still should have taken the time to listen and offer his expertise and advise on what was possible. This woman engaged him for a reason, and in the most critical phase of their relationship—private opportunity—he closed the door, not just to her immediate desire, but to her and anyone connected to her in any way. Private opportunity is ever present. It exists to give satisfaction to the individual interested in your services and to those connected to them.

IN PRIVATE

How do you rate in your timing and action of private opportunities, where conditions are private and favorable to build on the success of your practice? Consider the following scenarios.

1. You are engaged to correct the poor outcome of a prior surgery that was performed by someone else. You:

   A. Ask who the prior provider is, examine and define what is wrong, and describe how you will make it right.

   B. Ask who the prior provider is, then state what is wrong and what you would have done in the first operation.

   C. Discuss with the patient what he or she finds unsatisfactory, examine the patient, offer your recommended remedy, and ask whether the patient will secure prior records so that you can review a full history of the case and confirm or refine your remedy.

2. You are engaged by a referring physician to treat a patient whom the physician labels as "difficult." You:

   A. Refuse the referral.

   B. Take the referral and judge this patient for yourself.

   C. Ask for a history on the patient and for the candid insight of the referring physician, review this, decide whether to meet with the patient, make your own judgment, and share this with the referring physician.

3. You consult with a patient who is clearly motivated by the desires of another, not her own desire. That other individual is present in the consultation. You:

   A. Tell the other individual that his desire is not something you are willing to impose on another person.

   B. Tell both individuals that they are destined for an unhappy outcome.

   C. Ask the other individual to step out so that you may privately examine the patient, then take the opportunity to candidly dis-

Continued

IN PRIVATE—cont'd

cuss her own desires and share your theory and mission on fulfilling the personal desires of appearance enhancement.

4. A staff member makes a mistake, whether it be logistical, clinical, or in manner. You:

   A. Demand an immediate correction of the error, and reprimand the staff member.

   B. Call attention to the error, correct it yourself, and fire or reprimand the staff member.

   C. Swiftly and quietly correct the error, then privately with the staff member or among a group of staff members evaluate what went wrong, why, and discuss how to prevent similar occurrences in the future.

5. A potential patient is accompanied by a friend or family member who spends most of the consultation asking questions about her own condition, not lending support. You:

   A. Suggest that person make an appointment on her own.

   B. Ask that person to leave the room.

   C. State that for the patient's best advantage, you will focus only on one case at a time, and that you would be happy to discuss the other individual's concerns at a time dedicated to that person, either at the end of this consultation or on another day, and you will extend that person education specific to her concerns.

6. A patient comes for a consultation wanting improvement but is unable to specifically define her expectations, realistic or otherwise. You:

   A. Suggest what you think she should consider improving.

   B. Examine the patient, offer suggested improvements, and ask for the patient's input.

   C. Ask her to look in a mirror and describe the features that she wants to improve. Ask her to explain why, and then ask how she wishes to see herself. Then offer what you can do to fulfill those wishes.

> The common link to all of these situations, and any private encounter, is simply to turn it into opportunity, even if opportunity is not immediately apparent. Recall the five things any private encounter should be and make certain every time you engage someone in private, you see the end result as one or all of those things that affirm or demonstrate who you are as provider. Clearly, the response that most appropriately and effectively exercises private opportunity in each scenario is *C*.

Knowing when and how to seize opportunity is only one factor of timing that you must carefully evaluate to advance the success of your practice. Your ability to act at the best possible moment to take advantage of opportunity requires that you identify when it can exist, act upon it before it acts upon you, fully understand how it can contribute to your success.

Only then can you identify cycles that contribute to timing your practice efforts and recognize the importance of when to exercise privacy in your role as provider and proprietor.

IN PRACTICE: Blended Opportunity

> I was out to lunch one day with the patient coordinator from a client's practice and we decided to do a little shopping. We headed to a well-known department store and went to the lingerie section. We noticed that a woman was being fitted for a prosthesis. The patient coordinator went about her shopping, and I decided to stay within earshot to see what I might learn.
>
> The woman was trying not to be emotional, but she was clearly seeking help and support from the salesclerk, who showed compassion and was endearing, but unfortunately seemed uninformed. She was comforting the woman by trying to share her limited knowledge of reconstructive breast surgery. When the woman left, I approached the salesperson and asked how often they fitted prostheses, and if the emotions and concerns of their clients were similar to this woman's. Yes, they were, she responded, and why was I asking?
>
> *Continued*

⚘ IN PRACTICE: Blended Opportunity—cont'd

Did many other customers confide in the salespeople at the store about the desire for other kinds of breast surgery? All the time, was the reply, and why was I asking?

I pulled the patient coordinator forward and told her that she must forge a relationship with this woman. What resulted from this private opportunity where I had eavesdropped was a professional opportunity for my client to meet with the sales professionals in the store to give them an informative and direct education on breast reconstruction and breast surgery in general. That translated to a public opportunity for my client to meet with and educate women who had bought prostheses from the store in a breast reconstruction seminar sponsored by the store and held in their private meeting room.

It also forged an ongoing and trusted relationship between my client and the department store. He provided store staff with an education on breast surgery, he provided store management with the opportunity to better serve their customers through cost-free, private seminars, and in return, what did he receive? Referrals, lots of referrals for breast surgery as well as many other procedures.

The moral of this story is that opportunity is everywhere. When you think you have found it, think about the appropriate way to act. Whether it is public, professional, private, or a combination of all of these things, when you act with integrity, compassion, and planning, opportunity can translate to value.

CHAPTER 14

When Do You Respond to Cycles?

Here she comes
Beauty plays the clown
Here she comes
Surreal in her crown
— U2 AND BRIAN ENO WITH LUCIANO PAVAROTTI,
"MISS SARAJEVO"

Time passes in cycles: minutes, hours, days, seasons, passages in life. Who we are and who we become evolves as we pass through multiple cycles in time. This brings to mind "Miss Sarajevo," the story of a 17-year-old beauty queen, a passage in life for a young woman in a war-torn period in Sarajevo, Bosnia-Herzegovina, during the longest siege in modern history. It is the ultimate example of how cycles can coincide or collide and how even the sweetest success is sometimes overlooked by that which is beyond our control. It exemplifies how every story, every cycle has a different view when seen through the eyes of another.

The patterns of cycles vary or repeat over the course of your career and throughout the lives of those you serve. Often these cycles present the opportunity for you to act and build on your success by fulfilling the desires of others. More often, you and your practice team may fail to notice these cycles until someone approaches your practice to fulfill a desire related to such a cycle, such as a personal milestone in life. What are the most common cycles and what advantage do they offer to your success?

- *Seasonal cycles:* Repeat regularly over a defined period, just as the seasons occur throughout the year

- *Clinical cycles:* Repeat over the course of treatment, either to maximize or refine results, maintain results, or to advance the treatment

- *Individual cycles:* Specific to one's course in life or in time

- *Social cycles:* Affect our culture; these may be economic, political, or tragic

The advantage of any cycle is that when you can define it, you can respond to it, thus creating opportunity and enhancing the care you provide and the productivity and success of your practice.

SEASONAL CYCLES

As each year begins, we are exhorted to establish New Year's resolutions. Typically, losing weight is on the top of the list. Most often the top resolutions include some form of self-improvement. Appearance enhancement can be one of those ways and may resonate for you as a provider. As each new year begins, the cyclical moment for reaching out to an audience that subscribes to a philosophy of "new year, new you" presents an opportunity to enhance your success. How do you use this recurring human impulse to your advantage?

In addition to using media tools to define your audience's interests, you can use these to define cycles. Seasonal cyclical opportunities include New Year's, with its message of renewal; Valentine's Day, when the focus is on sensuality and passion; spring, a time of rejuvenation; summer, when clients prepare for bared limbs and cope with sun-exposed complexions; then there's the vigor of autumn's back-to-school rush, October, with its emphasis on breast cancer awareness, and the need to look and feel your best for the holidays and winter getaways. Seasonal cycles are defined based on society and our calendar, but they can also be individual. And any cycle will vary somewhat each time it repeats.

Consider a seasonal cycle specific to your market. Are you located in a Sunbelt state, where your community in winter is full of snowbirds who have migrated south? This demographic is likely an aging population whose members have the disposable income and desire to engage an aesthetic medicine provider so they can look as young as they feel. Their arrival may be a cycle that presents opportunity for you to increase productivity during the months they are in town while also looking for other traffic opportunities during the slower summer months.

Consider a seasonal cycle specific to your patients. Do the summer months allow teachers to use their down time to undergo aesthetic treatments? Does summertime prevent young mothers who are busy with their children's summer vacation activities from undergoing treatment? These individual seasonal cycles present an opportunity to better focus your messages and outreach.

Just as engaging opportunity requires that you act rather than react, using cycles to your advantage requires you to:

- Identify cycles before they occur

- Determine the strategic value of those cycles before they occur

- Plan how you will respond to or use those cycles to your advantage before they occur

Much of your success simply boils down to researching, identifying, and planning your efforts so you can target and time them to your fullest advantage.

⚡ IN PRACTICE: So Slow

My least favorite call, the one that absolutely riles me, is when I hear a provider state, "Things are very slow right now; we need to do something to increase traffic." The first question I ask is why the provider believes things have slowed. The response varies from "It usually gets slow this time of year," to "Economic conditions are awful," or "The competition has really eaten away at our client/patient base."

If you wait until things get slow, I will tell you that you are out of luck; you've missed the boat. Your timing is poor, and you have already missed the opportunity to advance the pace of things, because by the time you define and enact your efforts and allow appropriate time for the audience's consideration and reply, the cycle will likely have rolled along to a new phase.

I had a provider get angry with me for such a reply. She thought I was mocking her and simply shirking the opportunity to offer my expertise. Instead, I carefully evaluated the practice's productivity cycles, looking for trends and patterns. I identified the likely cause of the trends and patterns and then set a plan in motion so that before a slow-down cycle was ready to hit again, measures were in place to heighten the practice's visibility, opportunity, and traffic.

I worked with the provider to identify targets in her market who would find these points in a seasonal cycle attractive, and we planned targeted messages to them. I suggested that the client use this slow time as an opportunity to evaluate where the practice was in terms of achieving its goals, to plan accordingly, and to revisit and refine operational issues. She thought I was kidding. She retorted, "I don't have time for that."

As a business you need to make time to evaluate and plan. How do you know when to plan? You must look at your data. If you know some months are busier and what procedures are more in demand at certain times of year, you can respond. If you know what times of year are slow, these may be the ideal times to use your human resources for planning. It is imprudent to overextend yourself in busy times to do this. When you have time, use it wisely to focus on all of the efforts that you want to or need to have in place throughout the year. Although your business cycle is probably tied to your tax cycle, your efforts do not all need to be tied to this; you must simply define and allocate your capital resources accordingly.

Some time later, the same provider called me to say, "Things are slow—" Yet what I expected to hear did not come. Rather, she said, "But not nearly as slow as we usually would be at this time, because we planned for it. Do you have time to come in and review goals with me? I have the time now and really want to make the most of it."

To Every Season, Turn, Turn

Don't assume the holidays and seasons are your only seasonal cycles. Anything that changes but comes back full circle is a seasonal cycle. It may not occur annually; it may occur daily, monthly, or in an undefined but recurring cycle.

In addition to communication, seasonal cycles apply to operational issues too, such as your hours of operation. Do not make the mistake of defining hours by your own preference. Know your market and its cycles and plan your operations to meet these accordingly. For instance:

- You will not get an active mom of young children to attend a seminar at 4:00 PM; her children are coming home from school at that hour. Plan your events accordingly.

- Does your physician assistant work while her kids are in school, and does this mean that all the acne patients who see her have to miss school to be treated? You will have patients who cannot break away to engage your services during school or business hours, so extend yours.

- Do you schedule surgery days to allow patients the advantage of a long weekend to recover?

- In the summer months, does everyone in your town spend the afternoon golfing or swimming to take advantage of the warm weather, or are they hiding from the heat in cool quarters or fleeing north?

- Between Christmas and New Year's, is the whole town off skiing? Or are winter vacationers coming to your area who might be looking for a little self-improvement during their holiday?

All variables regarding seasonal cycles are specific to your practice location, demographics, services, and to you. One of the benefits of being a proprietor is that you make the rules and set the standard. Although you want these to be to your personal advantage, they will not be advantageous to the success of your practice if they do not take into consideration the cycles and preferences of those you serve.

CLINICAL CYCLES

Many providers are offering the less-invasive treatments that are growing exponentially in demand; these require multiple treatment cycles to achieve results or ongoing treatment cycles to maintain. If this is the case in your practice, you'd best accept the fact that keeping clinical cycles active—known as retention—is imperative to your success and likely your easiest reliable measure of productivity. Clinical cycles are where retention should thrive.

Clinical cycles can also range across treatments—leading to extension of services. For example, an individual who has undergone injection of tissue fillers to reduce wrinkles will eventually be a likely candidate for more comprehensive treatment. This patient is more likely to be interested in adjunct clinical care such as skin care or other noninvasive antiaging therapies. And this patient will need to return for repeat treatments to maintain the results of the original injection.

When you recognize that retention and extension of services are closely tied to clinical cycles, you need to identify how to use clinical cycles to your advantage. Clinical cycles require:

- Tracking

- Maintaining communication and outreach to keep them active

- An attractive appeal to your target

- Easy access and service that is easy to subscribe to

Unless the services you provide are purely surgical and you do not offer noninvasive services, personal services, or retail, you must actively work to maximize the contribution of clinical cycles to your success.

Do not make the mistake of believing that the only advantage of a clinical cycle is to generate repeat service. Repeat service requires repeat traffic, and as demonstrated in communication, transmitting your messages to current patients offers your greatest opportunity for acceptance of those services.

Repeat service translates to retention, and retention affords two advantages: it affirms that you are doing something right by building loyalty among your patients, and it affords predictable productivity and revenue streams. Add to this the extended value of loyalty from a patient with whom you have an ongoing, trusting relationship, and your practice now has the advantage of added sources for referral and future treatment potential from someone who is actively interested in and subscribes to aesthetic medicine.

Research shows that patients today are seeking their first aesthetic treatments at a much younger age and that more than 78% of patients who undergo treatments would do so again. Thus the value of actively nurturing clinical cycles in your practice is clearly a great advantage in outreach and communication. Clinical cycles offer:

- Predictable productivity and revenue

- Repeat traffic and visibility to your practice

- Ideal, targeted opportunities for hand-to-hand delivery of practice communications

- Loyalty and confidence to support and encourage referral

- Loyalty and confidence to maintain a lifelong provider-patient relationship

For clinical cycles to work to your advantage, you must identify the services and patients who subscribe to them and plan the timing of those services. If you directly remind a patient that the time for another treatment is approaching, there is a greater likelihood of booking that appointment. You can also immediately track a lost repeat service and can inquire why a patient has chosen not to continue or maintain treatment.

Maintaining active communications is the second requirement in using clinical cycles to your advantage. You must maintain communication, continue to act, and either book the appointment or discover why service will not be repeated now or in the future. That discovery is essential to improving quality of care.

Continuing to act can be complicated. First, the staff members doing the tracking must develop manageable systems specific to your office and keep those systems active. It also requires continual monitoring so that no cycle goes unnoticed, yet your repeat contacts do not become bothersome to the patient. Finally, it requires repeating the cycle continuously until the cycle of treatment is completed, or when the patient chooses not to renew. Even when the cycle of treatment is completed, do not overlook follow-up as a means to measure satisfaction, to refine results through adjunct treatment, and to maintain visibility for potential referral and future services.

Making cycles attractive and easy to subscribe to is what some may call marketing; I call it customer service. When someone already wants something, making it more attractive through price, convenience, or incentive is customer service. It is not playing on one's emotions to get the individual to act on something he or she otherwise might not initiate.

Package prices are clearly an advantage in clinical cycles. This can apply to any treatment that requires repeat cycles to achieve or maintain results. Packaging works well with personal services, such as hair removal or clinical skin care. Your flexibility and methods for making cycles attractive must be inviting, convenient, and must fit the expectations of your patients and be congruent with your image, brand, and mission.

❦ IN PRACTICE: In Pocket, at Hand

In helping a young provider establish some operational parameters for his practice, I suggested that he package certain clinical services that required repeat visits. Services offered to maintain results should be packaged based on the number of treatments one might need over a defined period, such as a year, or in a defined number of treatments. Those which required a defined number of treatments to achieve results should be packaged by the optimal number of treatments.

He objected vehemently, saying this was a marketing tactic and he would not have it in his practice. Further, he felt that this would require cumbersome administration to track and that it would appear that he was discounting. It just was not right for him.

Before I accepted his position, I shared with him the following: First, he would not be discounting. An initial visit requires more time for informed consent. Subsequent visits are shorter and should be billed at a lower rate. He agreed. Second, he would be collecting fees in advance and fueling capital resources. To discount only allows the patient the advantage of reduced fees for an up-front financial commitment from which a provider garners the cash at the outset to pay off young-provider debt. He agreed again. Third, he would be making it convenient for clients not only to commit to service initially, but also to commit to maintenance appointments, so the likelihood of satisfaction would be higher and the provider would be appreciated for a skilled job. Agreed again.

In addition, the likelihood of someone returning for something he or she has already invested in is higher. Through each visit that individual makes to the office, the provider gains more visibility for the practice and has an opportunity to extend education. Each time he serves that patient, he further fuels the patient's acceptance of him, thus generating referral or added service. Agreed once more.

Finally, people who commit to packages or subscriptions are very likely to renew without much forethought. This gives the provider a very good basis for predicting revenue from these patients and services in the next year and thereafter. He did not agree. He asked, "How can I expect that a year or more from now, the same services will be attractive to the same people, and that they will want to receive these services from me?"

If you do not have the confidence to believe that after a year passes you will remain an attractive provider of services to your patients, you have a big problem. Thoroughly examine your image, brand, and mission. If you are not confident that patients will want to repeat services to maintain benefits over time, do you really believe in the value of the services you provide?

When you are confident of yourself and your services, you convey this and others accept it. When you lack confidence you convey that, and your efforts will not just falter once, but will continue to slide.

Know your patients and market. Know their expectations. Meet these with confidence, and the advantage is yours. Moreover, if you are going to offer "flavor of the month" services, realize that you'll lose out on something very important to building a successful practice: consistency.

INDIVIDUAL CYCLES

People go through phases in life: we grow, age, graduate, marry, have children, age some more, our children grow, we age some more, we have grandchildren, we age further. A large component of aesthetic medicine is the treatment of the visible signs of aging, so the inevitable cycle of aging offers an advantage to the success of a practice in aesthetic medicine. However, there are caveats:

- On an individual level, the cycle must be one attached to someone you are already familiar with, namely, a loyal patient to your practice.

- On a targeted level to specific population groups, an interest in your services must be proven or must be measured.

The signs of aging are not the only cycles we go through as individuals. Women give birth; their bodies change. Men and women both change careers, partners in life, or motivations. Along with such alterations, individuals may want to improve their appearance, to make a fresh start in a new cycle of their lives. Cycles of aging require knowledge about the group in that cycle, and an individual patient's cycle requires careful discovery, planning, and a thoughtful approach.

Recognize too that individual cycles are linked. A young mother who comes to you for breast augmentation suddenly finds that her mother desires facial rejuvenation, her spouse wants to chisel his love handles, and her sister hopes to feel the same satisfaction the patient felt as a result of your care. An adolescent whose acne is cleared by your care finds that his mother wants the same hands to improve her acne scars or that a close friend wants her acne treated. The young woman who finds new freedom when her saddle-bag thighs have been reshaped has a sister who wants her leg veins treated, a mother who wishes to have her neck rejuvenated, and an aunt who desires a tummy tuck.

So how do you use these linked cycles to your advantage? Through the same methods you use to make every private opportunity advantageous. Practice with as much skill and excellence as you put into communication and compassion. Make education accessible, unique to your practice image, brand, and mission. Extend education at every possible opportunity. Build practice relationships not just for immediate satisfaction, but also for long-term satisfaction and trust. These efforts will translate to making you the one and only choice for many links in individual cycles and will bring you the advantage of trust, retention, and traffic through referrals.

Although ads can enhance your visibility, you cannot achieve such results through advertising alone. You cannot garner success through media relations alone, although that can enhance your visibility and credibility. However, through outreach efforts within your office and with the individuals you treat, you can effectively convey these things and discover some of your greatest opportunities for growth.

🌿 IN PRACTICE: Exclusively Yours

I know a provider who excels at turning individual cycles into service. He may not personally initiate the opportunity, but he contributes significantly. His practice is notable for its belief in and nurturing of long-term relationships. Paired with his attention to individual service, this approach continues to enhance his success.

He never allows a patient's birthday to go unnoticed, sending key patients messages directed specifically to that individual's stage in the life cycle. At age 30, the birthday message includes a gift certificate for personal service in skin care. At age 35, it includes an incentive for noninvasive rejuvenation. At age 45, he sends well-loved patients a book on aging. At age 55, he sends another.

When younger patients expand their families or older patients become grandparents, he takes note. He invites mom and baby to come in, and he personally takes great joy in the presence of children. This works to his advantage, because mothers and grandmothers revel in the attention he extends this new little person. They also take in the self-enhancement messages that his office very strategically displays.

When personal cycles present, this provider's actions are as unique as the man himself. He might not acknowledge an opportunity when it appears, but within a few short days, he acts in a most dignified and caring way: with a personal note and direct education that addresses the needs of the individual. He takes every opportunity to personally connect, which necessarily includes his services as a reason or a benefit of the connection.

Continued

IN PRACTICE: Exclusively Yours—cont'd

He also shows care and compassion beyond individual cycles of aging and linked cycles. His practice is not solely dedicated to aesthetic medicine; he treats cancer patients as well. We all know that cancer can have hereditary links, and in the case of skin cancer, behavioral/lifestyle links also exist. He takes every opportunity to address his patients' individual health cycles as well as those of their families.

For some this approach may seem extreme, and there are certainly some delicate issues of tact and privacy. The efforts of this practice may not be appropriate for you. However, this provider's methods illustrate that every practice can find a niche in which to serve the interests of its patients and target audience in a manner that is welcomed.

These examples also demonstrate that when you are fulfilling the most personal desires of others, you have the opportunity to do more than just provide medical treatment. You can build an enduring and very personal relationship founded on that care. Personal trust, desire, endorsement, and devotion—it is all attainable, and essential to your success.

Cycles perpetuate, but do not make the mistake of letting your wheels spin. Although cycles can define when some of the greatest advantages to the success of a practice exist, over time they evolve and change. How you address cycles must meet that evolution and address change. Further, cycles are only one component of when advantage exists. If you do not plan for and maximize all of your efforts concerning cycles, you will not maximize the value of your abilities or your success.

SOCIAL CYCLES

Social cycles are the positive and negative events that repeat themselves, sometimes predictably, sometimes seasonally, sometimes unexpectedly, and often with a great impact on the way we do business. Social cycles can have an influence on your practice's balance sheet, if you let them. But if your practice is truly focused on care of the individual, your practice will thrive on attracting and reaching the individual, regardless of the social cycle.

Business and Economics

The stock market, interest rates, consumer price index, the price of gold, gasoline, and even groceries are often used as indicators of cycles of prosperity, growth, recession, depression, and recovery. Business and economics influence your practice not through the need to adjust prices to meet a standard, but through the need to adjust your expectations, exceed the expectations of those willing to invest in your services, and to realize that at no time is excess pessimism or greed appropriate.

Politics

Right or left, liberal or conservative, conservationist or consumptionist, capitalist or socialist, just as political views change, so too do the cycles that accompany them. You don't need to change your views or your political preferences, but realize that these cycles can and will influence your practice.

Entertainment

Actress Angelina Jolie is popular, so women patients often request that their lips be shaped like hers. Actor Hugh Jackman is seen on the big screen shirtless, flexing his muscles, and therefore men want their pectoral muscles to resemble his. When "Baywatch" aired weekly on television, everyone wanted a hard body; today's "What Not to Wear" fans are more worried about clothing than what is underneath. Entertainment has cycles. Hollywood and the media go through alternating periods of attention to skin, faces, breasts, and bodies, and cycles of emphasis on twig-thin shapes followed by years in which voluptuousness is extolled. Celebrities are applauded for the things they do to look fabulous at a given age, while others announce their intention to age sensibly and gracefully.

The cycles of what is in vogue are difficult to predict and may change overnight. It is best to avoid being associated with the trend of the moment and simply focus on the needs of the individual. Because tomorrow, it may be Miley's lips instead of Angelina's.

🌾 RELATIVE WISDOM: The Cycle of History

Historic events may not relate directly to your practice, but they can influence existing cycles and certainly can hinder or create opportunity.

I was not born when President Kennedy was shot, but those who were alive remember the day well. My first memory of any historic event is of seeing President Nixon get on a helicopter making his famed sign of victory and my father trying to explain to a 5-year-old what had transpired. The day the Berlin Wall came down was the only time I ever saw my grandfather cry as he watched in disbelief and relief that the world he ran from to save his family and his life was once again a united world. September 11, 2001, was my eldest son Nicholas's first day of preschool, and although I should recall that day for the cycle in my son's life, I will never forget the cycle it began for a nation and for our world.

The day I spoke in Chicago before the plastic surgery assistants group was election day 2008. The city was abuzz, preparing for Barack Obama's election night rally that would become his victory celebration. As I write this book, the country and the world teeter on an economy built on pillars of salt and pillars of sand.

These events in history are memorable, but they also can influence society, the economy, the interests of individuals, and certainly your practice. What is significant in these cycles is that as a provider you must be alert to the way they influence your patients. As a proprietor you must make certain these cycles do not adversely influence your practice and operations. In fact, some may present opportunity, but be careful of how you spin that opportunity.

Earlier in this book I referred to an ad for aesthetic medical services that touted discounts on service to stimulate the economy. A poor approach, but not in theory. Certainly economic theory implies that if one sector gets moving, others will begin to rebound as spending stimulates spending. But do you discount medical service to get an economy moving?

You might use the opportunity to encourage your audience to invest in themselves when other investments offer little return. You would not directly communicate this in your message, or you could be perceived as an opportunist by your target audience, but such messages can find their way to help fuel an interest that already exists.

After 9/11, the concept of cocooning became a comforting idea. We all retreated into the safety and privacy of our homes; home and family became a societal focus. There are theories that those who were children at the time of this event will use their experience as a basis for defining their generation as one that is very private and individual.

Did you, your practice, or your patients use this experience, or any other experience, to shape the efforts and direction of your relationships? Should these types of events influence your practice? Do you need to recognize when they have the potential to and when they actually do influence your patients?

When history influences individual behavior, and your practice is devoted to serving individuals' most personal desires, you can be certain that history will influence you. However, using this to visibly play or prey on how history has influenced others is simply wrong. You cannot pretend history has not influenced circumstances, but you can and should only address those circumstances individually. Do not specifically address the cycle in history, because when you look at any historical event that truly changes people, it probably carries some negativity. And negativity does not belong anywhere in the practice of aesthetics.

The greatest example of this as it applies to aesthetic medicine is a cycle in the late 1980s and early 1990s: the silicone-gel breast implant crisis. Media and our society, and even medical societies, called it that—a crisis. And calling it that made it that.

It created alarm where alarm was not needed. It raised public outcry that could have ruined an industry, but when providers, medical societies, and the implant manufacturers took the stand early on to address this, they did absolutely the right thing. They avoided the negativity of this historic moment in health care. They focused on the desires of the individual, and they emerged to find themselves in an era in which the core of their practice, aesthetic medicine, is held in higher regard, is more accepted, and its services are growing in demand so rapidly that this may soon exceed the specialty's ability to serve it. Now, one decade later, silicone breast implants are no longer news; they are a choice for women in personal cycles of makeovers or breast cancer reconstruction, or in clinical cycles in which prior implants need to be replaced.

CHAPTER 15

When Do You Practice Privacy?

Show me someone who never gossips,
and I will show you someone who is not interested in people.
— BARBARA WALTERS

Humans have a need for privacy that is physical as well as emotional. We need private space, our own emotions, and issues and agendas that are ours alone. A physician must recognize, respect, nurture, and most of all, practice privacy. Despite Ms. Walters' amusing quip above, a physician is in the business of fulfilling people's personal goals, and although you should be deeply interested in your patients, you must *never* gossip.

When do you practice privacy? All of the time. Why? Because you are in a specialty devoted to serving the individual and his or her personal desires. That in itself is a very private matter.

We all require privacy: we protect the space around us, into which we allow only those we trust. The desire for privacy includes the need to sometimes guard our true feelings from others. We all have secrets that we keep about ourselves or one another—not things we are ashamed of, just matters we choose not to share.

Although we cherish privacy, we live in an information age where gathering private information about others is easy to do. Protecting privacy is more difficult today than ever before; therefore its value is even greater.

The U.S. Health Insurance Portability and Accountability Act of 1996 (HIPAA) imposed the Privacy Procedural Enforcement Rule, which took effect on April 15, 2003. This rule left medical practices scrambling to enforce new procedures and process paperwork designed to protect patient privacy in a provider's office and govern the use and transfer of information in patient records.

Although you may practice only nonpayor services and do not deal with any health care insurance, you are still bound by HIPAA regulations. For example:

- You prescribe a preoperative or postoperative medication that is narcotic. When the prescription is filled at your patient's pharmacy, the transaction is automatically reported to his insurer based on a prescription drug plan. The insurer later contacts you to find out why the drug was prescribed.

- You require preoperative HIV testing that could result in your obligation to report findings to health services agencies.

- A patient has complications that result in the need for emergency care.

These are all examples of cases in which the HIPAA rules apply and why, although you may not accept or provide payor services, you still must respect and practice privacy as it relates to health care information.

In aesthetic medicine, however, protecting a patient's privacy encompasses more than HIPAA regulations. Recognizing, respecting, and nurturing privacy is essential to your success and to your existence as a provider of medical treatment. Whether a procedure is simple and noninvasive or is surgical and intimate in nature, you and your staff must foster an awareness and respect for patient privacy, specifically with regard to:

- Direct encounters
- Consultation
- Treatment
- Communication

Although every patient has a different need for or expectation of privacy, it would be a grave error to take any aspect of privacy for granted. Further, privacy does not apply solely to the individual you are treating at the moment. Privacy must apply to any individual your practice has served or encountered in any way.

DIRECT ENCOUNTERS

When two or more individuals connect in some manner—visually, verbally, or physically—the encounter is direct. Direct encounters may occur in your office or in public places. They may occur between you and prospective or existing clients or patients, between you and your staff, between staff and clients or patients, and between clients and patients themselves.

Any direct encounter, particularly in your office, must foster privacy. Walking in the door, checking in with the receptionist, and even being seated in the waiting area should allow an individual to remain anonymous to anyone other than your staff. Of course, you cannot protect the privacy of your patients if you schedule them so that multiple patients are waiting at the same time; therefore adjust your scheduling practices or have patients escorted to a private room on arrival. This should provide individuals with a comfortable space to distance themselves from others and a private moment in which to complete or review documents. In some cases you may even need to provide individuals with a discreet, private entrance to your office. Likewise, leaving your office should afford the same respect for privacy.

Outside the office, you may encounter a past or current client or patient, as might members of your staff. Should you acknowledge the individual? To ignore the encounter is rude; to acknowledge it might violate privacy. A subtle smile and a nod of the head is something we direct even to strangers we pass. In doing this, you are not violating privacy, nor are you being rude. You are letting the client or patient choose how to respond.

How do you preserve privacy in direct encounters when they progress to conversations? Again, by letting the other party take the lead. It is reasonable to return a greeting or ask how the other person is, but do not go beyond that with anything other than small talk, even if the client or patient leads you there, because others around you may be listening. Do you want them to think that the discussion you are having as a result of a direct encounter in a public place is acceptable and common in your standard of privacy?

RELATIVE WISDOM: An Enthusiastic Crowd

A provider of aesthetic medicine belongs to the same fitness club I do. Some of his patients work there, and work out there as well. However, many of those who work and work out there would never be his patients.

Why? Because every time those patients who adore him (and they should; he fulfilled their personal desires) stop to say hello, the conversation leads to private details about that person's case or current phase in life. He is very social and is complimentary to these people. He loves the attention, and so do they, but his volubility makes many people question his standard of privacy.

There is another provider of aesthetic medicine at the same club. He is a model of discretion. He nods and says hello cordially to many people, goes about his business in a very polite but private manner, and no one could guess who among the crowd are his patients and what he has done to improve their appearance. I often wondered what would happen if someone approached him to engage in a conversation about his profession, but I never saw this happen. So one day, as we were both walking out the door, I decided to ask.

His reply was an indicator of why he is successful: "I keep my private and professional lives separate, and when I am in public, I mind my own business," he said. "My patients know and respect that." This is a man who is very clear about his image, brand, and mission as it relates to privacy.

Relative wisdom: While a public persona is important to let others know who you are, protecting the privacy of those you treat is an even more important message.

PRIVACY IN CONSULTATION

Although a consultation takes place in a closed, private room, very significant privacy considerations are involved. From the moment an individual enters that room, he or she will be sharing with you and your staff details of a personal desire to enhance appearance. The entire encounter should support the privacy the person has a right to expect in entrusting very personal information to you.

Consultations include three specific privacy considerations: those for the individual, the examination, and photographs. They also require that you ensure privacy for the individual physically, emotionally, and with regard to any information that person shares with you or that you discover.

The fact that medical information must remain private except when the patient signs a specific release is an industry standard, but other information may be discovered during consultation, such as the individual's motivation, expectations, outcomes, personal issues, agendas, and insights. This information requires even greater respect for privacy, because it is relative only to you and the patient. Rarely does such information need to be conveyed to anyone else, except perhaps a referring physician.

The emotions patients attach to the desire for which they have engaged you as well as the emotions attached to the consultation itself need to remain private. I do not know how many times I have heard practitioners discuss the emotions of their patients, although they do not mention names. A consultation is designed to focus on the desire of the individual; therefore you should focus on that individual's emotions and needs. Although you may find that examples from similar cases are beneficial to share, it is inappropriate to share anecdotes about other patients' emotions. Feelings are highly personal; no person's experience should ever be shared with another.

Physical examination requires that you enter someone's personal space. You must touch the individual, and this is an intimate and intimidating experience for some people. Examining a woman's breast or a man's love handles may be routine for you, but she or he might find the experience very uncomfortable. To ensure privacy in examination, you must:

- Allow patients to dress or undress in private; they should be undressed only during the examination portion of the consultation.

- Exhibit good manners. Knock on the door before entering, ask patients if you may touch them to examine them, and look at them when you speak. Keep a chaperone in the room to take notes, to hold a hand, or to simply be there to assist if the physician requires it.

- Set an appropriate tone. Do not use the examination for anything other than that—a discovery of the physical conditions present. Do not discuss anything other than what you find on examination; wait to discuss a recommended course of treatment after the examination. Do not try to use small talk to make an awkward situation a little less tense.

Taking photographs as part of the consultation invades the patient's privacy, yet it is necessary. So how do you nurture privacy when photography requires intimate documentation? First, explain why the photographs are necessary: they aid the patient to understand the goals of surgery and provide a baseline against which postoperative results can be seen. They benefit the provider by tracking treatment that requires multiple cycles or function as a reference during a surgical procedure. Second, be very specific about photographic releases, allowing the patient to determine whether photographs can be used for specific and clearly defined reasons other than for patient benefit and provider reference. Third, use existing patient photos to demonstrate outcomes with candor, respect, and in a positive manner. Do not use patient photos to point out what is wrong; use them to illustrate improvements and positive outcomes. Respect the privacy of the individuals who do allow you to use their photographs for patient education. In doing so, you will demonstrate your standards, and others will not hesitate to allow you to use their photographs for patient education.

Today imaging and video are being introduced to support the consultation. Video in particular allows a 360-degree view of the individual preoperatively and postoperatively. Imaging must be clearly defined as a communication tool, not as an approximation of results. Video must be defined as a means of documentation. The same standards of privacy must be ensured as with still photography, and equivalent consents must be documented. If the patient's preoperative photos are used to produce computer simulations to demonstrate the planned changes as a part of the consultation, it must be clearly stated that these images do not represent an approximation of results.

Whatever imaging method is employed, realize how vulnerable patients feel in this circumstance; do not ask them to walk them down the hall in a state of semidress to a room with glaring photographer's lights and unnerving flashes. If the patient must be photographed with intimate parts of the body exposed, explain the reason for such photos. Do not physically touch patients to move them where you need them; instruct them gently as to the appropriate positioning. If you know the lights will flash and the documentation does not require seeing the patient's eyes, suggest that he or she close the eyes. If you must photograph the individual in paper panties, keep these on for the shortest period of time—not for examination, not for any reason other than for taking the photographs.

IN PRACTICE: Mean Old Lady

I had a client who attached descriptors to some of his patients' photos. He labeled one preoperative photo in particular as a "mean old lady." Every time he said this, I cringed. What were those he was speaking to thinking?

When I approached him about this, he first said that no one seemed offended by his actions and that the woman herself labeled her appearance as "mean" in the preoperative images. As we discussed it further, though, he realized my alarm was well founded.

Although others might not immediately express an objection to such labels, at some point they would think it. That moment would likely be when they were about to sign a photo release form and were pondering how this provider would label their photographs. Name-calling is immature at best. What is most important, through his words this provider was violating something essential to fulfilling his vocation in aesthetic medicine: he was being negative.

This woman allowed the physician to include those photographs as a patient education tool, yet the provider's words lacked even a modicum of respect for that woman's privacy. You are the guardian of your patient's privacy, even in the use of photographs.

PRIVACY IN TREATMENT

Your patients are most intimately exposed and vulnerable when you are directly treating them, whether the treatment is invasive or not. During the course of treatment, the patient is never in an attractive state or position. Obviously, appearance is something that is of value to that individual, or he or she would not have come to you for appearance enhancement. How do you make your patients comfortable, less anxious, and help them feel less exposed? By ensuring privacy.

Privacy in treatment requires a greater effort and a more sensitive perspective than privacy in consultation, because any course of treatment is more intimate and intimidating than consultation alone. First, by accepting treatment the individual has acknowledged personal dissatisfaction with some aspect of his or her appearance, and that can weaken self-confidence. Second, by accepting treatment the individual is empowering you to alter or improve appearance in some way. The person is risking more than a bad haircut that will grow out or a poor fashion choice that can be returned or discarded; the results of an aesthetic procedure can be permanent, and outcomes are never fully predictable. Even if you have done an excellent job of educating the patient so that he or she confidently accepts treatment, there is still a bit of uncertainty that can make the patient feel even more vulnerable. Third, in many cases there will be people present during the treatment other than you, the trusted physician with whom the patient has built a relationship. To protect privacy and support the connection you've made with patients, all of these individuals should be introduced to the patient before treatment, and each of these individuals needs to respect and nurture your patient's need for privacy and comfort.

Invasive Treatment

In cases in which anesthesia is involved, a patient will likely not know the process that occurs during treatment. Nevertheless, you should respect this individual's privacy, even though he or she cannot hear you and is not aware of your actions. Your staff can hear and see you, and you must set an example by exhibiting the same standards of respect and privacy in this circumstance.

A patient should not awaken to find a urinary catheter in place that he or she was not told about in the preoperative preparations. Patients should not be dressed or undressed or have to wait, awaken, or recover in common areas or be in visual or auditory proximity to other patients. Before, during, and after treatment, and if necessary, on the way out the door, the patient should be isolated from anyone or anything not directly connected with that treatment.

Noninvasive Treatment

Even when a treatment is noninvasive and the patient is fully ambulatory before, during, and after treatment, you must still protect privacy. Allow the individual a quiet moment or two before treatment to collect his or her thoughts. While preparing for treatment, discuss with the patient what you are doing. While administering treatment and as you discuss the course of treatment with your clinical staff, do so in a manner that the patient can understand. Finally, when treatment is completed, allow the patient a few private moments to dress, groom, or apply makeup. Allow the patient to exit a treatment room when he or she is prepared to leave, not simply when your job is done. With any form of treatment, invasive or noninvasive, a gentle but firm touch of the hand, kind and encouraging words from you and the staff, and a direct focus on the case at hand will demonstrate your commitment to the individual and privacy.

EXPERIENCE MATTERS

Did you ever wonder what patients are thinking as they prepare for treatment and what cues they pick up from the environment?

Do the fast movements of staff, the disconnected conversations, the clinking and clanging of instruments, the unfamiliar smells, and the echoes of treatment rooms resemble an automotive repair shop?

Are instruments laid out—shiny, sharp, intimidating metal objects, including needles—right before your patient, with no explanation of what the instruments are for, and no notice to an awake patient before you use them?

Do you mark your patients preoperatively without telling them why or what you are marking? Do you describe the markings as you do them, but

Continued

EXPERIENCE MATTERS—cont'd

address only clinical staff, as if the patient were not there? Do you mark them when they are sedated so that when they awake, they wonder what all the ink is for?

Do you sedate patients and then strap them to the table? Do you catheterize them but fail to tell them beforehand? Are they semidraped and chilly when they awaken?

Do you make certain that waiting loved ones are updated as treatment progresses, even if the procedure is going well and is on track? Do you speak to their family members as soon as the treatment is completed and your patient is moved to a recovery area?

Are you the last person your patient sees before he or she leaves the facility? Do you reinforce all of their responsibilities that are essential to good outcomes and safe recovery?

The best way to judge just where you succeed and where you fail in preserving privacy and upholding individual patient respect and comfort is to measure patient satisfaction in all these areas, to encourage direct feedback on their experiences, and to use this information effectively. How can you improve without feedback from those you serve? The best means to continually improve your practice is to ask patients whether their expectations were met or exceeded—or if and how you failed.

PRIVACY IN COMMUNICATION

When you communicate with your patients one-on-one behind closed doors, you may suppose that privacy is not an issue. Maybe, maybe not. Ask a staff member to sit in an empty room adjacent to the room in which you might typically conduct consultations or examinations. Can he or she hear what is transpiring in the next room, or the room directly behind that room?

Medical practice examination rooms notoriously echo. Footsteps and voices in the hall carry. Might these have a significant impact on your practice? Probably not, but they will be something patients remember and carry with them, and it may inhibit them from freely expressing their desires, objectives, and motivation.

When is it appropriate to carefully evaluate the need for and influence of privacy in your communication?

- When communication is specific to the individual and exists anywhere other than behind closed doors

- When communication is specific to a case and is directed toward anyone including the subject of that case

- When communication is directed to an audience with whom you do or do not have an established relationship

Patient-Specific Privacy

Respecting and upholding privacy in communication with an individual begins the moment he or she engages your practice. As soon as the person introduces himself or herself, it is your responsibility to immediately obtain this individual's contact information and the method and manner in which that patient prefers you to communicate with him or her, such as the best phone number to reach the patient, where messages can be left, and with whom and at what time it is best to call. This is as essential as knowing that individual's name and how he or she prefers to be addressed (Mary? Mrs. Smith? Ms. Jones?). This information is as essential to protecting privacy as it is to maximizing the value of your communication efforts with this person.

However, gathering information, recording it, and using it effectively are three different issues. In many practices, patient information is collected, then placed in a hanging file. If the information is not recorded electronically, it has no value for use in building a database.

If retention is essential to your success in continued or added services and in referral, and the core of this is visibility through ongoing communication with those who know and trust you, how will you succeed if you do not communicate with existing clients and patients in the manner they prefer, such as email, telephone, or direct mail, or solicitation preferences. The communication efforts you plan will fail if they do not meet the audience's communication preferences, including their desire for privacy.

Case-Specific Privacy

Communication specific to a case exists between the provider and patient, between the provider and staff, between the provider and a referral source when it is another physician, and between the provider and patients other than the individual you are treating.

To educate other patients, you need to communicate information about specific cases to them about other patients' cases. Speaking in generalities and presenting an overview of a procedure is important, but direct examples, including patient photos, are the most effective means of illustrating your skills and demonstrating theory and potential outcomes.

Respecting and ensuring privacy in these situations requires that you focus strictly on the relevant clinical facts as they apply to the individual in consultation or the case you are illustrating. Educational tools such as patient photos must be displayed in a manner that does not reveal the patient's identity. For the use of such teaching aids as photos, you must have signed releases on file, because photos and case histories must be completely anonymous.

Upholding privacy also requires that you transmit only essential knowledge about the case to staff members, other providers, and patients you are educating. Do not editorialize or offer an opinion unless that opinion is a professionally recommended course of treatment. Do not characterize the case under discussion by using labels such as "clearly overbaked" regarding someone's sun exposure, or "nice grandma" to refer to a woman in her senior years. Sometimes we casually use labels to categorize things in our own terms of judgment or familiarity, but using such labels in your practices is a breach of privacy—and good taste.

Audience-Specific Privacy

You and your staff should not send messages that are highly personal to people you do not know. You do not want your practice or your communication to be unwelcome or to appear misguided. Make certain you respect your audience's communication preferences and privacy. For example, if you send all patients in a certain treatment category a relevant clinical update, make certain the information is correct as to target and substance. Build a database on individual patients' communication preferences and apply these when you target patients as a group.

IN PRACTICE: Messy Matters

The relationship a patient develops with you is personal and based on trust; the foundation on which you provide care is built on that individual's personal desire and the trust he or she has in you to fulfill that desire. There are times when that trust transcends the immediate course of treatment, and as a caring provider, you might find yourself caught in the middle.

A young woman and her much older fiancé arrived in a provider's office. The woman was seeking a specific treatment. Both were candid by all appearances: she in her desire for treatment and he in his support of her personal desire.

After the consultation, she agreed to treatment. Several days later, she called the office wanting to speak to the provider. She was having second thoughts. She left a message with her cell phone number for the doctor to call her back.

The provider called her back on her home phone as listed in her chart, rather than on the cell phone. Her fiancé answered. The provider asked to speak to the woman, but she was unavailable. The fiancé asked the reason for the call and if he could take a message. The provider noted that he was returning her call. As a cautious and caring provider, he wanted to discuss her concerns with her.

Two weeks later, the provider was slapped with a lawsuit. The woman's concerns were that she was not certain if the procedure was right for her, and she was being pushed by an adamant partner's desire, not her own. By speaking with the fiancé, albeit briefly, the provider unknowingly came between the patient and her fiancé and violated the woman's privacy.

The lesson here is one I know you recognize right away. Never discuss a patient's case with anyone but the patient. The provider here thought his actions were innocuous. The couple seemed to be a happy and mutually supportive couple. Their initial visit presented no hint of the woman's true feelings. Regardless, the damage was done.

SECTION V
Why

First, have a definite, clear, practical ideal; a goal,
an objective. Second, have the necessary means to achieve
your ends; wisdom, money, materials, and methods.
Third, adjust all your means to that end.

— ARISTOTLE

CHAPTER 16

Why Do You Practice? Your Business, Your Goals

I want to be remembered as the guy who gave his all on the field.

— WALTER PAYTON,
NFL HALL OF FAME RUNNING BACK

Your practice is your vocation; it is also a business, and its success is a goal you set for yourself years ago. You found the money to pay for your education, earned your credentials and perfected your skills, and gathered the wherewithal to open your practice. The materials and methods you use daily to attract, educate, and treat your patients are collectively aimed at a single goal. Your goals may include personal and professional fulfillment, money, celebrity, survival, commitment to your vocation, or the satisfaction you receive in seeing the happiness of those you treat. There are times when you must adjust your goals because of economic conditions, limited resources, or a transition in your life or practice.

Goals are essential in business and in life to give us direction and a benchmark against which to measure our ambitions and accomplishments. To set unrealistic goals is to guarantee failure. To define realistic, attainable goals you must be candid, objective, and pragmatic.

In aesthetic medicine, each goal achieved through traffic, conversion, retention, and revenue contributes to your success. Measuring your progress toward achieving your goals is of little value if you do not focus on the core goal of aesthetic medicine: fulfilling the desires of individuals to improve their appearance and enhance their life.

Your broadest goal is likely to be to run an active, lucrative practice. How you define "active" is subjective, based on the amount of time you wish to and need to work. Work encompasses the time you spend providing care and service as well as in administrative and nonservice functions. It is the total commitment of time and labor you are willing to make to your practice.

You may think that the first goals you set relate to traffic, conversion, and retention, but initially you must define your ultimate goal: what your expectations are for your practice as a whole. You may measure this in revenue, or in productivity. Goals may also be defined by growth, pace, personal fulfillment, research, and innovation, perhaps even in an arc of time culminating in retirement from active practice to allow you to pursue other goals.

IN PRACTICE: A Different Game

When I was 5, I met a man who would one day provide a valued lesson to my professional life. He began his career as a medical specialist in the 1970s, when aesthetic medicine was a novelty. He and his practice have matured and evolved, keeping pace with technology, innovation, and patient demands. In writing this book, I asked him how he developed into a provider in an almost purely aesthetic practice. What were his goals, and what did he value most?

High-priced leases, high-pressure staff, and high visibility were not part of his image, he told me. They were not essential. High revenue was not his main goal. Revenue comes with commitment and skill.

I wondered, what then was his ultimate goal? He told me it was the smile of every patient whose life he had enhanced through his skill and care. Where others defined goals in terms of revenue and productivity, he defined his in pure emotion. His commitment to the joy and satisfaction of helping others fulfill their goals was all he needed to fuel his practice. His game was won not by numbers, but by smiles.

What I learned from this man is something no practitioner of aesthetic medicine should ever allow to wane. First, your goals must be uniquely yours. Although practice success is commonly defined in revenue and personal success in wealth, not everyone values these goals similarly. Moreover, whereas the ultimate business goal of your practice may be a measure of profitability or a defined number of procedures or hours billed, you must never lose sight of the reasons you chose to become a provider of aesthetic medicine: to enhance the lives of those you have chosen to serve by fulfilling their personal goals.

BENCHMARKING

The process of comparing the volume, cost, traffic, retention of one practice, provider, or product against similar entities is *benchmarking*. A number of benchmarking studies exist, and many doctors hire consultants to benchmark, or evaluate, how well the practice is performing against others. Benchmarking has great value when it is used to measure vital elements of the practice, such as adverse events, good outcomes, repeat procedures, or even selection of one product or procedure over another.

However, benchmarking can be counterproductive if it leads you to feel less than adequate and stressed by supposedly underperforming—not meeting or beating the competition by some arbitrary number that has no direct relation to good outcomes and patient satisfaction. Benchmarking has been used to compare overhead, salaries, revenue, retail sales, retention, and more. Although this can provide useful comparative data, where it falls short in every case is in pointing to the source of discrepancy. If you don't collect data specifically about your own practice, you may receive an indicator that you don't measure up by some generic standard, but that won't give you the reason, or help you correct the problem.

TRAFFIC

Traffic refers to anyone who comes in contact with you and your practice. It is essential to understand this general definition; your image must be consistent in every contact. As has been stated, the greatest opportunity to build an aesthetic practice lies in referrals. Referrals can come from planned or unplanned exposure, from resources and sources, and from your clients, patients, accompanying friends or relatives, staff, sales reps, service reps, and neighbors. Those people will carry an image of you and your practice that must be congruent with your mission in providing care. Everyone in your practice must treat all traffic in a manner consistent with your image and mission.

Measuring Traffic

Your greatest measure of traffic is of individuals who have expressed a direct interest in your practice or services. This traffic is measured first, quantitatively:

- How many calls of interest are received daily, weekly, and monthly?

- How many consultations are scheduled daily, weekly, and monthly?

- How many consultations are held daily, weekly, and monthly?

- How many consultations are cancelled, daily, weekly, and monthly?

- How many are existing patients, how many are newcomers?

This provides a quantitative assessment. Today's sophisticated scheduling software can be used to measure and provide reports on consultations. Staff members should have a standard procedure for gathering information on all serious inquiries into your practice data software to measure legitimate traffic inquiries about services.

If the number of calls of interest is disproportionately high compared with the number of consultations or initial office visits, you have identified a problem. The problem may be rooted in any number of areas: staff response, scheduling, pricing, or misinformation. These are all likely but not exclusive sources. Find the reason for this problem and correct it. Likewise, the number of consultations or initial office visits scheduled compared with the number of appointments kept should be relatively consistent. A high number of cancellations requires investigation as to the cause so you can correct the problem.

Daily, weekly, and monthly traffic can be tabulated to monitor trends and measure performance. Monthly trends can be compiled into annual cycles to track broader trends. Interest and traffic may have established patterns from year to year. Addressing these patterns through communication with target populations and with existing clients and patients can further enhance the level of traffic and service at peak times and build interest during off-peak times through targeted communication efforts.

Monitoring quantitative traffic trends is most beneficial in determining what external communication and outreach your prospective patients either noticed or sought out; measuring performance is most beneficial to assessing internal communication and operations. On a daily basis, measuring traffic provides valuable information about:

- The performance of key contact employees, such as receptionists. This is essential to identify the strengths and weaknesses of those who provide the first impression of your practice. For example, if you notice that each Monday and Wednesday you schedule more appointments than on any other day, could the reason be the person answering the telephone on those days?

- The influence of any external communication, such as the public's response to advertising, media coverage, or other outreach efforts. If you notice more calls on Monday and Wednesday, is it because you run ads on Sunday and Tuesday?

- Scheduling preferences and conflicts. Knowing when your traffic expects you to be available is an essential component of productivity. If Monday afternoon office visit and consultation schedules are never full, schedules should be revised to increase productivity.

- The effectiveness of cross-promotion. If the practice has more than one service sector or outside source for referral and with whom there is cross-promotion, you must identify which of these efforts or relationships has the greatest value. If you send every postoperative patient a gift certificate for aesthetician services or skin care, how many are using it, and if not, why not?

These are simple examples of quantifying traffic, but they demonstrate a means to measure the performance of your staff as well as your efforts to connect with prospective patients and current patients. When used in conjunction with a qualitative analysis of traffic, such measurements can create opportunities to improve performance and productivity.

Once individuals expressing a direct interest in your practice are quantified, they must be qualified.

- What source or resource prompted the client to contact you?

- What sources or resources provided the client background information on you?

These data are useful for tracking the source of interest in your practice. Other patients, other providers, advertising, outreach, and patient relations efforts are the most likely sources. Qualitative data also give you a sense of what tools your clients use to learn about you (such as websites, referral services, and directories). Rarely is only one source involved in connecting a prospective patient to you; even if someone receives a glowing recommendation about you from a satisfied patient or another physician, chances are that individual will research you on the Internet, look in a directory for your contact information, recall a media story or ad that featured you, or speak to another patient about you.

Qualifying the sources of traffic lets you know whether your efforts are succeeding. You can then redouble the efforts providing the greatest traffic and reevaluate efforts that do not provide consistent traffic. It is also vital that you show your appreciation to individual sources for referrals by other patients and physicians.

Part of achieving your goals requires collecting data to determine outcomes:

- How much interest should your practice generate?

- How much of that interest should result in a connection—a consultation or office visit?

- How much interest should referrals generate?

- How much interest should paid sources generate?

Determining answers to these questions will help you to model the communication vehicles, methods, and messages your practice uses to generate traffic; these answers will also help to establish communication goals and maximize your efforts. You will learn where time and money are profitably spent on your efforts.

Measuring traffic requires more than just determining what works. Without a measure of traffic, you do not have a basis for gauging conversion or retention, leading to a calculation of revenue and productivity and your ultimate business goal. Reaching your ultimate business goals requires assessment of multiple practice goals, beginning with traffic goals.

YOUR TRAFFIC EQUATION

No traffic equation, and no practice goal, should come from an outside, predefined standard. Specific benchmarks offered by consultants and accountants, unless they reflect the nuances of your practice, market, and goals, are useless at best, and counterproductive to your success at worst.

I don't know why almost all surgeons completing a fellowship believe their goal should be to spend half of their productive time in the operating room. I cannot find that equation in any medical book, yet I seem to find a lot of standardized equations and goals like this one that medical professionals take as gospel and struggle to accomplish. Just as you and your practice are a unique model, so should your equations and goals be defined by your individuality.

First, as a medical provider, you are not required to also be a detailed expert in practice development and management. However, as a provider and proprietor, you need to be savvy enough to hire the right people to help you build your success. Therein lies the key: your own model of productivity, revenue, and success—not an arbitrary standard.

Next you need to understand that your ultimate goal will be achieved through compounding goals of:

- Traffic
- Conversion and retention
- Productivity
- Revenue

Although these goals are achieved in this order, they are determined in reverse order.

Your traffic equation, or quantity, which will be determined last in your business plan, is simply the amount of interest your practice must generate to result in a connection—a consultation or an office visit—that will lead to conversion of a patient. You must have a traffic goal. The success of where and when you generate quality traffic is crucial. It is the most simply stated equation, yet it has a complex set of variables and opportunities that influence its attainment.

Tracking

I am often asked about software or systems for tracking traffic, conversion, and retention. The most sophisticated software systems are meaningless unless they are programmed and used correctly and applied consistently, and analysis of the data is essential.

Maximizing the function of your billing software will yield valuable data about your practice. All services, including nonpayor services, must have a numeric billing code, and in some cases, multiple codes. For example, treatment that requires multiple cycles to maintain results can have code modifiers to delineate what is the initial (xxx.1), second (xxx.2), or subsequent treatment, and so on. A clinical service that requires continuing cycles to maintain results again has its own code and modifiers for the first and subsequent visits.

Reports generated by sorting billing codes with these modifiers will indicate which patients have come in for initial treatment and have returned. This will pinpoint any weaknesses in your patient retention or communication systems. Data extracted from reports allow you to plan treatment cycles based on the average number of treatments patients undergo. You can also plan for productivity and budget for purchasing pharmaceuticals and supplies.

Any tracking system must be consistent and compatible to avoid duplication of tasks and data collection. All staff members should understand and consistently use tracking devices and procedures and keep data current.

IN PRACTICE: Traffic Lost and Found

It happens all the time. Someone calls the office asking for a specific procedure or treatment, and the person who answers the phone says, "No, we don't do that." I was visiting an office and standing near the phone when a staff member got one of these calls, and before she could say "Goodbye" after saying "No," I snatched the phone from her hands and completed this call. The caller was asking for a dermal filler that was not available in the United States. The staff member answering the phone had not heard of this filler and stated "No," because it was not on the fee schedule of the practice.

I asked the caller where she had heard of the filler, "I read about it online."

I asked, "What did you want this filler to achieve for you? There are several great options that are safe, approved, and that Doctor regularly uses, for which we have many happy patients."

"I want to reshape my butt; it's flat and it makes my thighs look big."

I responded, "You realize that dermal fillers to inject in the buttocks are costly, have not been tested for that purpose, and are far outside the scope of what is appropriate or safe use for these injections; in fact, they may be dangerous. Doctor prefers to shape buttocks with your own fat, in a process called fat grafting; the results are far more natural."

"I'm very thin; I don't have a lot of fat," she responded.

I told her, "Then an injected filler could give you a terribly unnatural result. By the way, how did you come to call us?"

"My mom has her lips done by Doctor."

This could have been traffic lost. It ended up being traffic found, because the thin young woman who wanted to fill out her buttocks actually became a

Continued

⚑ IN PRACTICE: Traffic Lost and Found—cont'd

thin young patient who had her thighs liposuctioned to bring a little more definition and balance to her otherwise small derriere and thin upper body.

Your staff should be taught to optimize each contact and opportunity. The treatment or procedure could be something unheard of, something you'd rather not hear about, or something you simply don't believe in. But if the person who called you took the time to seek you out and ask if you perform a specific procedure, doesn't he or she have a little more value to you than to simply respond with a flat "No"? Taking a few moments to explore the person's reason for contacting the practice not only projects your interest in the individual but also can lead to conversion to a satisfied client or patient.

When your office receives a call inquiring about a procedure or treatment, the person answering the phone should respond as follows:

- Never say "No" if you don't offer a specific procedure or have never heard of it; instead, ask about the caller's goals or desires.

- Never say "No," even if the procedure is something outlandish and out of the scope of your practice; ask how this person learned of your practice.

- Always inquire about where the person heard of the treatment and what he or she hopes to accomplish; there could be misinformation about your practice or the procedure that you can correct.

- Always ask where the person calling heard about your practice and what motivated him or her to connect with your practice.

- Always be polite, patient, and ready to educate, even if the call is the strangest you have encountered.

I know, calls can be startling. I've been there when a transvestite calls and asks if you will perform laser hair removal on his entire body. I've been there when someone asks if her 12-year-old is too young for lip augmentation. I've been there when the call comes asking if you carry "those candy implants" or the laser that shrinks skin. No matter how bizarre the call or the caller, find out why he or she contacted you. Then, with no other patients in earshot, and without judgment, have your laughs. Traffic lost can be traffic found, just make certain it is you who is laughing not your competitor down the street who took the time to listen and say more than "No."

CONVERSION

Conversion occurs when a client accepts your service and agrees to undergo aesthetic treatment with your practice. Conversion is quantified when someone converts to patient status—the individual agrees to your recommended course of treatment and price. However, conversion is not documented at the time of informed consent or actual treatment—conversion occurs at the time of acceptance. Why? Because when you quantify conversion at the time of treatment, you overlook the individuals who have accepted your service but for some reason declined to follow through. Tracking these individuals is essential to confirm that your conversion and retention methods are effective. If you experience more than a few instances of lost conversion (instances where an individual accepts and later declines your services), you must look for the cause in each case and the commonality among them.

Conversion must also be qualitatively measured; this is the most often overlooked goal or measure of nearly every practice. Qualitative measurement of conversion involves gauging patient satisfaction. It is the individual encounters that cumulatively shape an experience. It requires a dialog, and your success requires that qualitative measures of conversion be positive, even when clinical outcomes may not completely fulfill a patient's goals.

What good is it to convert a patient, only to have that conversion or course of treatment fall short on patient expectations? Not clinical *outcomes,* but *expectations of care.* The three greatest factors that can have an impact on your bottom line require that you consistently meet positive, qualitative measures of conversion:

1. *Patient satisfaction:* An unhappy patient may reveal more about you than a happy patient

2. *Opportunity for referral:* A patient who is fully satisfied with the outcome and experience has a greater potential to refer you than one who is just happy with the outcome

3. *Opportunity for retention:* A patient who is fully satisfied with the outcome and experience is more likely to return to you than one who is just happy with the outcome

It cannot be repeated enough: referral is the greatest resource for building your practice. If the result of your client-to-patient conversion is measured as a positive conversion, meaning your patient expresses fulfillment by undergoing treatment as your patient, you have likely won yourself a positive referral source. If the result of your client-to-patient conversion is measured as anything but a positive quality conversion, this patient will probably not recommend you to others. Only the most satisfied clients and patients will refer others to you, and personal referral by someone who has had a positive experience in your practice is better than any other source or resource for building your business.

Your Conversion Equation

Ideally, your conversion equation is 1:1, meaning that every individual who comes to you and is an appropriate candidate accepts treatment and converts to patient status. However, research indicates that most consumers of aesthetic medicine seek out more than one provider before making a decision; therefore projecting a 1:1 conversion for your practice is highly optimistic.

Your conversion equation should define a goal that compounds traffic through to productivity rather than simply serve as a ratio of individuals you should be converting to patients. The individuals of your traffic stream have varying interests and personal goals. The more comprehensive your personal goals are, the greater the likelihood that the time you invest in the conversion process, as well as the time you spend providing service, will be greater, thus generating revenue.

The time required to educate and convert an individual to patient status is in direct proportion to the amount of time the actual procedure requires and the amount of time an individual will invest to make a decision. For procedures that are less invasive, require little treatment time, and offer a short recovery period, your time investment to convert patients is limited, but the likelihood that the person will sign on should be higher. Few clients will invest a large amount of time in consultation with multiple providers for more limited procedures. In addition, many who request less-invasive procedures are seeking instant gratification.

For procedures that are invasive and require a greater client/patient invest-ment of discomfort, recovery, and money, your time to convert patients will be greater, and the likelihood one will sign on is lower. Most individuals in this category will invest as much time as necessary to feel completely as-sured that the provider and procedure are right for them. Therefore your conversion equations begins by defining the following:

1. The number of individuals who consult your practice for noninvasive, limited procedures in relation to the number of individuals who sign on to these procedures with your prac-tice. The equation is:

$$LPC : LPP$$

[limited procedure client : limited procedure patient]

Convert this ratio to a percentage by dividing your LPP by your LPC to get a limited procedure percentage, or LP%, of conversion. Do this by procedure, by provider, and by pro-cedure/provider, and you may learn who has strengths and weaknesses and in what areas.

2. The number of individuals who consult your practice for comprehensive, invasive procedures in relation to the num-ber of individuals who sign on to these procedures with your practice. The equation is:

$$IPC : IPP$$

[invasive procedure client: invasive procedure patient]

Convert this to a percentage by dividing your IPP by your IPC to get an invasive procedure percentage, or IP%, of con-version. Do this by procedure, by provider, and by core com-municator if you have more than one patient coordinator involved in the education of patients. It is important to know the reason someone did not convert; this will uncover weak-nesses in your process, in education, or any other variable that lends to making a conversion.

Now weigh these percentages against the relative value each has in your practice mix. For example, if your mix is 50% limited procedures and 50% invasive procedures, your final percentage of conversion will be simply an average or:

$$LP\% + IP\% \div 2$$

If your mix is 30% limited and 70% invasive, your final percentage of conversion will be:

$$3 \, (LP\%) + 7 \, (IP\%) \div 10$$

What this final number tells you is how productive your educational efforts are overall:

> If the number is 50%, then half of those you see in consultation convert to patient status.

> If the number is 80%, then four of every five you see in consultation convert to patient status.

> If the number is 20%, then one of every five you see in consultation converts to patient status.

Is there a measure of what the conversion percentage should be? Yes. It is, just like any component of the aesthetic medical practice plan, an individualized number that takes into account:

- The type of practice
- The maturity/reputation of the practice
- The practice's market location
- The practice's demographic target
- The practice's competition
- The provider's objectives
- Market cycles

Take all of these factors into account when analyzing your conversion percentage. You must ask yourself: Does my conversion ratio leave me as productive as I feel I can be? If it does not, then you need to determine where the problem exists:

- Is traffic too low to generate enough clients for conversion?

- Is conversion low—not generating enough patients?

- Is conversion volatile—patients not following through on treatment?

There is no magic equation for conversion, and although your goal for conversion is qualitative, it is the consistency of that numeric value and its comparison to your own internal expectations that has value rather than the number itself. Numbers are not answers; they provide clues to what may be right or not so right, and what needs to be assessed and improved. If you draw the line at measuring numeric nonconversions without finding out at what point there was a disconnect or for what reason the person chose not to convert, you'll miss an opportunity to evaluate your approach. You simply cannot become better if you don't know why you are not where you should be, and you cannot appreciate meeting your goals if you don't recognize how you arrived.

RETENTION

Retention is as important as referral. If a positive conversion is likely to generate referral, it will also likely result in future service to this patient. Consider these factors of consumer research that validate the importance of retention to your success:

- The majority of individuals who have had one aesthetic procedure will likely undergo future aesthetic procedures of the same or a different nature.

- Overall, the population of individuals undergoing aesthetic treatment is growing in range, particularly among younger populations.

- Noninvasive treatments are rapidly growing in demand and most often require repeated treatment to maximize or maintain results.

A patient whose quality of conversion was not positive will not remain with you. No patient will willingly pay for and undergo elective procedures with you a second time if the experience the first time is not a rewarding one; they will likely seek out your competition.

If patients are young, they will continue to pursue practitioners of aesthetic medicine who provide the quality conversion they seek, and they will likely remain with that provider in what could be a 40-year cycle as a consumer of aesthetic medicine. Moreover, if treatment is noninvasive with a repeating cycle, what likelihood is there that a patient will return for future treatment if the experience is not of high quality? Results with noninvasive procedures have limited variation in the hands of skilled practitioners. Therefore it is *the quality of the overall experience* that will define whether you retain a patient or not.

Measuring the quality of conversion will tell you if and where you fall short of providing a positive experience, even when clinical outcomes are favorable. This measure is your greatest indicator for improvement and your greatest indicator for referral and retention.

Your Retention Equation

The retention equation is not one simple measure and it is not necessarily simple to compose, because there are four categories for retention:

1. Completed services of multiple-cycle treatments: treatments that require multiple procedures over time to reach a final result

2. Ongoing services of nonpermanent treatments: treatments that must be repeated over specific intervals to maintain results

3. New or additional services recommended to patients who have completed a related course of treatment with your practice

4. New services to patients who have completed a nonrelated course of treatment with your practice

The goal is 100% retention in the first two categories. If retention is not complete, you need to find the cause:

- Is it incidental, such as a patient relocating or becoming ill?

- Is it procedure related—resulting from a poor result or unmet expectations?

- Is it practice related? Has a service failure occurred, and what specifically is that failure? (For example, is it difficult to book an appointment at a time that is advantageous for the patient?)

Once you identify the cause for lost retention, you must act. When it is incidental, find out how you can help, such as by referring the individual to a colleague in the new market or by expressing your concern for your patient's overall health. You are always a physician first; despite your specialty, your primary concern is the individual's health. If the lost retention is procedural, review the cases and correct what you can. When it is practice related, find the source, evaluate the impact it may have on your practice overall, and modify policy to address this.

The third category, new or additional recommended services to patients who have completed a related course of treatment, should also yield 100% conversion. However, the likelihood here is not as great. Why? Because recommended added services can sometimes be perceived by patients as salesmanship or as efforts to amend or improve poor treatment outcomes. Allaying this perception requires recommending any added services at the time of initial consultation as a component of treatment, not after treatment has occurred as an adjunct. Make it part of your initial-consultation agenda to discuss potential outcomes and added services that may be necessary following treatment to fully achieve the patient's goals; then a later suggestion regarding additional services will not come as a surprise during posttreatment evaluation.

The fourth category of retention, new services to patients who have completed a nonrelated course of treatment, should also be 100%. However, this category is very difficult to measure unless you maintain an ongoing relationship with patients after their course of treatment is complete. An ongoing relationship is best achieved through communication, personal services, and retail complements.

Even with an ongoing relationship, it takes a lot of effort to determine your rate of retention in this category. Rather than exhausting resources for what may be a very small margin, use your resources to maintain a relationship with your patients throughout their cycle as potential patients and potential sources for referral.

⚜ IN PRACTICE: Last-Minute Jitters

Every practitioner of aesthetic medicine has heard this, but when it happens to you, you may be blind to it.

A client of years past called me. His practice was doing so well that he had hired a second patient coordinator and was bringing on a new surgeon to help him manage his patient load. However, what was a booming patient load soon became a loss of conversion; numbers were below what the practice had experienced even in the toughest of times.

My first thought was to look at traffic and conversion trends. Recent traffic was high, as was conversion. However, productivity and conversion did not correlate. Cancellations were unusually high.

The cancellations had one commonality: they were all consultations with the new provider and his patient coordinator. I asked the office manager to spend some time making a few random calls to the cancellations to discuss their experience with the practice. "Why?" she asked. "They are already lost."

First, I said, they might not be lost. Second, even if they are lost, you need to find out why. Something had to happen to result in more than random cancellations.

It took only three telephone calls and three candid discussions to discover that each patient who cancelled experienced the exact same thing: anxiety. The patient coordinator was telling clients that the new provider was quickly gaining popularity and things were beginning to book quickly. Through these statements, individuals felt pressured to sign on quickly, which generally results in one of two things:

- Stress on the patient, who wonders whether he or she has acted too quickly

- Dissatisfaction among patients who did not take (or were pressured not to take) the time to fully consider and accept all possible outcomes

Had the practitioner measured conversion at the time of treatment rather than acceptance, these cancellations would have been overlooked. The resulting low conversion rate would likely have been attributed to poor education, not to pressure. Without qualitatively reviewing the lost conversions, the source for poor performance would have continued unnoticed, and the likelihood of success would have been threatened by pressure, undetected.

The lesson here: Conversion numbers are goals that compound to productivity. They should be measured at the time of acceptance, not at the time of treatment. Qualitative measures of conversion are greater indicators for improvement than numbers alone.

WHAT YOU KEEP

I know an accountant whose mantra is, "Wealth is not measured by what you earn, but rather by what you keep." Of course he is referring to money, but I apply this precisely to the practice of aesthetic medicine today, and I believe that the patients you keep are far more lucrative to your practice than the money you make, or the expenses you are able to contain.

In an era of noninvasive procedures requiring either multiple treatments to achieve optimal results or continuous treatment to maintain results, retention is an immensely profitable and highly overlooked component. An initial visit for wrinkle reduction by injection or for enhancement with an injectable filler requires consultation, evaluation, informed consent, and treatment.

Consider the fee for initial treatment relative to the productivity and time investment required of the provider and staff. Now consider the repeat visit and the productivity and time investment required of the provider and staff on this and each subsequent visit. Add to this the value of someone who has made the commitment to retain your services as an ongoing provider of aesthetic service and thus is a potential source for referral and added service. Now consider the value of the patient you simply gain versus the value of the patient you keep.

Retention has limitless value. Track it, measure it, and build on it. Make retention easy for your patients by reminding them to maintain treatment. Make buying appropriate and individual to each patient, provide single treatments, package treatments, and easy-to-follow options for your plans. Always measure satisfaction with every phase of treatment. If satisfaction wanes, so too will retention and the benefits of what you keep.

The person who starts out simply with the idea of getting rich won't succeed; one must have a larger ambition.
— JOHN D. ROCKEFELLER, FOUNDER OF STANDARD OIL

PRODUCTIVITY AND REVENUE

Any business must produce goods or services to generate revenue. Ours is no longer a society of barter; you expect payment for your productivity or services rendered. In an aesthetic practice, productivity is commonly prioritized and measured in these categories:

- Treatment or surgery

- Consultation and office visits

- Posttreatment follow-up care

- Administration

- Outreach

Providers and staff must have individual goals for productivity; it is these revenue-earning areas of productivity for each provider of services and for retail sales that compound to define net practice revenue goals.

Is there value in looking at these productivity goals quantitatively and qualitatively? Absolutely. Although productivity and revenue are inherently defined only as quantitative measures, without quality measures of productivity, one might not attain defined quantity goals of productivity. Also, without quality review of the factors that diminish gross earned revenue, you will not attain your goals for net revenue.

Goals for provider productivity should be set first. The most valuable time you have as a provider is productivity that directly generates revenue. Your greatest productivity or time investment is providing treatment or surgery. These, however, would not be possible without investing time in consultation and office visits. This time is necessary to educate clients, convert them to patients, and clinically manage the individual case through to treatment or surgery and beyond. Quality and safety issues require that you also spend time in posttreatment follow-up and care. Your second greatest investment in productivity is consultation, followed by office visits and follow-up care.

Administration is commonly the next priority for a provider, but it should not be. Too many providers choose to control administration on a micro level rather than empowering capable staff members to carry out and manage all levels of administration and the practice's business operations. You should set productivity goals for administration in terms of quality and quantity. Capable staff members must be empowered to manage daily business operations as well as to propose and carry out appropriate long-term plans. This allows your time investment in administration to be minimal.

Administrative micromanagement by the provider most often results in a drain of any available time for outreach. When outreach suffers, inevitably overall productivity will suffer. Understanding why is simple:

- Outreach can generate more business for you, whereas administration is simply taking care of business.

- Providing and generating services must be your greatest priority of productivity to attain your revenue goals.

Once productivity goals for the provider are set, they should likewise be set for staff. Staff goals depend on the role each person plays in operations. Goals should support provider goals in these clinical and administrative areas. Goals should also contribute to these overall practice goals in complementary operations, such as personal services and retail, even though an individual's function may not be directly related to revenue (such as providing a service or selling a product).

In theory, when productivity goals in clinical operations, personal services, and retail are met, gross revenue goals in these areas should be attainable. In theory, each of these three goals, when met (less the expenses tied to each operational function and administrative expense), will lead to attaining net revenue goals. Why only in theory? Several factors can have either a positive or negative impact in the progression from attained productivity goals to gross and net revenue goals.

Fees   Productivity generates revenue only through fees charged and collected. With elective services that are not reimbursed by insurance, you may encounter difficulty in collecting fees from patients. With fees that are reimbursed by insurance, there may be adjustments or delays in the length of time it takes to be paid. These things cost you money. In addition, discounted fees create the need for greater productivity to meet revenue goals. This is most relevant with promotions and packages for personal services or retail.

Direct Expense   Clinical, personal service, and retail staff and operations (including inventory, supplies, and other direct operational expenses) are likely your greatest variable in the progression from achieving productivity goals to achieving revenue goals. A positive impact on net revenue requires that you carefully plan and minimize your direct expenses.

Overhead   Your operational expenses in clinical, personal service, and retail functions—all administrative expense and debt—are considered overhead. Some areas of overhead are in your direct control, such as practice communication, patient education materials, and added amenities; others are not, such as utilities, insurance, and taxes. The expenses in your control are most often the things that individualize and support your brand and mission and must be first qualified (do not sacrifice quality) and then quantified. Expenses not in your direct control can still be wisely contained.

Practice goals are ultimately achieved in a progression in which:

- Traffic goals lead to conversion and retention
- Conversion and retention lead to productivity
- Productivity leads to revenue
- Revenue is qualified in terms of gross (overall revenue earned from services) and net (gross revenue less all expenses)

No goal can confidently be met without first achieving the goal before it. However, goals are defined in an inverse relationship to which they are achieved. They are defined in this order:

- Ultimate practice/business goal

- Net revenue (what you want left after all expenses are paid)

- Gross revenue (what you will need to collect in order to cover expenses and make the money you expect to make)

- Productivity (the amount of service it will take to bill and collect the fees needed to achieve revenue goals)

- Conversion and retention (how many people you will need to treat, or how often)

- Traffic (how many people you will need coming through your door interested in treatment)

The ultimate goal aesthetic providers set for their practice is simply what they want the practice to achieve as a medical service and a business. In some cases this may be defined in terms of revenue, in others it may not. Revenue, however, will inevitably define the survival of your practice as a business enterprise. It will also define what you personally gain in income from your efforts. Consider all of these factors as you define your ultimate practice/business goals and your net revenue goals. As a provider, you are the greatest source for revenue in your business, but as a proprietor, you are the last to be paid.

In an existing practice model, goals may be based on continuously improving performance. In a new practice, goals may be based on more long-term projections of building a brand than on immediate returns. In a practice retooling to increase the aesthetic or nonpayor component, goals may be based on a combination of improved performance and long-term growth.

Just as no practice should be modeled after another, no goal should be stated in terms of an industry standard or the competition. You must define your goals by what you wish to achieve in your business based on what is realistic for your market, maturity, and productivity.

Macromanaging

Although you must be an expert at the medical specialty you practice, you need only understand the broad basics of the nature of the business you practice. Empower your accounting and operations team and consultants to manage your business, or replace them. Use your time providing service on a micro level and managing business on a macro level; this is the opposite of what most active service proprietors practice in the business world at large.

Productivity

Productivity is the most complicated of all equations in the aesthetic practice business plan. It's also the most variable. Factors of variability include:

- Your practice mix

- Available productivity of direct revenue function

- Actual productivity of direct revenue function

Aesthetic services are nonpayor. They should be defined separately from payor services in a practice that is not wholly aesthetic. This is essential to your revenue goals. Available productivity creating direct revenue includes the total number of hours any direct revenue producer is able to provide services. This includes:

- You, the provider

- Employees such as aestheticians, dieticians, and massage therapists who provide personal services that directly generate revenue

- Any retail sales personnel

Actual productivity is what is realistic for each employee who directly generates revenue to generate in the time he or she is providing service. In any practice, these factors can have a significant impact on defined productivity of each individual and the practice as a whole.

In a small practice, clinical support staff to the primary provider may also provide personal services as well as retail sales. A larger practice may have several individuals fulfilling each of these functions. The small practice may have more varied productivity goals per revenue producer, with lower output expectations per goal. The larger practice may have fewer productivity goals per revenue producer, with higher output expectations per goal. What matters most, however, is not the size of your practice or the nature of your goals; what matters is that you maximize your practice's productivity.

Therefore your practice productivity equation is defined as the sum of maximum time available for billable direct service by each service provider and revenue function. Don't try to compile the individual productivity of all revenue functions into one productivity goal. A compilation of productivity only has meaning when translated into revenue. Translation into revenue requires the following:

- Each service provider has maximum productivity defined for each revenue function he or she fulfills. This, multiplied by the related service fees, will define that provider's maximum potential for individual revenue.

- Nonservice revenue (such as retail) has a defined maximum productivity measure (sales volume). Sales volume (units) multiplied by pricing will define that function's maximum revenue potential.

The sum of maximum productivity, when translated to revenue, is the maximum potential your practice has to generate revenue. This is your gross, or revenue before expenses.

Revenue

You make money by billing for the services you provide and the products you sell, and that money is used within your practice to operate the business and to make your practice function. Money in, money out. It is a simple equation that governs any business.

Patients or clients will pay you by one or more of these means:

- *Cash:* Green is gold, except when it goes into someone's pocket and is kept off the books. It's easy, when a patient or client pays cash, for an employee to avoid recording a transaction. This is a loss to your business. It's easy to hide cash paid for services with low cost of treatment, such as procedures outside the OR, that need no clinical support, or peels and microdermabrasion, waxing, and massage. Cash becomes an even greater liability when it is used to pay for skin care or cosmetics; if the employee pockets the money, you lose out on revenue as well as the value of your inventory. Most staff are trustworthy and few actually steal, but the easiest thing to take without being noticed is cash. However, you cannot banish cash from your practice. Patients will sometimes want to pay with cash for convenience, to avoid debt, or to avoid any trace of the transaction. If you recognize more or fewer transactions or erratic cash flow, start looking for a cause.

- *Checks:* Personal checks are still used in business, although in a much smaller portion of transactions today. The beauty of personal checks is that electronic banking now allows immediate deposit of funds into your account. The disadvantage is that if funds are not available in the patient's account, you will need to collect. This takes away staff time, and it will cost you money while you wait to get paid or if you must go to collection. Allowing checks as a form of payment presents a smaller percentage in the cost of doing business to a greater percentage of risk to actually collect payment. Expect that fees be paid at the time of service and that deposits for surgery clear days before surgery. Define a collection policy for returned checks, or do not accept personal checks in your practice.

- *Credit and debit cards:* Miles, rewards, financing, and convenience are among the reasons your patient or client may use a credit card. These transactions add security for you as well as your customer, but they also come with a cost of doing business (fees to the credit card company). It is naïve to think that there is no risk with credit and debit cards: identity theft is rampant, and your business may suffer if a scammer uses stolen identity or other tactics to exploit your practice. In addition to theft losses, disputed charges represent a loss to your business. Unhappy or debt-ridden patients have been known to dispute charges in an effort to avoid paying. While this is in resolution, you don't get paid. Enact security practices with credit cards: instruct your staff to discreetly pay attention to the name on the credit card, and match signatures.

- *Gift certificates:* Your practice or medical spa may sell or issue gift certificates. The practice of selling gift certificates is big business. It allows either a particular service or a specific dollar amount to be given. Laws regarding gift certificates or gift cards and their expiration vary from state to state. In general, never allow gift certificates to be issued for surgical procedures, and never limit gift certificates to a specific procedure—the recipient may not be interested or may not be an appropriate candidate, and as a result you will be viewed as restrictive and the gift-giver will be unappreciated.

- *Patient financing:* Options abound, and practices regularly offer financing programs to patients on high-ticket items such as surgery. But given the cost of doing business, administrative time, and fees paid, there is a value judgment to make in offering patient financing for fees in the hundreds, rather than thousands of dollars. Set a limit, or define a policy on when patient financing is offered and what it can be used for in your practice.

- *Barter:* Quid pro quo is the oldest principle in business. You provide my skin care services, and I'll refer patients to you, promote your spa in my salon, do your floral arrangements, babysit your children. The question becomes, does barter benefit the practice or the provider? Barter can be beneficial, because without collecting cash you are reducing taxable income. Although barter is easy, don't diminish the value of your services—barter for what they are worth. Set rules for barter so providers are individually benefitting at your expense. Proper accounting for barter is essential, or any analysis of your model will be flawed.

Money-in is what you collect for the services provided and products sold. It is something you must account for daily. A daily closing not only maintains balance, but also provides important tracking data. With daily closings you'll notice discrepancies sooner, such as cash transactions rapidly falling off. From daily closings you can chart the trend of your most productive days in procedures and product sales. From this you can plan staffing more productively. And if you look closely, you might even determine whether busier days can be attributed to more productive staff, or simply the trend of time your patients like to schedule services or make purchases.

Money-out is your cost of doing business. It involves much more than what is typically considered overhead: rent, utilities, salaries, marketing, and capital equipment.

- *Cost of treatment:* The cost of treatment includes single-use items for the cost of treatment such as breast or other implants, units of botulinum, syringes of dermal filler, and single-use packaged chemicals for peels; these are easy to allocate to each procedure performed. Technologic devices must also be considered a cost of treatment; however how you allocate that cost is a calculation you must make.

- *General supplies:* General supplies include gauze, needles, cold packs, alcohol, gloves, and other disposables. It's difficult and time consuming to directly assign these costs to a treatment, so estimate, and from that define a global supply cost to assign to treatments.

- *Back bar:* Cleansers, volume chemicals, masques, massage oils, and skin care products used during the course of treatment. These items cost you money and may be a source of waste or an easy target for theft, so maintain an inventory and account for the use of all products. Either estimate a global cost to apply to each treatment, estimate a specific cost depending on the type of treatment, or include this as part of overhead, but either way, attribute it to cosmetic medicine and keep an inventory.

- *Complimentary treatments:* Whether testing a new treatment, treatments for staff, as a thank-you, as a touch-up or for any other reason, complimentary treatments cost you something. Record this and compare what complimentary treatments cost you to the value they bring you. Complimentary treatments are an important part of demonstrating the value of treatments, creating walking billboards for treatments, testing new treatments, and showing favor or reward. I favor complimentary treatments or added value far more than discounts.

- *Discounts:* Procedures must always be recorded for their full price; discounts must be recorded as cash-out. You must have a measure of how much discounts truly cost your practice to determine whether they really have value, as in generating increased sales.

Money-out also includes what you pay providers and staff. There are multiple models of compensation, and combinations among the models:

- *Hourly wages:* Wages are paid for time spent on-site, whether productive in treatment or not. This is most often the least expensive model, but also the most likely to result in non-productive time. When paying wages hourly for providers of cosmetic medicine, make certain the job description includes duties in addition to performing procedures that are beneficial to the practice.

- *Commissions:* Commissions can be paid on product sale. It is unethical to pay a commission to someone who converts a patient to accept treatment. You've now made a medical treatment a commodity; this is not a car, a pair of designer shoes, a vacation, a stock sale, or a real estate transaction. Therefore you must not commission booking procedures. Higher commissions are typically paid for commission-only models; lower commissions are commonly coupled with hourly wages. Commissions can be individual or team based. Com-

missions can drive people to sell, compete for sales, and up-
sell. Carefully consider the relationship of commissions to
your image and your client base and determine whether commissions create incentive and value, or pressure.

- *Direct percentage or set fees:* Direct percentage or set fees are
more common with contractors than with employees. The
provider receives a direct percentage of the revenues collected, or a set fee for specific treatments provided. Or the
contractor may actually make the collections and pay you a
direct percentage or a set fee.

Whether money-in or money-out, tracking dollars is more important than
simply an accounting function—the empirical characteristic of financial matters allows you to make some important business decisions about how you
practice cosmetic medicine. Tracking dollars provides a basis on which to
develop and revise policy, procedures, or pricing, identify losses and gains,
and make valid business decisions. Tracking dollars is also essential for
tracking value.

REVENUE EQUATION

Gross revenue is the first component of your revenue equation. It is quite
simply all the money you bring in: service fees plus retail sales. It has value
in illustrating exactly what your practice's maximum output is at present—
not always an ideal, but a maximum. Although your goal for gross revenue
may be your maximum, your revenue goal is more appropriately defined by
your ultimate practice goal. Your ultimate practice goal may be to generate a
certain amount of revenue for yourself, or it may simply be to be as productive as you can. Whatever your ultimate practice goal is, your business's
gross revenue is the first measure of meeting that goal.

Gross revenue should be defined for each service provider or revenue function and compiled to reflect gross revenue for the entire practice. All expenses directly attributed to a revenue source must be deducted from the
revenue generated by that function to determine net revenue. This is not
practice net revenue, but the individual net for each revenue function.
Then, from the sum of net revenue you deduct all practice overhead to ar-

rive at net revenue for the practice. The equation, beginning with productivity through to net revenue, is as follows:

$$SPP \times SF - ERF + RV \times RP - CG = Net$$

- The sum of provider productivity (SPP), multiplied by

- Service fees (SF), minus

- Expenses directly attributed to the revenue function (ERF), plus

- Sales (retail volume [RV]), multiplied by

- Fees (retail price [RP]), minus

- Expenses and cost of goods (CG) sold attributed directly to the revenue function

The sum of each function's net revenue minus administrative overhead (expenses), interest, depreciation, and taxes is your net revenue. The value of looking at gross versus net revenue for each provider allows an evaluation of:

- Weakness in productivity

- An imbalance in fees associated with productivity

- High or imbalanced expenses among like providers

- High or disproportionate practice overhead

Review of the bottom line will indicate only whether you have failed to meet your revenue goals; it will not show where in the revenue equation you fell short. If you cannot define this, you will have difficulty attaining your practice goals. You may attempt correction by increasing productivity goals without a concrete basis, or you may attempt correction by cutting expenses without basis. Either could have a negative impact on revenue if not carefully examined for the source of the shortfall and the associated cause and effect.

It is unlikely that all goals and projections for productivity or revenue will be precisely met. Business can be unpredictable. By monitoring things across general streams of revenue and expense, it is more likely that your business will provide predictable returns.

🌾 RELATIVE WISDOM: Adjusting

There is a new trend in movie theaters in our town. Once going to the movies meant standing in line to buy buttery popcorn, sticky candy, and frozen sugar-laden beverages; now we have multiplex cinemas where you can purchase a glass of wine or a cappuccino, a plate of fruit or even sushi, find a comfortably upholstered reclining seat reserved just for you and your party, and be served your snacks before the movie begins.

At a time when the airlines are cutting back on service, movie theaters are adding on. Why? Adjustments. Air travel became expensive, and the airlines cut amenities to offset their loss of revenue. The little things people enjoyed when they flew are nostalgic memories now. Among most airlines, flying has gone from glamorous to being mass transportation in the skies over a few short decades. But the theaters have done just the opposite, going from pleasing the masses to offering the expensive amenities that people enjoy and are willing to pay for. The choice in our town is simple: the mass theater for a $12 ticket, or a little luxury and comfort for a few dollars more. Guess what business is booming, regardless of economic conditions, at least among adults and among young families? The luxury theater. As a result of the added cost and amenities, the audience consists of well-behaved adults who are engrossed in their entertainment experience. There are no ticket lines to pay for tickets; you reserve your spot online in advance. There are no lines to wait for Junior Mints or a Slushee; a server comes to your seat before the movie. Teenagers on budgets avoid these theaters, and adults are finding going to the movies is fun again. How did this all come about?

The motion picture industry evaluated where they were making and losing money. Concession items were already expensive, so why not kick it up a notch and offer something better for the price? Rarely are all seats in a theater filled, so why not make them more spacious and charge a little more? The cost of dinner and a movie can start to add up, so why not wrap the experience into one?

Relative wisdom: Review your goals, not just to pinpoint where you fall short, but to identify opportunity. Don't merely look at the numbers, or follow the business trends. Look at patterns, consider demographics, talk to your patients, and garner their feedback about expectations and value. Revenue may have fallen as a result of fewer procedures being performed, higher expenses, and a plethora of other factors. If you have a historical basis on which to compare, and you have qualitative input from your very best customers, you just might find that it is not your ability to serve; it is a better service model that will help you attain your goals.

✿ IN PRACTICE: Measuring Up

You are a practitioner of aesthetic medicine who is appropriately trained, skilled, equipped, and ethical; you believe that by virtue of who you are and the practice you have built, success will naturally follow—but you are wrong. Who you are and the practice you operate will not by itself draw in clients or generate traffic. You must reach out, be visible, and remain connected. Doing this requires resources (expense).

A young, aggressive practitioner was not meeting her goals for revenue; they were nowhere within reach. However, she seemed immensely busy all the time. After the first year in practice, she decided that to meet her goals she needed to eliminate some expenses: no more advertising, outreach, media relations, or directory listings. She eliminated everything except her website; it was the only thing she was willing to expend resources on, because she felt that a website is your link to the world. She did not think about how interested clients would find her or the website without communication and outreach. In addition, she cut back dramatically on staff, leaving only a skeleton of clinical and support staff.

I asked what her goals were, what she wanted her practice to attain, and how she expected to connect with the audience that would become traffic and eventually translate to patients paying fees for services. She told me they would come through referrals. That being the case, I told her she needed to take the time to actively establish and maintain relationships with potential referring physicians, and the practice needed to maintain communication and goodwill with existing patients for their referral. "No time," she told me. Her plate was full because she had cut back staff.

So here we were: She was not generating fees, but she was busy. So we looked at conversion. Conversion rates in the practice were great. Productivity, however, was low in service time, whereas consultation and administration time was high.

This tale bears three immensely important lessons. First, traffic, conversion and retention, productivity, and revenue are all interrelated and interdependent. They all carry some expense of capital and time. If you do not evaluate and measure each component individually but rather just review the bottom line, you are likely to overlook the cause of your shortfall. Additionally, you may make an adjustment that results in a further impediment to your goals rather than a correction.

Continued

🦋 IN PRACTICE: Measuring Up—cont'd

Second, when you do not set goals, you probably have no measure of success for your practice and no measure of operations to guide you as a provider, the single greatest source for generating revenue in your practice.

Third, when you do not empower others to manage the myriad small details of your business so that you can focus on direct patient care, you limit your ability to practice.

We set goals for this practitioner and practice, found balance in what revenue was generated from current productivity, and built on that for a consistent, balanced climb. Regular review of all these measures led to this provider's ultimate measure of success: a lucrative practice, a balanced workload, and a positive, solid basis for the future.

Once you set goals and establish means for measuring your revenue stream, following a system will help you keep your finger on the pulse of your money, time and services. These are not absolutes, but they are the foundation for making adjustments, decisions and noticing when things are going well, or going bad.

Take, for example, the stock market; it is just one measure of how the economy is responding at any given time to specific conditions. Unemployment, interest rates, and consumer spending indexes all contribute. What are your indexes? What must you measure in a "snapshot" view, or in weekly, monthly, and annual detail?

- *Per provider:* Surgical and nonsurgical services, in numbers of procedures and dollars

- *Per procedure:* Surgical and nonsurgical services, by numbers of procedures and dollars

- *Per source:* Surgical and nonsurgical, the most direct reason this patient came to you (you will not learn this on a form you will only learn this through direct, face-to-face inquiry)

- *Comparatives:* The past 1, 2, and 5 years; the past 1, 2, 6, and 12 months; the past 12 weeks

- *Method:* How did you collect this? (If you have recently changed practice software, the parameters for software, added or removed procedures, or adjusted classifications for procedures, this will have an impact on your numbers)

You may find that the trend-of-the-moment laser you purchased is now costing you money without making you money. You may find that older or abandoned technologies are again new and useful in your practice; learn why. You may find you are more efficient in your time or less efficient because you have more time. It takes a qualified person a few moments to run these reports for you, and it takes you only a few moments to read the data, look at the trends, and make adjustments, just like you might read the data of your own stock portfolio, consider the trends, consider whether you need your money to grow now or whether you can wait, and make the adjustments necessary to measure up to your goals.

RELATIVE WISDOM: I Will Remember You

Early in the learning phase of my career, I had the opportunity to be involved with professional football and to get to know some true champions of the game, and of life. Walter Payton was one of them. What I remember most about Walter was not his days as a running back for the Chicago Bears, but his days connecting with people. I grew up in the community Walter called home, where he and his wife, Connie, raised their children. When his children were young, I recall reading them stories in the grammar school library. When my son Nicholas was just a baby, I would run into Walter often at the club when his daily workouts coincided with our "mommy and me" swim class. Walter never failed to smile at a child, to touch a hand or cheek, to hold open a door, to make small talk. He was a private person, a man of few words, but sincere in his connection. He was a celebrity not only for who he was on the field, but for his warmth off the field. "Sweetness," as Walter was nicknamed, had a greater ambition than to be remembered and giving his all on the field; he gave his all off the field.

After his retirement from football, Walter was a successful businessman, in race cars, restaurants, and real estate. In 1999 Walter developed a life-threatening illness and desperately needed a liver transplant. During his wait he became ineligible for his desperately needed organ. In the last few months of his life, he did not become bitter for his personal loss; he became a crusader for organ donation. Organ donation at this point would not save his life, but perhaps he could help save the lives of others in the very few weeks he had left on earth.

Continued

✿ RELATIVE WISDOM: I Will Remember You—cont'd

The day he died, in his home just down the street from us, I had my own memories of Walter, and then I began thinking about how Walter would be remembered. Even today, every football game, every Super Bowl, every time my son dons his Number 34 Bears Payton jersey, I stop and think of this man who gave so much of himself to others.

Today Walter's legacy on the field remains with his record. Off the field, his legacy is instilling in others the desire for the very difficult life-changing and life-giving opportunity to be an organ donor. It is the single most successful organ donation program in history, and it lives on today. Long after his football records are broken, as they will be, Walter will remain a hero, a champion of life.

Relative wisdom: You never know who you will touch in life, or for what reason. You may believe you will be remembered for your patients, for your work, for your success and the wealth you amass, but equally you may be remembered for who you are outside of medicine. Live your life for how you want to be remembered, not what you want to achieve.

CHAPTER 17

Client and Patient Goals

The pain passes,
but the beauty remains.

— PIERRE-AUGUSTE RENOIR, PAINTER

To measure success solely by achieving your own goals overlooks the highest purpose of your practice: fulfilling the personal desire of others for appearance enhancement. Your patients come to you with the hope of improved appearance, of beauty. The path to achieving that beauty for your patient involves an investment of money, time, and tolerance of pain. Success is not measured by your patient in the beauty achieved or the absence of pain alone, because as Renoir so eloquently expressed it, the pain passes.

Why are people motivated by appearance? Time and again we hear about studies that illustrate discrimination against people with certain appearance traits, about various perceptions of what beauty is, and about the relationship between attractiveness and success. Is there value in such research? There certainly is value in understanding the general concepts of appearance in our culture as well as in other cultures, but such research cannot help you understand the individual motivations of your potential patient population. Understanding their motivations is essential to serving their needs and communicating your ability to meet those needs. Your success as a provider is as much a measure of practice goals as it is a measure of:

- Client/patient goals

- Their acceptance of you as potential provider to fulfill their personal desires

- Their acceptance of the services you recommend, and all of the outcomes and risks associated with a procedure, through informed consent

- Satisfaction with the service you have provided and the entire experience with your practice

Accomplishing all of these things may not be central to how you define your practice goals, but it is essential to how your clients/patients view your success. Whether you meet your practice goals of revenue, traffic, or conversion is not apparent to your clients/patients, nor is it important to them. They will not choose you based on your ability to achieve these goals; what they see and measure your success by is the satisfaction you are able to provide to them and others.

Physical Satisfaction   Although a pleasing, attractive outcome is the ultimate goal for the patient's physical satisfaction, the process for achieving that goal and the physical experience also contribute to satisfaction. Pain, recovery time, social down time, and self-consciousness are also factors in the patient's total experience. Whether the desired physical change is achieved immediately or takes time to develop, and whether the change is to the extent the patient hoped for or is within the range that is acceptable to the patient are all factors in the physical satisfaction you can provide your patient.

Consider not only the patient's body, but also the physical environment the person is in during consultation, treatment, and recovery. Are the surroundings warm and soft against the skin? Is the patient touched in a soothing, confident manner, or with hands that are cold and clammy? Is the patient made comfortable while sitting and lying down? Does someone speak reassuringly to forestall anxiety? Do staff members do all they can to alleviate the patient's discomfort? Or will the whole experience be remembered in a negative light for its discomforts rather than for its positive outcome?

From a physical perspective, your patient wants to look younger, happier, and less scarred, as well as more attractive, normal, proportionate, unique, or conventional. Your patient's physical needs for this procedure must be considered as representing more than just the final outcome; you must factor in the person's reason for wanting that physical change.

When evaluating patient goals and satisfaction, you must consider:

- The visible outcome

- The patient's physical experience and environment, before, during, and after treatment and recovery

- The patient's physical tolerances and limitations

- The patient's physical desires

- The physical environment in which the patient experiences a greeting, a consultation, education, photography, treatment, anesthesia, surgery, recovery, and follow-up visits

Emotional Satisfaction   Whether an individual's desire is purely to look younger, fresher, or just a little better, or to restore a lost appearance, to improve the scars of injury, to erase the physical signs of pregnancy or weight loss, to correct a nose broken in a football game, or to erase a gang tattoo, your patient's goals for the physical outcome always carry an emotional component. You must learn not only about your patient's emotional aspirations, but also his or her emotional state. Some may be frightened; some may be naïve; some may be exceptionally modest; others may be completely unrealistic or may purposely ignore the emotional issues that are tied to their physical wants and needs. Evaluating a patient's emotional needs includes:

- Feelings, current and desired

- Exposure to information

- Exposure of oneself

- Privacy from the initial point of contact through to the examination or treatment room

- Expectations, whether extreme, real, or accepting

- Influence: Who and what the patient looks to for support, or to diminish the negative aspects of the experience

- Stability: Whether this person's emotions are consistent, controlled, and healthy responses, or whether his or her reactions seem excessive or extreme

Experiential Satisfaction   The course of treatment is not measured as one single event; it is a series of experiences to achieve the ultimate goal. At any point you may fail to meet your patient's needs and expectations, resulting in a service failure that makes the overall experience less fulfilling than it could have been.

Experiential satisfaction encompasses the wait times, the music, the tone of voices—the total physical and emotional experience wrapped together. It includes the amount of time necessary to connect with the office or the number of connections that need to be made. It involves the paperwork, education, and simplicity or complexity of everything your patient encounters in your practice. Measuring your patient's experiential journey through your practice requires:

- An awareness of the physical and emotional factors the patient encounters

- A measure of the purpose and success of each connection in the patient's experience

- The impact of some experiences over others in influencing the patient's overall satisfaction and ability to achieve goals

Specific Satisfaction   Specific needs and goals are immediate; these may be as simple as changing an appointment time because of a conflict, or as complex as desperately wanting a major procedure now, for some known or latent or motivating physical and/or emotional reason. Specific needs are the imperative of the moment and may or may not be important when weighing the overall satisfaction of this patient's experience in your practice. Specific needs may be long remembered or easily forgotten, making their ultimate significance negligible. The only way to measure whether specific needs are fulfilled is to ask the patient, "Did we meet all of your needs today?"

Sustained Satisfaction   A sustained need may be how long the physical outcome you can achieve for your patient will last; it may be how long you will be in practice to fulfill your patient's needs. Sustained needs may involve the emotional and physical support and environment and the privacy the patient experiences each time he or she comes to your office, or knowing that you will always have evening hours to accommodate a busy patient's schedule. Sustained needs arise over the course of your relationship with your patient, and the only way to know whether you are able to meet sustained needs is by meeting the needs of the patients you retain.

Unless you understand and satisfy a measure of client/patient expectations, whether physical, emotional, experiential, immediate, or throughout your relationship, your practice goals will never be achieved.

If you were to define client/patient motivation and goals (acceptance, informed consent, and satisfaction) in terms of quantity or place a numeric value on satisfaction should always equal 100%. When satisfaction is not consistently achieved, there is a greater potential for dissatisfaction, disconnection, or risk. In practice, no matter how skilled you are, satisfaction will not always be accomplished, but you must strive to provide it.

EDUCATION

To meet patients' goals you must teach them what to expect, what they need to know about the procedure, and what can help them to be better patients and have safer outcomes. Without education, your patients simply cannot legitimately accept what you offer, nor can you accept the responsibility to provide a service.

Education includes all the elements of a patient's experience:

- Initial contact and screening of the prospective patient's reason for contacting you.

- Exchange of information about the prospective patient and his or her goals, and about how the practice works to achieve those goals.

- A consultation to learn more about one another. Patients must express their goals, share their expectations, history, and health, and ask questions. The provider must listen and share what the patient needs to know about the practice, the procedural options, the experience, and the expected outcome. The physician must answer the patient's questions and propose a plan of treatment that will lead to acceptance, or not.

- Acceptance is the formal process of informed consent and subsequent treatment. It is the patient agreeing to follow directions as given and agreeing to undergo the treatment as proposed.

You can control one-on-one education in your office and through written or electronic instructions provided by your office. However, patients may also be gathering information outside your office over which you have little control. There is no foolproof system, but there are some very important steps you must take to ensure that your educational efforts have the best possible chance to lead to acceptance:

- Printed or electronic information should not conflict; it must be up to date, consistent, and clear.

- Education should be customized to the patient, your practice, and your preferences. Use line drawings, work sheets, and digital means of collecting or conveying information, such as photographs or electronic imaging. Document your findings and share your recommendations clearly with the patient.

- Timelines should be used whenever possible to help put the treatment process into proper perspective. This is especially important if the proposed procedure requires time for results to be optimal, or multiple treatments are typically needed.

- Questions and answers must be documented. Add follow-up questions to ensure clarity. Track the overall trend of questions you receive; those that come up frequently may be topics that you should strengthen in your consultation discussions.

- Details are important to the patient and to his or her ultimate satisfaction with the process. The time to tell a patient what he or she needs for aftercare in terms of garments, skin care, diet, or behavior changes is before the procedure. The particulars of the treatment process and the posttreatment effects may seem routine to you but are entirely new to the patient. There is nothing more disconcerting than to have something unexpected happen and then to learn that it is to be expected. Even minor details count in the patient's overall experience.

Whatever vehicles you use to educate, no matter how many visits or how much time it takes, do not seek acceptance until you have fully educated the patient.

IN PRACTICE: How Annoying

I am utterly surprised by how many practices do not prescribe or recommend an antiitching cream for postprocedural and surgical patients who will experience the itchies.

A friend confided that she wanted a breast augmentation and tummy tuck now that she was planning no more children. I gave her a few names of physicians in town to consider and told her to please ask me any questions, but to communicate more with her doctor than with me. As I tell friends who ask my advice, I am not a doctor, and I don't play one on TV; I'm just the reporter.

A few weeks later my friend called, excited to have surgery scheduled. She shared a lot about her experience, and she had a lot of questions.

One week after her surgery she called me, desperate. "My chest and my breasts itch so badly I want to tear away at the skin. I know that sometimes stitches can itch when they are healing, but this is my entire chest. It's maddening. What is going on? Could I be allergic to my implants?"

My first step was to explain to my friend what was going on, and to offer her some comfort in compresses and creams. I provided the reassurance she needed about the horrible itching. Next I visited her and reviewed all the material the surgeon had given her. Nowhere did it say anything about itching, she told me, and she was right. My next step was to contact the physician, who was not a client of mine—just someone in town who I knew had the credentials and talent to treat my friend, and who she chose at my suggestion, but without specific advice. He was happy to receive my call, thanked me for the referral—and then he wasn't so happy, because he took the free advice I gave him as a criticism: "I suggest that you get your materials up to date and realize that for every patient who isn't fully educated, despite the perfect outcome from the procedure, you have created a less than perfect experience."

ACCEPTANCE

Your market, clients, and patients all have differing interests, educational needs, and levels of comprehension. While these differ among individuals, they are consistently the three things that clients need to make an informed decision to undergo treatment:

1. Interest in themselves and a specific goal or treatment to enhance their appearance

2. Education about the process, procedure, risks, and recovery—the experience—and the alternatives

3. Comprehension of their goals and all the information necessary to accept what is possible, what it will take to achieve those goals, the expected outcome, associated risks, the potential for an unexpected outcome, and the nature of that unforeseen result

Realistic goals and expectations are the two things that you must be able to document and understand about your client/patient to fulfill desires. Further, you must avoid any inappropriate messages when communicating your value.

Acceptance means that the patient has agreed to undergo the treatment recommended based on:

- Confidence in you

- Unwavering personal desire

- Personal motivation to act on that desire, not based on influence by others

- A consistent expectation for the outcome

Did a client/patient choose you because you offer the treatment at the lowest cost? Offer the best financing? Are the closest to home? Because someone else claims you are the best? The only reason clients/patients should choose you to undergo an elective procedure to alter their appearance is because they feel you are the most qualified person to perform the procedure and to meet their expectations in the course of treatment. If not, acceptance is not 100%, and you are at risk.

Is the client/patient absolutely certain this is what he or she wants? Is he or she fully committed to something that may be irreversible? If not, acceptance is not 100%, and you are at risk.

Is the client/patient motivated only by his or her uninfluenced desire, not by spousal, family, or peer pressure, not by trends or a need to conform to the norm? If so, you are one step closer to 100% acceptance and one step further from risking unfulfilled patient goals.

Does the client/patient clearly and consistently express the same realistic desired outcome? Does he or she fully and consistently understand and accept the process necessary to achieve that outcome? If so, you now have 100% acceptance. If not, you should not proceed unless you feel that the risk of an unfulfilled patient is less important than the revenue treating this patient will provide your business.

Complete and unquestioned acceptance is essential, in theory. However, in practice it is a challenge. You hope that your clients/patients are sincere in what they express, but they may not be. Can you always recognize such individuals? No. It is for this reason that you must follow established process and procedure for treating the patient, such as complete informed consent. It is also why you must carefully evaluate the patient's physical, emotional, and experiential needs so that you know he or she sincerely accepts all that the treatment entails, and so that you can be confident of what it will take to fully satisfy this patient.

✂ IN PRACTICE: Price Versus Service

I often lecture about the differences among brands and the expectations those brand names carry. For example, high-end retail stores carry clothing, personal care items (cosmetics), tools and gadgets, and even food. Walmart carries clothing, personal care items, tools and gadgets, and even food. What makes the $300 jeans at a luxury store different from the $30 jeans at Walmart? The label, the fabric, the quality of construction, or where the item was constructed? The exclusivity or the mass availability, the service that goes along with the sale of those jeans, and even the marketing? The glossy catalog and chic display, or the stack of folded Wranglers?

Your practice may be no less or more different from others than a luxury store is different from Walmart.

One provider's fee schedule was the highest I had ever seen for certain services that are known to have a generally accepted fee range, such as cosmetic injections. He was trying to grow this part of the practice and related his injection fees to his surgical fees. We discussed at length that he didn't need to compete with the "Walmart-style" shopping mall franchise medical spas of the world, but that by pricing his treatments too high, his service menu would be rejected by patients who could get the same treatment with a similar experience elsewhere, although with fewer amenities, and not performed by a physician.

He argued that his outcomes were unparalleled (physical). His practice afforded greater amenities in privacy and comfort (experiential). His relationship and the time he spent with patients was an important personal touch, and his patients accepted this (emotional). He felt there was absolutely no problem with his patients accepting the new fee structure, and if they disliked it, they were free to go elsewhere.

I countered that he needed to consider whether over time patients would continue to accept paying more than what they knew they would pay elsewhere. Would the value of their going elsewhere for their injections expose his practice to those of other physicians and lead to a loss of retention?

I asked that over the next week the staff members who answered the phone conduct a simple study, letting me know how many current patients delayed booking their injection appointments when they heard the new prices, and let me know how many prospective patients calling for injections did not book. At the end of the week, we reviewed the numbers. There was a small percentage of new and existing patients who booked treatment despite the higher rate. There was a higher percentage of prior patients who did not book treatment, despite their prior experience. The bottom line: He was losing not only revenue, he was also losing loyal patients.

The lesson here: Whatever your service model and what you believe your patients are willing to accept, consider what has value. Surgery is a much more involved experience than an injection, and the outcomes and experience are highly variable among practices and surgeons. A limited procedure such as an injection has fewer variables, requires less time, and is more contained, but is nonetheless an important experience for the patient. You cannot relate your fee schedule for surgery to a fee schedule for an injection or other procedure that can be more easily compared among providers. Understand what physical, emotional, and experiential elements your patients are willing to accept, and then make the experience specific to that treatment and what has value. Kiehl's lip balm purchased at a high-end department store or at a drug store is a Kiehl's lip balm for which you will pay $6. The jeans at a luxury store are not the jeans at Walmart. Acceptance must have value.

Accepting Responsibility

When you agree to treat a patient, you are accepting responsibility for the clinical outcome and for endeavoring to fulfill the patient's physical, emotional, and experiential needs. It may not be your business to learn why a married woman does not want communications sent to her home, wants to pay only in cash, and will not divulge her spouse's contact information for emergency purposes. But will she be fully satisfied with you and your services when her marriage fails despite her aesthetic enhancements, or because she had the confidence to lure a lover after her aesthetic enhancements? You are not an internist. If you agree to treat a woman who desperately wants a face lift but should not undergo general anesthesia for health reasons, or a morbidly obese individual who thinks liposuction will reshape his life, are you ready to accept the responsibility for what the outcomes may be?

You are not the department of children and family services, or a family therapist, but will you allow an individual to stint on essential family needs to fulfill his or her personal goals? Do you accept responsibility and tell the patient "No," or do you try to find a way to address the person's desires without causing financial hardship?

There are countless times when you must choose to draw the line, where you feel it is not your right to judge, or when you feel that this person's desire is so strong that you must overlook the caveats and agree to satisfy this person's need for appearance enhancement. Why do it? You can weigh revenue (money for you) and desire (the goals of the patient) against risk, and accept the responsibility that comes with it. But if something goes wrong, will the fact that you crossed the line to make someone happy be an acceptable response? Think not only of the impact on this one person; think of how an adverse outcome would affect your other patients, your staff, your family, and your community. Nevertheless, there are cases in which your compassion and your passion for making others happy leads you to respond to a patient whose need is so compelling that you feel you cannot let this person down. Then you have three choices:

1. Accept the responsibility to offer an alternative if one exists, and define explicitly why the patient's goals cannot be met.

2. Accept the task of refusing treatment and disappointing the individual, and offer a sincere explanation why, or simply state you cannot meet this person's goals.

3. Take the chance, accept responsibility for your actions and your patient's goals and expectations, and hope for the best.

How do you choose which path to take: Intuition? Experience? Careful consideration? A calculated equation to balance risk, outcomes, and rewards? Accepting responsibility is the one case in patient satisfaction and in practice where there is no single correct answer. Clearly, there is a likelihood the patient will go to a less skilled provider who is willing to offer treatment. But there can be a means to arrive at an answer that is correct for you and your practice, and ultimately for the patient:

- You are not the only individual who has encountered this patient in your practice and has an opinion on this patient's goals and satisfaction. Discreetly get others' input, but realize you have to make the decision and accept responsibility.

- Talk to a mentor, a colleague, a peer. Be objective, look for input, but realize you have to make the decision and accept responsibility.

- Talk with the patient if you believe he or she has the ability to separate his or her desire and the strength of that desire from the realities of the situation. Be objective, look for input, but realize you have to make the decision and accept responsibility.

Realize that accepting responsibility is not about dealing with unrealistic goals or poor candidates. It goes much deeper, to determining how or whether you can satisfy this person within your practice: the education, the experience, whether you are able to meet his or her goals, or change his or her goals, or simply accept the reality that you cannot accomplish what this person expects or wants. Equally important, how you can educate this person so that he or she doesn't leave your office only to be injured, or at the very least unfulfilled, at the hands of a less ethical, less skilled provider?

SATISFACTION

A patient's joy and confident smile when the results of an aesthetic treatment begin to take shape are a significant measure of satisfaction. But the only true measure of satisfaction lies in direct feedback from each patient. In some cases, this is voluntary; in other cases, accreditation, certification, and risk-management issues require that this be measured with formal surveys. I urge providers to measure the satisfaction of every patient. Surveys are becoming increasing popular, because they can be easily translated into quantitative data for benchmarking and other comparisons.

Whether you use a satisfaction survey or administer one in dialog with your patient, whether you gauge satisfaction through conversation or in numbers, measure satisfaction in every case.

- How can a practice feel confident that it is achieving satisfaction if satisfaction is not directly measured?

- How can a practice improve on its service to clients/patients if it cannot identify that expectations are met in all areas of operations?

- Why should a practice be concerned when patients do not respond to satisfaction surveys or questions?

Quite simply, ask and you will be told. If you don't ask, you'll be guessing about the single greatest *measure* of success for your practice: client/patient satisfaction. To determine that your practice is achieving satisfaction among clients/patients requires a direct response that qualifies such satisfaction. A patient's failure to reply is not a neutral measure; it is in fact a negative. Why? When you have provided treatment to fulfill an individual's deepest personal desire, he or she will likely be very vocal about satisfaction and either vocal or silent about disappointment. Rarely is someone without an opinion about the outcome of an appearance-enhancing treatment. If the individual is indeed neutral, it is cause for concern. No effort of your practice to build and grow can succeed without a solid, reliable, and vocal measure of patient satisfaction. Why? Patient satisfaction translates to patient referral and patient retention, and as stated previously, referral is the single greatest *source* of success in your practice.

Conversely, when patients are not fully satisfied, they may be vocal about their treatment experience simply as a means to vent their disappointment. Just as positive word of mouth or referral is your greatest source for building a successful practice, negative word of mouth is your greatest liability. In fact, criticism can be much louder than praise. If you do not measure satisfaction, you may not know where it potentially exists or falls short.

Ask each individual you serve about his or her satisfaction in every area of your practice, including communication, education, staff, operations, administration, comfort, privacy, characteristics that define your brand, clinical outcomes, and overall expectations. You will use this information to address any shortcomings directly with the client/patient to try to resolve dissatisfaction, and you may turn a potential negative into a positive. Determine whether this was an isolated shortcoming or has occurred with other clients/patients and requires correction. Continued measurement of satisfaction is a necessary affirmation of the value and validity of your practice. If your value is questionable or satisfaction is low, you must identify the cause and correct the situation.

Building a Survey

The outcome of any survey is a measure in quality or quantity. The validity of that measure requires two things: a valid number of replies, and a valid measure of the replies. There are several different ways of conducting a survey.

In Person   There is no better way to learn something than to ask. Feedback has no value if you don't document it. You should not get defensive when patient critiques of your practice are not glowing. Pay attention: listen and be grateful for honest feedback.

Electronically   There are anonymous survey sites that allow your patients to leave feedback about your practice; there are also doctor-rating sites that you can encourage happy patients to visit. The trouble with doctor-rating sites is they are highly optimized, so if an unhappy patient decides to use this method, the complaint will be widely distributed online.

Alternatively, you may choose to build your own electronic survey, whether for overall satisfaction or for clinical studies. *SurveyMonkey.com* is just one of several inexpensive and easily programmed means to create your own survey. The caveat is that it is easy to get carried away with extensive surveys. Keep it topic specific, easy, and brief, or no one will respond.

By Mail   Paper surveys are easy to send and have the patient check off responses, but someone has to tabulate the results. Reading these comments can be enlightening, but wouldn't you rather hear these comments first hand?

Over the Telephone   Calling with survey questions or just to ask patients briefly for feedback can be a valuable endeavor, but it can also be annoying, especially when it happens time and again after every visit.

Building a survey and using it effectively do not require that you be a statistician. However, you must develop a survey that is user friendly, with comparative measures, and that you use consistently. Patients are more likely to respond if they are assured that their response is blinded. Begin your survey by identifying what it is: an individualized measure your practice has developed to maintain consistency and gain patient feedback to provide a consistent, high-quality experience. Put your logo and name on it. State your practice's service mission, and indicate that the survey is an important means for you to measure whether you are meeting your mission and achieving patient satisfaction. This, along with an easy-to-complete format, will make it more likely that patients will comply with this voluntary survey, and you will receive a valid number of replies on which to formulate results.

The easiest means for categorizing responses is to provide a numerical or rating scale that is consistent across all areas queried; for example, "Rate your satisfaction with the information and education you received about your procedure: 1 through 5 (or poor through excellent)." It allows tabulation, and a quick glance will identify where satisfaction is low. In addition, it is quick and easy for patients to respond to; therefore they are more likely to complete it. But in itself, a sliding or numeric scale does not allow comments or the detailed feedback that can help to identify shortcomings.

Define exactly what you will ask, being certain to cover each area of your practice.

- *Communication:* Is it accessible and understood? Has it provided all the information a patient expected? If so, it is effective.

- *Education:* Is it accessible and understood? Has it provided all the knowledge patients needed to make an informed decision? If so it is effective.

- *Staff:* Are they helpful, courteous, and supportive? Do they fully respond to patient needs within a reasonable amount of time and with clear, complete responses? Do they define their obligation to the patients and fulfill these? The provider should be included in this measure. You may wish to identify all providers individually, as well as patient coordinators and clinical support staff. Although the expectation is that the patient knows who was involved in his or her care, indicate directly on the survey who the patient is asked to evaluate.

- *Operations:* Is procedure clear and timely on every occasion the patient engages your office? Is the location and facility convenient and inviting? This means every facility, including your office, surgical facility, postoperative recovery care facility, and any location outside your office that you generally refer patients to in conjunction with care.

- *Administration:* Is it orderly, concise, clearly communicated, and accessible? Include outside administrative services, such as patient financing, where appropriate.

- *Comfort:* Do your office, consultation room, examination room, and surgical facility meet the standards of comfort the patient expects?

- *Privacy:* Does the patient feel that you, your staff, and your physical operation value and protect individual privacy?

- *Characteristics by which you define your brand:* Were the patient's expectations of your practice met, based on how you have defined your practice and its quality of service and experience?

- *Clinical outcomes:* Were the clinical outcomes based on education and informed consent met? Were clinical outcomes based on personal goals met?

- *Overall expectations:* Were overall expectations with the collective treatment experience met?

Responses to these questions will help you determine where your practice is consistent, where you need improvement, and where you excel. In every case that you are able, immediately address low satisfaction directly with the patient. First, resolve any dissatisfaction if possible and/or demonstrate your commitment to satisfaction. Second, retain this patient as a possible referral source (if that opportunity still exists), or at least avoid an unfortunate situation in which the patient broadcasts dissatisfaction through potentially damaging channels.

The factors measured by the rating scale can be long term or cyclical. The scale allows you to easily compile results in a defined cycle, giving you the ability to compare certain periods of time against others.

Along with questions that measure satisfaction on a rating scale, surveys should directly request specific feedback by allowing space for comments. Most comments will come from patients who are exceptionally pleased and those who are not satisfied. Both have value.

First, determine whether comments are isolated or repeating, positive or negative. The comments do not have to be of the same nature, just the same value. Next, respond directly to the negative comments immediately. Do this for the same reasons you would address low satisfaction. Then determine whether specific comments are repeated. If people take the time to consistently offer the same comments, positive or negative, you have identified a strong trend. Build on the positive and correct the negative.

Patients are required to complete significant amounts of paperwork, and survey responses are voluntary, but for your practice they are just as essential as any other forms completed by the patient. Emphasize the importance of this tool to enhance the total quality experience that the patient can anticipate in all visits to the practice. Show appreciation for candor and the time taken to complete the survey. Actively use the satisfaction survey to build a successful practice of satisfied patients.

IN PRACTICE: Your Daily Pulse

- How do you learn what your patients want? Ask.

- How do you learn what your patients expect? Ask.

- How do you learn what your patients will endure? Ask.

- How do you know what your patients are thinking, feeling, what their motivations are? Ask.

- How do you know what your patients experience? Ask.

- How do you know if your patients have questions? Ask.

- How do you know if your patients will refer you? Ask.

- How do you know if your patients are happy, fully satisfied? Ask.

The pattern here is not meant to be sarcastic or arrogant. It is genuine. If you want to know something, ask.

A practice that was doing well invited me to consult with them. The physician had just hired a new practice manager and felt there was a real disconnect in the way she was focused on practice management and client service. As many of us will do, he compared his experience with this new, very qualified practice manager to his prior experiences in life.

She wanted data, lots of it, to track things and run a tight ship. He was successful and happy in practice, and he felt he didn't need data; the smiles and happiness of his patients and a healthy bank account were all that he needed to know he was doing well. He felt surveying patients was a nuisance. As I spent time with the practitioner and the practice manager, I learned they both had their strengths, and very valid points. How could I bring these two talented individuals together to understand and appreciate one another? When you want to learn something, what do you do? You ask. How would I help these two learn about each other? Through the very reason the practice existed: a patient.

I had the practice manager do something she had never done: shadow the doctor for the day in every consultation, in every postoperative check. She saw how he would lean in to a patient, make eye contact and say, "Tell me what questions you have." "Tell me what you have learned." "Have I given you everything you need to know, everything you came here to see me for?" "Is there something more that you need?" "I want you to be happy." She walked out of the room impressed. "What I learned in there I could never learn from numbers," she stated.

I sat down with the physician and practice manager and had them go through some very simple numbers. By glancing at recent expenses, she found that the cost of providing certain treatments had gone up, but the fee schedule had not. She found that an expensive device the practice leased had lost its luster and was not even paying for itself. She conducted a survey of past patients to find out that laser just didn't meet the expectations for outcomes that were purported in the media and by the manufacturer. She was smart, and she collected data to learn why no one wanted that treatment any longer. Her means of doing so was identifying a problem before it had a big impact on the bottom line.

The true value and validity of patient satisfaction is that it will inevitably make or break your practice and that you must look at it, measure it, and ask for feedback at every appropriate opportunity. If the physician were not a master at asking, connecting, and serving his patients, the practice would not have been succeeding. If the practice manager could not find the source for a downfall in treatment of a specific procedure, the practice was losing patients, money, opportunity, or a number of the little things that inevitably contribute to success.

Patient satisfaction is not determined through a survey or a number alone. It is not measured by a smile alone. It is part of the daily pulse in all the little things that happen in your patient's experience within your practice: in the physical and emotional, in acceptance, and in articulating satisfaction or the lack of it from which you must ask questions, make modifications, grow, and learn.

CHAPTER 18

Safety:
The Ultimate Goal

Even if you're falling or you're struggling
There is still beauty, in what we do
So que sera, let's go sailing on
There's a wise man in everything
— DIDO, "FEELS LIKE FIRE"

In the practice of medicine, as in any other business, things can go wrong. Events can occur that affect the safety of your patients and any person on the premises. If safety is breached, there is potential trouble for your business. Practice safely, and be prepared for any event.

Safety is vital to your success. I am not a physician, so I will not address clinical safety. If it were up to me, no one would be permitted to practice outside his or her specialty, and everyone would be held to the highest standards of training, board certification, and accreditation. It would be much easier to rescind the medical license of anyone guilty of clinical or ethical malpractice, whether an incident occurred from intent, malice, or blatant stupidity. This chapter is not for those who practice recklessly; it is for providers who believe in acting ethically and responsibly and protecting their investment in their practice, reputation, and the people they serve. Even if you have unstinting standards of clinical safety, risk and danger still pose a threat to the success of your business every day, often simply by chance. The wise physician who plans for success also develops safety strategies.

DATA

The detailed information you have about your patients is an inestimable resource for your practice. It contains private and sensitive information and the history of your relationship with the satisfied patients who are your most valuable asset in growing your practice—those who will potentially return for additional or repeat services or may refer other patients to your practice. Such information is essential in devising schedules, accounts receivable and payable, supply orders, messages, and inventory of products. These data help you project future appointments and formulate strategic plans, contracts, insurance, and credential certificates.

Data can be stored on paper, electronically in information technology systems, or both. Data may be in active use, in temporary storage, or may be archived. How do you keep your data secure and accessible, and which data are vital?

- All data must be securely stored with safe, predictable backup or duplication.

- Vital data must be maintained and accessible, with safe, predictable backup or duplication.

- Emergency data must be collected, current and secure, with safe, predictable backup or duplication, and must be immediately and easily accessible to multiple individuals in the practice.

Storage and Security

In the blink of an eye, whether through a power surge or a simple technical glitch, all of your data can be lost, corrupted, or become inaccessible; this will inevitably disrupt the practice's daily routine. Data storage requires more than enough room on the server; it is how the data are stored and the means by which data are accessible. If you have more than one program to encompass your scheduling, patient data, electronic medical records (EMR), electronic prescriptions (ERx), financial, marketing (such as your website, if you are the host), and other key data, or if this is all in one program, you must have backups of the system and data, as well as the templates and preferences. When weighing the time and cost of backing up, consider that if the whole system goes down, a significant amount of time may be required to bring it back up as well as to make the data operational. In addition to protecting your data, you must carefully consider who has the ability, access, and expertise to evaluate and upgrade your IT function, including security and backup. This may be a staff member or a trusted outside resource.

It is prudent to store or archive duplicate data off-site. In the event that your office systems and location are not operational (such as after a fire, hurricane, blizzard, or any unexpected event), having complete, current backup data available off-site will facilitate your getting up and running in another location.

If you keep paper or hard copy files, store them in a fireproof, waterproof storage system; do not house them in the same location as your electronic backup. Instead of trying to manage all this on your own, research data-management and storage companies. You'll be surprised how economically and swiftly they can archive your data.

Security involves more than password protection on your wireless system, on specific programs or accounts. Security on your data and on your storage system must be absolute. If hackers can access retail and credit card company data and steal what they need, imagine how damaging it would be if the personal records of your patients were pirated for profit, or even worse, for publicity. Have firewalls and pass codes, and frequently update or change passwords. I like to rotate two or three relevant passwords, which is a little easier than always making a change. Although this may seem a nuisance to operations, the greater nuisance would be to have your valuable data illegally accessed and stolen. If you offer wireless connection to your patients within your office, make certain the network they can access is different from the network you use for your practice operations.

Licenses and Certificates, Account Numbers, and Passwords

Active licenses and certification and accreditation documents for your practice as whole and for every provider in your practice must be current and kept in an accessible but safe, fireproof place. Consider the danger if someone acquired or stole your DEA number. Never allow these documents to expire, and keep track of expiration dates so there is no rush to renew.

Account numbers and their passwords are equally vital to keep current, accessible, and safe. Limit the access to account numbers and highly sensitive documents to need-to-know personnel, and do not allow these numbers or passwords to be carelessly jotted down on Post-its at work stations or on hard drives.

Keep an electronic file with scans of documents and a duplicate electronic file on a portable data storage medium, as well as a paper copy that includes vital information, such as license numbers and contact numbers for state medical boards or licensing organizations. It's unlikely that someone will question the validity of your credentials, but credentials or identity can be stolen physically or electronically. Accounts can be easily tampered with or accessed to steal vital information. A catastrophic event that causes damage to your office could irreparably damage important documents or account statements on which account numbers and passwords may be found. Keep current copies safe, secure, and off-site.

Licenses and certificates are vital to the legitimate operation of your practice; so too is all supporting documentation, such as operational and accreditation manuals. Maintain these digitally so they are easy to update, but keep them in print so that if data systems go down or your office facility is displaced, you have all the operational information you need to operate seamlessly and successfully. The same is true for credit card accounts, supply accounts, bank accounts, insurance, utilities, anything that is important to the day-to-day operation of your business.

In Case of Emergency

Data required in case of emergency (ICE) are vital to have on hand and up to date for every patient, employee, and contractor associated with your practice. If someone has an accident or emergency health problem, whom will you contact? Direct emergency medical telephone numbers and 911 information are essential to summon help, and this information should be posted by all the phones in your practice. Also essential are the personal contact data for patients and staff.

Although patients always come first, accidents, emergencies, and adverse events may occur in your office that do not involve people. Devices fail to function, safety equipment, information technologies, even utilities can malfunction or go down, suspending your operations and threatening practice productivity at any time. If there is a power failure, generators fail (because they haven't been tested?), and the phone system is electric, how will you contact the utility or a generator service? How will you collect the data for upcoming appointments and contact patients to reschedule? An inability to communicate with your patients may not only inconvenience and annoy many individuals; it can also cast doubt on your practice's ability to anticipate and handle unforeseen events.

FACILITY AND PROPERTY

Whether you own or rent your facility, and whether you are the owner, a contractor, or an employee of the practice, the safety and security of your patients and practice are closely tied to the safety, security, and functional status of your office and surgical facilities. Violent weather or accidents such as fires that can destroy a building are beyond your control, but providing for the well-being of all individuals on-site is in your control.

Security

If intruders broke into your home when you were not present, whether they destroyed or stole your possessions or simply broke in to cause damage, you would feel violated. If someone broke into your home when you were inside, you would feel your safety threatened. The same is true if the security of your facility is breached; the security of your place of business must be maintained whether there is anyone on-site or not.

Alarm systems are only deterrents. They must have a fail-safe backup system in case of power interruptions and be monitored 24 hours a day. Although they are important to an overall security plan for your office, equally essential is the need to secure drugs, medical devices, equipment, and your data. These must be locked and properly stored when not in use. Labeling a drug cabinet is simply inviting someone who has broken in to explore the contents. In addition to alarms and locks, some security systems include cameras, but these are of no use if the cameras are not maintained. With any security system, a panic button should be available in multiple locations within the office to alert emergency services if you and staff members are unable to use the telephone or an emergency is in progress. The ideal place for a panic button is within easy reach of the individual who monitors the front door.

It is critical to test the security systems regularly. Often security, fire, and panic alarms are tied together in one system and operated through a phone line. In the event of a fire, explosion, or power failure, will the system work? You must have locks as well as alarms and alerts to secure your office.

Access

Keep careful track of who enters and exits your office through front or back doors. Cleaning crews, maintenance staff, delivery people, mail carriers, building managers, and your staff must all be carefully tracked if they have access to or are in the office when you are not. Everyone, including those who service your office in your absence, must keep doors that are not attended locked at all times and keep all doors locked when the office is closed. A staff member should be designated to keep track of who has keys to specific doors, storage, medical devices, and who has access and pass codes to specific data. If an employee leaves your practice, their key or access device must be reclaimed.

In public areas, during regular business hours, nearly anyone has access to your office. Today more than ever, buildings have more sophisticated security measures, but this may not protect you from someone who truly wants to gain access to your practice or to disrupt operations or cause harm. The front door should be monitored continuously when it is unlocked, and a window should be positioned next to or in the front door so that people entering can be seen before they step into the facility.

For the safety and privacy of your patients, maintain a strict policy that office hours are by appointment only. Schedule maintenance and sales calls by appointment, and limit access (such as a particular day for calls). If you have a retail segment to your practice and invite the public to stop in at will for products or service, make certain office hours are defined and that you are adequately staffed to have at least one person to mind the store, and another to mind the practice. If the retail operation is open when the practice is not, make certain there are distinct means to keep the practice closed to individuals who should not have access.

Hazards

Slippery floors, obstacles in front of doorways, broken lights or ceiling tiles, defective alarms or equipment, chipped mirrors, or splintered counters all pose hazards. Leaking toilets, rattling pipes, arcing electrical switches, or frayed electrical cords are all dangerous. Leaving equipment or medications unlocked or unattended is a serious hazard. Medical equipment and biohazard materials must be properly labeled, stored, or disposed.

Serving alcohol at a function on the premises is a hazard, whether you are treating individuals or not. The people you serve may get in the car and, legally intoxicated or not, may cause an accident. If a staff member is driving and texting or talking on a cell phone owned by your practice and an accident happens, you may be liable. If a vehicle owned by the practice is involved in an accident, you may be liable.

Hazards may seem trivial or perfectly innocuous until someone gets hurt. Regularly survey your facility for unsafe situations, perform regular safety checks, and address or prevent dangerous conditions. Make certain your office policy defines how to deal with hazards and how to avoid them. Even if the hazard is not within your control, such as a dangerous intersection in front of your building or inadequate lighting in a stairwell, bring it to the attention of those who do have the authority to address this, and warn those who may not be aware of the hazard.

Equipment

Sterilizers, lasers, lights, tables, telephones, fire extinguishers—your office and surgery center are filled with equipment. Faulty equipment is a hazard. Equipment that is not tested regularly can jeopardize safety, particularly if it is designed for safety, such as a generator or fire extinguisher. Even a coffee maker in your office that is overheating presents a safety risk to someone.

It is a good policy to maintain a log of testing, service, and maintenance for all vital medical, treatment, and operational equipment. You don't want to find out the laser is misfiring after your patient develops second-degree burns. You don't want to realize you don't have a Banyan Stat Kit after someone passes out. You don't want to learn the backup generator has no fuel or the gas line is not working when the power goes out. You don't want to address the burned-out parking lot lights after someone gets mugged. Even if you are not responsible for the generator or the parking lot lights, take the responsibility to get those who are responsible to act immediately, and take the precaution of monitoring all equipment and its service. A designated staff member should be responsible for following up on such details as noting that a light fixture's bulbs are burning out too fast, and getting that fixture checked.

Maintenance

A physician does not perform maintenance in his or her office, but those who do provide your safety checks and maintenance must understand your standards and expectations for the cleanliness of the floor and mirrors, and the reliable function of the lights and equipment. The designated staff member should monitor this and see that actions are documented and reported accordingly. Set standards high, be observant, and make certain that those who are given these responsibilities realize the seriousness of keeping your property and facility well maintained.

 RELATIVE WISDOM: Slow, Children Playing

We've all seen the signs on the road that warn us "slippery when wet," "curve ahead," "no parking, fire lane" or "slow, children playing." I have a friend who owns a martial arts center where the parents regularly drop children off at the curb and go about their errands. Located in a busy strip mall, parking is always an issue, so parents regularly pull up to the curb that states, "no parking, fire lane" to drop off and pick up their children.

It was the very first warm sunny day of spring and just as class times were changing. As usual, the parking lot had a line of parents' cars waiting to drop off and pick up students. A police officer decided that day to start giving tickets to those who disobeyed the "no parking, fire lane" sign, and the parents were furious. It caused a flurry of parents zooming around looking for a place to park to avoid a ticket while they collected their children. Some walked to the sidewalk to collect their kids; others simply parked and waved and called the kids to their cars.

Then it happened. The screech of tires, the loud thud that makes your heart stop beating, and the screams of panic. While the officer was busy writing tickets and parents were scurrying to get their children, someone new to the area, just stopping in to the sushi restaurant next door to pick up some dinner, hit a child as he stepped from in front of a car parked at the curb that was being ticketed by the officer. After that incident, the school implemented a system: no dropping students at the curb; parents had to sign their children in and out. But the school did more—they persuaded the mall owner to post multiple signs stating, "slow, children playing."

Relative wisdom: The unforeseen can happen inside or outside, when you think all is safe and secure. The safety of your patients and anyone visiting your office is critical; you must think not only about your facility, but about the boundaries, corridors, driveways, and streets that lead to it.

HUMAN SAFETY

Your practice exists to serve people who have aesthetic desires. You want them to have safe, happy, and fulfilling experiences. But people by nature are unpredictable. Unforeseen intentional or unintentional actions by people may put everyone on the premises at risk—as well as jeopardizing your practice. Safety is fundamental to your continued success. Being cavalier about established precautionary procedures may result in a total disruption of your ability to practice.

Although you cannot control others' behavior, you can establish your expectations for your employees and contractors, publish policies to protect those you serve, and set an example of how to respond appropriately in any unanticipated event. Although it's easy to say you must be prepared for anything, it is difficult to be prepared for everything, particularly when the unpredictable human element is involved. Plan and practice how to respond, and in the unlikely event you must respond, the entire team will be better prepared.

Protecting the Provider and People

You are vital to your practice and need individual protection, as does any true revenue-bearing business owner. You must get an annual physical examination without fail; no excuses that you are healthy or feel well. Address health issues immediately. You may be a physician, but remember to practice within your specialty and go to colleagues in other specialties when you have health issues, as you would expect them not to self-treat in aesthetics.

Make certain to have adequate key-man and disability insurance to protect your practice and your family if you are ill or become unable to practice for a time.

In addition, you must protect your practice, staff, and patients from the potential risk of someone who is either abusing prescription or recreational drugs or is under the influence of any substance that can modify behavior or judgment. Random drug screening is only a problem for those who have something to hide. It is a small investment in the security of your practice. Protect your practice, staff, and patients from contagious illnesses; you can require annual tuberculosis screening for staff and enforce a strict policy that keeps people with easily communicable illnesses such as the flu at home, not at work.

HEALTH INCIDENTS

Whether a cardiac event or appendicitis, a bout of vertigo or a debilitating migraine, health incidents can happen unexpectedly to you, your staff, patients, or visitors. Although the diagnosis and treatment of such health incidents are not part of your specialty, you are a physician, and your staff probably includes trained medical professionals. Make certain everyone on your staff knows how to respond to a health incident. Teach nonclinical staff to recognize the signs of a potential problem and to alert the appropriate team member. If a visitor to your office who is accompanying a patient or delivering the mail becomes ill, the staff members on hand must know how to deal with the situation swiftly, calmly, and appropriately. The practice of aesthetic medicine is a relationship-based business, so even if you don't provide the treatment to anyone who falls ill, follow up with any individual who has a health-related incident in your office.

ACCIDENTS

Although it is true that most accidents can be avoided, people will stumble, slam a door on a hand, or have other mishaps. Accidents can happen in your office even if you have the very highest standards of safety and facility maintenance. Address any accident, no matter how minor, by ensuring appropriate care for the injured individual and filing an accident or incident report within your practice. In the event this accident becomes a contentious issue in the future, or a similar accident happens, having the details recorded can be beneficial to recall the events precisely as they occurred. This will also help to find the cause of the accident and remedy the situation before it happens again.

EMOTIONAL ISSUES

Emotional issues can be obvious, or very difficult to predict. It may be evident when an individual is anxious, upset, or confused, particularly if you know this person's usual demeanor. A person who has a clinically diagnosed mental illness may seem perfectly normal if receiving the appropriate medications but may be prone to outbursts of inappropriate behavior when he or she is not medicated. If an individual's behavior becomes agitated or erratic, you must handle the situation calmly, rationally, and firmly to prevent the individual from harming himself or others. At the same time, you must not let the individual disrupt your practice. You have every right to dismiss a staff member who has emotional issues that affect the harmony and safety of your office; you have every right to dismiss a patient or visitor whose behavior disturbs your practice. When emotional issues cannot be contained, controlled, or removed, call for help.

INTRUDERS

Any person who walks into your practice may be an intruder: someone who is unexpected, unwelcome, and there to cause a disruption. You may tell an intruder to leave, that he or she is trespassing, but beyond this, don't try to handle matters on your own; call immediately for help. Make certain all patients and persons in your office are safe and isolated from an interloper, and if possible, keep an eye on the person until the proper authorities arrive, but above all, keep yourself and others safe. I know of an office that "buzzes" people in simply to prevent the entry of intruders and the need for security in their practice location. Your patients will not find this to be a nuisance if they know it is in the interest of their personal safety.

RANDOM ACTS

Random acts are not restricted to television programs; they happen in real life, and they can happen in your facility. The security of your practice may be breached by an addict searching for drugs, an emotionally disturbed person who wanders into your office, a person making a bomb threat, or a bank robber who has decided to use your office as a hiding place. You have two equally important immediate actions: to notify the authorities (use that panic button) and to move others to safety if possible. Random acts are unpredictable, but if you keep your facility safe, if you keep your awareness up at all times, random intruders may choose a more vulnerable target.

IN PRACTICE: Don't Talk to Strangers

A doctor was at a social function when an unknown man engaged him in conversation. The man introduced himself and began to make small talk. They discussed the event they were at and the World Series, then the stranger asked about the doctor's occupation. He responded that he was an aesthetic surgeon. The man asked casually about breast implants, about liposuction, and about the people who undergo these procedures, wondering whether it changes them more than physically. Proud of his profession and his patients, the physician told him that even very minor procedures can have very positive results in self-confidence when individuals are realistic.

Two weeks later, the same man walked into the surgeon's office and told the receptionist he was a friend who had met the doctor at a social function; he dropped a few names of others who had been there, then said he was just passing by and wanted to say hello. He had really enjoyed meeting the doctor. Unsuspecting, the receptionist called the doctor, who came out to see the man. The doctor barely had a chance to say hello when the man pulled out a gun and shot him.

Random acts of violence happen anywhere, any time. But this was not a random act. It was learned shortly thereafter that this man had recently divorced. His wife had undergone plastic surgery and was moving on to date and enjoy life again. The man, in his emotional distress, blamed the profession of plastic surgery and decided to take out his anger and his anguish on this physician, who was not even the surgeon who had treated his ex-wife, but one he met casually at a party.

Could this incident have been avoided? The physician might have been more curious as to why a casual exchange at a reception had resulted in an unannounced visit to the office. The receptionist could have asked whether the man had an appointment. Everyone could have been a little more observant, but the reality is that this man knew the harm he wanted to inflict, to retaliate for his personal circumstances against anyone he could find to blame. While you do what you can to reach out and be visible among others, without question our world requires that we exercise caution when we talk to strangers.

The surgeon recovered, but his practice was never the same. He didn't have the procedures and plans in place to keep his practice functioning while he was disabled, and gossip surrounding the shooting affected his practice. He decided to retire early. Through no fault of his own, except perhaps a lack of a heightened sense of caution, a random act of violence ended his successful career.

SAFETY PRACTICES

Your practice must have a plan for any event that may jeopardize the safety of your practice and those in the facility. Like any liability, you must have insurance to protect those who may be hurt, to restore your property and facility and to cover your expenses if your practice is disrupted. Insurance can be expensive, but the only time you truly realize its value is when you don't have the right coverage or enough coverage and wish you did.

A well-developed response plan is another form of insurance. You must ponder the imponderable in advance: What happens if there is a sudden fire or an act of nature? When must you evacuate? Where will you direct patients to go? Who will take responsibility for the patients in the practice, and who will contact those on their way to your practice to let them know that you have evacuated? How will you account for all people? When will you decide it is safe to return? The answers to all these questions must be defined in a comprehensive evacuation plan.

Shelter is the alternative to evacuation; you hunker down, lock up, and don't move. My children's school is in the quietest, prettiest, safest part of our community. Yet because of our unstable world, they practice lockdown drills. The children learn where to hide, who to respond to, and how they must not react. Just as the school is responsible for those children when they are in the building or school grounds, you are responsible for the people in your facility. You too must determine what your lockdown drill will be, and make certain your office is equipped with the communication, food, water, and protection necessary for as long as you must seek shelter from a storm, a threat, or a disaster. Determine what will signal the all-clear so you can unlock and leave your shelter. Practice unannounced safety drills with your staff to ensure that every team member knows what his or her role is in case of evacuation or lockdown.

With all the planning, procedures, safety measures, drills, insurance, and more, things that can affect the safety of your practice can still happen. How do you respond so that you do not jeopardize your success?

- *React:* What immediate action must you take? Call for help, lock down, evacuate, remove an individual calmly from public areas. There are as many logical and appropriate reactions as there are unpredictable events. Most important to your reaction is calm, focus, and strength.

- *Act:* Remain composed, demonstrating leadership, whether the situation escalates or is controlled. Begin to give directions, or take direction from the individual most capable and responsible for taking control of the situation. Give instructions, look for comprehension and compliance, keep others calm, and act to bring the situation under control.

- *Regroup:* After the incident has been resolved, regroup. Bring together those involved, those who witnessed the situation, and make certain everyone has their physical and emotional needs met. Offer appropriate resources if individuals need further assistance. For example, if there is a fire and you must evacuate, when you regroup let everyone know where and to whom they may turn for help if they feel anxious or have health questions.

- *Document:* As soon as possible, and among as many individuals who were involved as possible, document the event. Try to remember details that contributed to the event and such data as date, time, and the individuals present. Document who responded to the event and how.

- *Learn:* Together with your team, review the details of the incident, appraise how you all responded, and analyze what you learned. This is not a time for blame; this is a time to become more aware and better prepared for the future.

- *Recover:* Give yourselves a little breathing space, a little peace—time to recover and come back to practicing as you would had this incident not occurred. The incident may not be forgotten, but you can give yourself and others a little time to recharge.

IN PRACTICE: Real Life

September 11, 2000. Hurricane Katrina. US Airways Flight 1549 lands in the Hudson. In my neighborhood, the name Laurie Dann is synonymous with a woman who entered an elementary school brandishing a gun. In real life, inexplicable, random, tragic events can happen that may turn your world and your practice upside down.

A plastic surgeon I know lost his entire practice facility to a fire that began in the neighboring suite. The resulting water, smoke, and structural damage required that the building be razed. The office staff recovered what they could, the surgeon managed his patients and his business, and the quickest location he was able to find to set up practice was to share space with his friend, a gynecologist, who offered him a temporary home. Two years later, the two founded a large women's health center, born from the tragedy of a fire and the friendship of two very different physicians who found they had a common ground in treating women.

Discussing their success, I asked the plastic surgeon what he had learned from the whole experience, and he replied, "Que sera sera, Marie. It is what it is. I could be angry about the fire, but I am grateful no life was lost. I could be angry about the disruption to my office, but I am grateful for the friend who gave us a home. I could have acted quickly to find a new office, but I took the time to seek out the right opportunity for my practice, my friend, my patients, his patients, and new patients. It is what it is."

The lesson here: You may not be able to change the events that have threatened the safety or security of your practice or yourself. It is what it is. But when the waters calm, be the wise man who takes what he has learned, and sail on.

SECTION VI

How

You have to learn the rules of the game,
and then you have to play it better than anyone else.

— ALBERT EINSTEIN

CHAPTER 19

How Do You Plan for Success?

So much of who we are and what we become in life is a result of how we approach and execute our plans. Rarely is success achieved by accident, and seldom do we fail to succeed when we employ skill, strategy, and passion. Providing service to patients is the reason your practice exists; it is not simply a part of your success, it is necessary to your existence. The elements you need to define to provide service and establish or operate a successful business include the following:

- Who your practice involves, serves, and competes against; you, your team, audience, and market

- What you must define and accept in your enterprise: image, the needs and expectations of those you serve, and risk

- Where you connect: your practice facility, goals, and purpose, externally and internally

- When you engage opportunity, act on cycles, and exercise privacy

- Why you are motivated to practice

- Why others accept your services

- Why you must have safety procedures

Although you can practice without considering these elements, how well and for how long? When you have invested so much in education, training, and attaining your credentials, should you risk your career and all you have invested in yourself on merely practicing day to day and accepting what comes? In medicine this is known as *triage,* and while you must prioritize, you must also plan.

Taking the time to review all of these variables is essential to a new practice, a practice that is changing in some way, or even a practice that remains consistent and successful. Review will show you exactly where you are and help you determine exactly where you should be or want to be.

PLANNING

Wouldn't it be amazing if someone invented a GPS-like device for the practice of aesthetic medicine? It would assist you to define your route to success, alert you to detours, accidents, and pitfalls along the way that might slow you down, reroute you if you got lost, and be reprogrammed to get you on your next journey to success when the ride was concluded.

However, such a device doesn't need to be invented—it already exists in the combination of your training, instincts, ambition, common sense, and a business plan that defines who, what, where, when, why, and how you will practice. These variables are all interrelated and interdependent in the success of your practice; together they are the basis for planning. Using these variables helps to define how you will get to where you want to be as a provider and proprietor of aesthetic medicine in plans that are:

- *Strategic:* Strategic plans include the predefined steps for all of the actions necessary for your practice to succeed, and the goals and objectives of these actions. This is the map for your intended journey.

- *Economic:* Economic considerations include what each step of the plan will cost, what you can afford, and where any tradeoff must be made with the resources you have available, including money and time.

- *Applied:* Tactical and economic planning that, along with outcomes and the influence of outside conditions, will be your applied plan, the course you actually take in building success. This includes the revisions, detours, and side trips necessary to respond to opportunities or unexpected potentially adverse events.

- *Planning for the future:* Steady growth, expansion, research, innovation, taking on partners, or retirement are all common agendas for the future. Plan not only for what you hope to accomplish in the near future, but also in a general way for the entire course of your career.

Strategic Planning

Strategic planning may seem at first a monumental task, and it certainly can be. By using an outline, what appears overwhelming can be made manageable, and by building a plan through an outline addressed in phases, what is manageable becomes straightforward. Each section of this book is your outline to building a strategic plan. It includes the things you must research, consider, define, carry out, and attempt to achieve to be successful in practice.

- *Evidence and data:* Research is needed to determine where you want to be, who you want to serve, and what they will expect. By gathering data you will define which people you will need to support you in this task and how you will function. You will explore the opportunities to connect with your market and patients and the vehicles you will use to make those connections.

- *Outcomes and recording:* The evidence and data you collect by being in practice are your outcomes, and to build a valid strategic plan, you need a record of what transpires: the actions you have taken, the people or strategies you have enlisted, and the resulting outcome. What is collected can be sorted and reported in multiple ways to help you define or refine your plan along the way.

- *Trends and cycles:* The data that you collect in your practice will reflect the trends and cycles of your own productivity, services in demand, patient demographics, and more. Identifying trends and cycles can be valuable in defining the preparedness you require and your response to anticipated needs or shortfalls for any given day, week, month, season, year, or period of time defined by outside pressures, such as economic, political, and social events or pressures and even disasters. For example, during hurricane season or winter snows, you must be prepared for potential cancellations, rescheduling, or other disruptions in service.

- *Disaster planning and recovery:* If you woke up tomorrow and for some unforeseen reason your practice was gone—simply nothing left, not a piece of paper or a bit of data, how would you go back into practice? Or would you go back at all? Some see starting over as an opportunity, but frequently the cause for starting over presents obstacles. Disaster planning and recovery limits the obstacles and recognizes that some things, such as your reputation, relationships, and even data, if duplicated and kept secure, are yours to keep.

- *Practice transition:* There may come a time when you wish to change, or things need to change. Practice transition affords you the experience of what you have already learned about the business of aesthetic medicine, and the opportunities to avoid past mistakes. Practice transition is something best achieved by reviewing past strategies, evidence, data, and outcomes and considering cycles and trends to shape your future.

WHO DO YOU NEED?

You cannot change the way you practice unless you update your skills and credentials or plan properly. You cannot be attractive to all defined groups in your market based only on the services you provide; you must also consider the image you project. Be brutally honest with yourself about this. You cannot be all things to all people, nor can you be one thing to all people, but you can be someone who provides a service that a defined group is likely to find attractive. Moreover, you cannot do this alone. Who comprises the team you must build for your day-to-day and strategic operations?

Who is the defined group that is more likely to find you attractive, and what do you need to know about them to serve them? Research is essential, but you don't need to bury yourself in statistics and variables. Learn what appeals to your market and why, and make certain that when you engage your market, you offer what is desired. Engaging your market also means identifying the most likely means this population will use to reach you or to learn more about you or a treatment that can fulfill their personal desires. Aesthetic medicine is very personal and private. Research indicates that those interested in it probably go to the media first to obtain information. Why? Not because media are the most informative tool; rather, the use of media allows an individual to remain anonymous while not yet committed to a procedure or a provider.

You want to be among the means by which individuals in your market can learn how to fulfill their desires. If the only means for you to be a source of information is for interested individuals to contact you directly, you may be missing significant opportunities. Know what vehicles and what channels your market uses to educate themselves and use these optimally to reach them.

The last component of *who* requires defining your competition; it is not about competing with them. You need to know who they are, what they do, and who they serve, not in order to compete, but so you can distinguish yourself from them. Build your model uniquely and precisely to target your market, not to outdo your competitors. Who you are, who you serve, and who your competition is all come together in planning to pinpoint the niche that is perfect for your practice. Your research will also help you determine whether there is a void or saturation of any type in the market.

What Do You Represent?

What you do is reflected in a visible, constant, and identifiable brand, image, and mission. It is how people find and recognize you. To understand the importance of brand, look at the clothing you wear, the car you drive, the restaurants you patronize, and anything you purchase in goods or services. How many of these do not carry a brand? How many of these did you choose by brand? A brand is essentially how one finds you among an array of providers. Image and mission are what make you stand out. Are you a "drive-through," or are you a "five-star fine dining experience"—or are you something unique and extraordinary between the two extremes?

What do you do? Certainly you provide medical services to enhance appearance, but a strategic plan requires more than just defining clinical services. It requires defining purpose, objectives, and goals for all of the support that clinical service and operations require and for all that enhances clinical service.

What do others expect of you? The answer is not as simple as the clinical service you provide. Define the purpose and objectives of all the factors that influence what you do in the eyes of those you serve: education, comprehension, and risk. These are as essential to doing what you do as defining what supports clinical service.

WHERE WILL YOU CONNECT?

Where will you welcome and provide services for your patients? Where will you perform surgery? Where will you reach out to those you wish to treat? Where do you maximize the value of those who support you in your outreach efforts?

Planning your location and facility requires defining access, structure, environment, and decor. Planning operations requires a service menu and how those services will be delivered.

Communication is as essential as planning operations. If you do not know what you want to communicate, if you do not know who to communicate with and how to deliver your message, how can you build a relationship based on personal service? No relationship can exist without some form of communication, and certainly no business as intimate as aesthetic medicine can exist without communication. So where do you communicate, with what purpose, to whom, in what tone, and with what call to action?

Strategic planning requires that you define the communication efforts essential to your ability to practice. Before creating and disseminating these efforts, you must define what you are comfortable with, what enhances your ability to practice, and what efforts are most appropriate for your audience. Moreover, second to operations, all of your communication efforts will cost time and money. What you must spend, what you are willing to spend, and your expected return tied to your goals are all essential to managing your communication efforts.

Why must communication be planned in such detail? Because if you do not time your communications strategically, they have no value, and timing requires planning.

WHEN WILL YOU REACT?

The timing of your communication and operations requires you to seek opportunity and use it to your greatest advantage. You must be able to identify and prepare for seasonal cycles, maximize your opportunity in clinical cycles, and seize opportunity in individual cycles. When you act is more important than how you act. If your actions are poorly timed, they may become irrelevant.

An essential component of any good plan is knowing when to act. However, you can only identify the appropriate timing after you establish who you are and what you do. You must define your communication preferences before you can plan when to use them. Above all, you must define the purpose and objective of your operations and communication and determine how you will employ these to meet the personal desires of others.

The timing of privacy is simple: always. Planning just how each element contributes to privacy and your goals for meeting privacy is a core component of your practice.

Strategic plans may have elements that change regularly and some that change as needed. These changes may be based on fiscal considerations or circumstances that arise when strategic plans are applied. A core plan that defines all of the elements and efforts of your practice is essential as a foundation to and as a means of organizing your practice operations.

Why Do You Plan, Why Do You Practice?

Define the purpose and objective of your goals. Why do you practice? Just because you love it, or because you are a passionate provider and savvy proprietor who wants to maximize the potential of a business enterprise? You need to know what it will take to allow you to survive and grow.

You must also ponder why your practice is able to prosper and what measures could improve your practice. At the heart of your success lies clients' or patients' motivation and acceptance of you, your services, and the satisfaction you provide. You need to know whether potential clients/patients understand all that you can do, including potential outcomes. If you do not measure this or have goals and objectives for patient satisfaction, how will you know where you excel, where to improve, or where patients' expectations are changing?

You provide medical treatment that carries risk for unexpected outcomes that may be permanent. Risk is ever present, underscoring the need for constant safety practices and precautions to protect what you have invested your money, time, education, and reputation to build.

RELATIVE WISDOM: Blueprint

Can you build an office without a blueprint? Certainly, but without a blueprint for your practice to review, modify, and implement, can you consider all the operational, health, and safety needs, such as administrative and storage space, water and electrical supply, and examination rooms? What about traffic patterns? What about privacy? Without a blueprint, do you know whether your facility will ensure privacy by minimizing sound transmission?

In addition to a blueprint, you will need a decorator or plan for decorating that includes everything from samples of cabinetry to wallpaper and paint. You will need to plan your office computer, telecommunications, and security systems. Will the community you are building this office in grant a permit to build unless you have a blueprint? Will the bank agree to financing unless they know exactly what the financing is for and what collateral value exists?

A mature physician who was a somewhat naïve businessman was opening his own practice. He boasted to me how much money he was saving by having his brother-in-law remodel and revise the location he had chosen for his practice as a side job. All in all, throughout this building process, he claimed to have saved more than $100,000.

When the doctor was ready to move in, a few things became obvious: The wiring would not support a laser—it kept shorting out and damaged the equipment. There was no data wiring either, and the existing wiring was too old to support more than two phone lines. There was no hot water. The walls dividing examination and treatment rooms were simply drywall, without insulation, and from room to room you could hear every conversation. There was no locked storage, and there was no overhead medical lighting. Furthermore, the facility violated local ordinances for a medical facility, because there was only one entrance and exit, and in an emergency this could hamper safety.

Despite all he had invested, he had failed to have a blueprint, obtain a permit, have construction up to code, or even have a facility up to par for his needs. Correcting all the structural problems cost more than the $100,000 he boasted that he had saved.

Relative wisdom: Building an office requires a blueprint and foresight, and operating a practice requires a strategic plan that provides the foundation for operations. This includes attaching a purpose and objective to everything you do through careful research and evaluation, and with defined, candid, and realistic goals. Without this plan, you are simply building from imagination. Can you trust your success to that? Although imagination can drive your vision, without planning, little of value is likely to materialize.

Economics

I am not an accountant, or a banker, or a financial advisor. You will need these individuals on your team, but you must also understand some basics regarding the economics of running your practice. Whether you are in a very lucrative practice or one that is just beginning and is heavily leveraged, you need to comprehend and participate in your financial planning. A financial plan in which you project, allocate, expense, adjust, and use all of these variables to set reasonable goals is the primary means to control the economic operations of your practice. You may trust your accountant to tell you whether you can afford to invest in a new piece of equipment or a new facility, but it is ultimately your decision, and therefore you must understand some basic concepts:

- **Assets:** Most often measured as tangibles that have worth, assets in your practice equate to property, equipment, and inventory (retail, drugs, and devices), your cash on hand, and the financial investments of the practice, such as retirement plans. Property, equipment, and inventory can all be financed, and they all can serve as collateral (used as security for financing these specific items or other endeavors). Assets in general can appreciate, as a retirement account would grow with interest income in a healthy economy. They also can depreciate, both for tax purposes and in terms of true worth. Technologies often depreciate quickly as they are replaced by newer and more powerful technologies. In addition to tangible assets, you have those that are intangible—your clients and patients, referral relationships, and your image. While these don't carry a dollar value on which you can leverage, they do carry immense value essential to your success.

- **Cash flow:** Cash flow is simply the amount of money you have on hand based on the income from services and what you must spend to stay in business on a daily basis. A healthy practice makes effective use of cash so that you are never out of cash, but also that you don't have large amounts of cash on hand uninvested in your practice or in other valuable ways.

- **Debt:** The total of what you owe in principal, interest, penalties, on your line of credit, on credit cards, or even in utility bills or property taxes constitutes debt. Debt, like financing, may be short or long term, but you are accountable for what you owe.

- **Leveraging:** The concept of leveraging is simple: You borrow money to fund your practice or practice growth, planning that what the business makes will cover your investment and interest. Taking it one step further, leveraging also means that the cash you generate will also be enough to fund new endeavors, technologies, procedures, practices, or facilities in the ever-changing and advancing world of cosmetic medicine. The art of leveraging is simple: Short-term borrowing is for things with a low cost, potentially a short life, but a high cash return. Long-term borrowing is for things with a high cost, a long life, and a predictable return. Leasing is for things with a high cost, a short life, and a predictable return.

- *Projections:* Generally tied to your tax cycle, projections are used to forecast what you might earn or spend in operating your practice. But projecting requires more than simply projecting your future based on the past year's taxes, or planning for the year ahead based on the outcomes of financial reports associated with your taxes. Projections must take into account your strategic plans for growth and what you must borrow, expense consolidation, economic cycles, or even new trends and opportunities. The past is a basis; projections are a forecast based on multiple factors including the past.

PLANNING INCOME

Projecting income is part of a strategic plan for success. Unfortunately, although expenses are generally detailed, budgeted, and allocated in a very defined manner, planning income is frequently overlooked. Commonly, practices use a historical basis and apply a reasonable increase based on economic factors or projected growth to arrive at projected and budgeted income. Rarely is income budgeted and broken down in an aesthetic medical practice as succinctly as in other industry segments. Why? It is not that this is unreasonable, it is just that it is not easy. You must budget income based on:

- *Clinical service fees:* Fees are broken down by reimbursed or insurance work, aesthetic surgery and aesthetic medicine, by service and by provider. Surgery and anesthesia fees, if collected by your practice, should not be totaled with your practice's clinical service fees. These are facility and anesthesia fees, even if the anesthesiologist is an employee. Revenue generated by anesthesia is an adjunct, not direct revenue to your clinical fees.

- *Personal service fees:* Aesthetician and other nonphysician, nonclinically generated revenue, by service and by provider.

- *Retail:* By each brand and product.

In theory, each has considerations for uncollected fees and returned retail; however, with a nonpayor service, all fees are collected in advance, so there is no need to account for uncollected billing.

Why is so much detail required? Before even applying direct expenses to each income line item, you will have an easy indicator of your greatest source of gross revenue. Then, once you apply direct expenses, you will have an indicator of all net revenue. Compare the two and see if your highest gross revenue is also your highest net revenue producer. If not, you must review the direct expenses attached to that revenue producer to find out why a disparity exists. You can also use these factors to:

- Build growth on your greatest source of net income, your cash cows (this is easy logic).

- Develop or retool those services where income and direct expense can improve (translate to cash cows).

- Retool or eliminate services where income and related direct expense result in a low net income. Retooling is valid if you can reasonably improve net income or if you cannot eliminate a service. Elimination of any service that yields a poor net income may mean a reduction of revenue, but it also affords greater productivity—an increase in time commitment to the services that result in a better return.

In addition, budgeting income in such detail allows you to plan your direct expenses accordingly and maintain appropriate inventory as well.

EXPENSE PLANNING

Direct expenses are relative to income. An increase in income or service may carry an increase in the expenses directly tied to providing service. For example, if you perform more cosmetic injections, you will need the drugs and injection devices in inventory, and your expenses for purchasing those increase. If you increase the income projections of personal services, such as clinical skin care, you must also account for the increase in related expenses, including all additional staff, supplies, and even the additional communication that will be necessary to grow that segment of your business.

Overhead expenses are those incurred regardless of the pace of your business or income projections. These can be variable for many reasons. For instance:

- Rent or mortgage is easily defined and likely unchanging in a yearly fiscal plan (unless you refinance or default on a payment and incur penalties).

- Compensation of salaried employees and benefits to those employees are also easily defined and likely unchanging, although a rehire at a different compensation level or change in benefit plans could result in changes to overhead.

- Insurance and utilities are easily defined and unchanging, unless you have a claim, the cost of utilities dramatically changes, or your utility consumption changes.

- Taxes and interest expenses are also easily defined and should be unchanged in your annual fiscal plan, unless your income changes, tax law changes, your write-offs change, the principal of your debt is paid down, you refinance, or you acquire more debt.

There are countless examples of just how easily defined overhead expenses in an annual cycle can be variable and how all of the variables tied to your business operations require a solid, detailed fiscal plan, including appropriate projections. So even though changes in direct expenses are theoretically relative to income and overhead is static, in reality, none of this is entirely predictable.

Operating where nothing is fully predictable without a plan or projections will result in outcomes that are unpredictable. Even if you practice simply for the love of what you do in fulfilling others' personal desires, you still must stay solvent—you cannot operate a business that continuously loses money. Without a plan, you will likely find yourself looking at an empty checkbook and an unexplainable balance sheet, unable to focus on what you do best: serving the needs of your clients and patients.

WHAT YOU MUST EXPECT OF YOUR ACCOUNTING TEAM

John N. Kuechel, CPA

For two decades I have advised closely held businesses and corporations as a CPA, many of those physician groups. As a physician you are unique—a business owner whose expertise is outside the scope of business practices. For this reason, it is imperative that the physician have not only a solid financial team to turn to for advice but also to fulfill your needs as a business owner or leader.

In residency, you spent all your time focused on learning your medical specialty. During a fellowship, you honed your skills to become a highly desirable specialist in your field. You were not taught the business acumen that you acquire—that is the function of the financial expert to whom you look for guidance and advice, a person with proficiencies as specific to finance as your skills are to aesthetic medicine.

It is imperative to have financial advisors from the moment you dream of your practice, until the moment you retire—and beyond. Generally, a corporate attorney or accountant is retained first; both must work as a team to establish your practice, develop a business plan, make recommendations for banking and financing relationships, and refer you to insurance brokers who you will need to get your practice running.

Although the corporate attorney's input may be infrequent during your entire practice life, your accountant will be closely involved throughout your practice. The scope of the accountant's expertise encompasses advising you on the implementation of your business plan and development of growth and tax-saving strategies as your practice matures. The accountant will counsel you in devising exit strategies when you decide to start a new chapter in your life, balancing it all with your personal financial needs and aspirations. Your accountant must not only be your business advisor, but also a personal advisor who understands your goals, such as retirement planning, estate planning, and asset protection.

Look to your accountant as the leader of your financial team, recommending the additional professionals you will need on your team for both business and personal needs: attorney, insurance broker, banker for daily needs and financing, and investment advisor. In addition, you may need the expertise of real estate professionals to acquire or sell property. Turn to your accountant as more than your tax professional; your CPA will be your long-term business and financial guide.

The principal things to expect from your accountant include:

- *A connection:* Expect and feel that it is an intrinsic part of your relationship that your accountant is always working in your best interests. Look for someone who is proactive for both your business and personal needs.

- *Proactive and reactive communication:* Your accountant should be one step ahead and should communicate at the same pace. Don't be afraid to ask if you don't understand a concept or calculation. Your accountant is there for you to clarify matters in a timely and consistent manner.

- *Inherent trust:* Your accountant is not only your financial advisor, but your business advisor. If you have an idea, a hurdle, windfall, or setback, keep the lines of communication open and trust that he or she will respond with your best interests at heart. Medical practice by law requires confidentiality; this is an essential part of the ethics of accounting. Trust that your accountant is an individual who holds your cards *within* the vest.

- *Innovation:* Whether dealing with electronic data, the latest tax advantages, or the realities of debt, your accountant must present ethical and innovative solutions for your day-to-day and long-term financial and business success.

Applied Planning

Even the best-laid plans may not materialize exactly as expected. Numerous outside factors can influence your ability to meet your goals: namely, opportunity and cycles that lead you to amend your plans to maximize their value. Your strategic plan is your roadmap or blueprint. Your applied plan is what actually transpires based on adjustments, reactions, accounting for evidence and data, outcomes, and recording; trends and cycles; disaster planning and recovery; and practice transitions.

Whereas a strategic plan is your map for meeting goals, delineating the approach or route you plan to take, financial planning is a means of measuring how and where you meet or fall short of your goals based on the single measurable variable that can be attached to any goal: money. Where these two plans meet will result in your applied plan—exactly what you do, based on the outcomes of your objectives and the influence of outside conditions, to continuously work toward meeting and exceeding your goals. It is where you identify deviations, unmet or exceeded expectations, and determine the source of these. Unless you do this, you cannot identify or build success where it flourishes and make changes where it is warranted. Without an applied plan, you have no basis for building, defining, or revising any future plans or goals. An applied plan is the course you actually take in building success; some see this as immediate, but it is not. The best-applied plans use the present to adjust for the immediate future.

An applied plan relies heavily on recording the actions taken; it is your tracking mechanism, your history. You can see what worked, what did not work, what it cost you, what you earned, and why. How you arrived from one point to another has little value if you cannot document the route taken and the outcomes of objectives. Your practice will grow, and change in cycles. Your applied plan is a key element to recognizing many of these cycles and anticipating their outcomes. It must include:

- Documenting the outcomes of specific goals in your strategic plan

- Defining any deviations from your strategic plan

- Documenting the outcomes of goals on your financial plan

- Defining any deviations from your financial plan

- Measuring goals and why they were met or unmet

Beyond the value of building on or repeating success, or of recognizing where you might be failing, an applied plan can give you direction by identifying strengths and weaknesses. Such detailed planning may seem unwieldy, but what is more cumbersome is failing to plan and then looking for the cause in unmet goals. If history is documented as it happens, it is more factual and thus more effective and flexible in helping you steer or alter your future course. If history is re-created after the fact, is it ever truly accurate?

You need to maximize your time providing service for your practice to succeed. Your business is built on the premise of your service. So how do *you* plan? Technically, you do not procure the details of the plan—you oversee, you direct, you empower others to effectively, candidly, and skillfully build, document, analyze, and revise your plans. You require these people to serve your interests and those of your practice, and you define your expectations of them. Your resources and relationships are as essential to the success of your practice as is having a plan that is directed and defined by you, built, carried out, reported on, and revised by those you have empowered and engaged to fulfill your goal of succeeding in your practice. It is not difficult. It may be time consuming initially, but without strategic, financial, or applied planning to define your goals and strategies and to measure success, how will you know where you are going, how you will get there, and how you determine whether your trip was worthwhile?

IN PRACTICE: Growing Pains

The members of the practice were excited; plans for a new office and a new service model were the focus of every discussion. It was time to move, to improve, to roll out the practice of the future for the doctors, patients, and community.

The very first time I met with the practice, I asked a few initial questions:

- Have you looked at the numbers with regard to what the new space will cost, what it will require to build out and furnish, and how your overhead will increase relative to your existing or projected income?

No, we are not worried; we can afford it.

- Have you met with your accountant to determine what you have to invest, how much you can leverage, or what ability you have to borrow?

No, we are solvent; that is no problem.

- Have you pulled together a market or feasibility study to determine whether the vision you have is one that your market will bear?

No, we know people will love it, and it is what we want.

- Have you looked at your current plans in terms of marketing, traffic, and productivity? Do you have financials, a strategic plan, something to help determine whether you can sustain this growth?

No, we are busier than ever; it won't be a problem.

Continued

✕ IN PRACTICE: Growing Pains—cont'd

- Have you defined a business or strategic plan for this new venture? If you expect financing, the bank will want this.

No, our banker loves us; this will be no problem.

A few days went by, and some real problems unfolded: A rough budget estimate of more than $1 million to finance the new venture was a shocker to the doctors. When they went to their accountant, they found they were highly leveraged, with little cash flow. There was little in terms of tangible assets. A quick feasibility study determined that within their market there was a saturation of aesthetic providers, yet they had not defined how they would differentiate their practice. Their current traffic, with aggressive marketing and overhead, was just enough to keep them solvent, but not making enough to invest or to grow into what would be needed for the future. Finally, when they met with the bank, they were met with a request for the past year's financials, a strategic plan, and 1-, 2-, and 5-year income projections. They were also told they would need to personally secure any additional loans— the doctors would be putting their homes up as collateral for the build out. What's more, during this entire process the lead provider in the practice, the one of four partners responsible for 50% of the practice's revenue, suffered an unexpected critical illness and was unable to practice any longer.

In this case, the partners were clearly naïve. Other than bank receipts and a checkbook and payroll record, they had few data to support their attempt to expand. It required serious research, many assumptions, and quite simply in the end, there were far too many unanswered questions for the physicians to be able to secure the funding they needed or to take on the risk they thought they could to fulfill their dream. Within the year, the partners separated and went their own ways.

The lesson here is simple: Don't be surprised. You may feel you have your finger on the pulse of things. But no matter what transpires, whether by your own motivation and desire or by a need that requires your practice to move, grow, or transition, you must always have a solid strategic plan, financial plan, and valid projections. This must be shared and understood by all of those who have an interest in the practice or business, and you must be committed to 200% of the projections it takes to make a plan succeed, because you simply don't know when circumstances beyond your control will impose hardship on you.

PLANNING FOR THE FUTURE

In practice, and in life, so many of us focus on today. We may plan in a general way for tomorrow, but with what goals to be accomplished and by what strategies? Where you are in your practice cycle may dictate how far into the future you can plan, and how much time your have to amend or accomplish those plans. Regardless of where you are in your practice cycle, you must have future plans.

Retirement   For some, this is an endpoint to professional life, a time when we stop working. For others, it is a time when the next adventure or career begins. Define not only when you wish to retire, but also what you will do after your retirement, and what is required to reach that point and beyond. In an ideal world, we all define our own retirement, but it is prudent to plan for an imposed retirement because of the unexpected, such as disability.

Growth   You may choose to grow from employee to partner, from partner to connecting with more partners . . . there are few limits. Goals for growth may be defined simply in financial returns, or they may be defined in terms of personal growth to keep pace and be fully viable in your profession. Goals for growth may be the most dynamic throughout your practice life, and they are the most important. Document the goals for your practice growth and revisit them once per year, or as often as necessary. Document your goals for your own personal growth and revisit them once per year, or as often as necessary.

Change   How will you plan for change, whether in your service model, your staff, your practice model, or your personal status within the practice? For every item in your strategic and financial plan, there is an opportunity for change, and despite full control, change you don't expect, whether major or minor, is in your future. It is simply inevitable. You cannot plan for future change if that change is undefined, but you must be prepared for change with questions, candor, and flexibility regarding your options to react and the potential outcomes of your actions.

You may have a multitude of plans for the future, but all of them in some way will influence or be influenced by your retirement, growth, or plans for change. Some say that you must have a 1-, 2-, 5-, and 10-year plan for the future. Although this is realistic and prudent, some may not be able to predict 10 years into the future. If you have practice plans that are strategic, financial and applied, you have all the evidence and outcomes of the past and present to help you plan and adapt for the future.

✄ IN PRACTICE: Left With Nothing

What you see is not always what you get.

A small practice had great success in building its reputation, facility, and services. Over time, the physician added new providers as employees who evolved to become partners to keep up with the growing demand. The continued trend was bigger, busier, more of everything. Bigger practice size, more office space, busier practice and staff, more investment in services, retail, and the practice in general.

As time when on, the physician who started it all stepped back and was pleased to see what had been built. Several offices, a dominant force in the market, an army of physicians, providers and staff—this was indeed a burgeoning business. Now it was time for him to retire; he was ready to sell his share in the practice. The problem, despite what he thought was careful retirement planning, was that the practice was so highly leveraged that there was no means to buy out the provider. Everything the practice had coming in was going out to cover operating expenses and loans; the younger remaining partners could not collectively take on more debt for the buyout. In fact, they were so leveraged, they borrowed against their own retirement plans for their continued expansion. The founding physician was left with nothing, except the nagging question: How did this happen?

This is a prime example of why you must plan not only for today, but for the future of your practice and your own future. Even if you are fully in control of your own private practice, or you are an employee of a large corporation, plan for retirement from the moment you begin working, and plan to reap what you have sown through your energy, commitment, and efforts.

CHAPTER 20

How Do You Manage Limitations?

*Everything has its limit—
iron ore cannot be educated into gold.*
— MARK TWAIN, AMERICAN AUTHOR AND HUMORIST

Limitations exist to define reasonable bounds, such as when we are reaching limits in our own abilities or resources. I've watched physicians consult, inject, or operate so many times that I can almost predict what their recommendations or next moves might be. But that doesn't mean I have practiced or ever will practice medicine; this would be an extreme exaggeration of my knowledge of the practice of aesthetic medicine.

You did not acquire your skills, credentials, and the respect and image you have by chance. Likewise, you cannot attain success as a provider of aesthetic medicine by chance. It is reasonable to accept that you have some limits and understand where those limits exist is reasonable and necessary in everything you do, including your practice.

- There are physical limitations in what you as a provider can physically accomplish.

- There are financial limitations in what you as a businessperson can economically manage.

- There are legal limitations in what you as a provider and businessperson are required and allowed to do by law.

- There are social limitations in what your market or your specialty will tolerate of your messages, methods, and motivations.

Although few truly ethical and conscientious business people or physicians would ever push the limits of people, money, the law, or propriety, recognizing standard limits and setting your own limits for your expectations within your practice are essential to your success.

Standard limits are those outside your control; they may be imposed by your resources, your specialty's governing bodies, the medical profession, or state and national government regulations. Personal limits are the standard limits that you further elevate to serve your expectations, image, and patients; that is, raising the bar—setting higher standards on limitations. It does not mean pushing your limits or extending them; that flirts with extremes. The only place extremes exist in medicine is in saving lives in emergent situations or in situations where all reasonable protocols have been exhausted. There is no room for extremes, or pushing limits of any kind, in fulfilling the appearance enhancement desires of others. The result of such action puts you, your practice, and your patients at unnecessary risk, and when life is not at stake, risk must be limited, not embraced.

PHYSICAL LIMITS

There are limits to what you can accomplish in any given period in providing service, managing your practice, and achieving your patients' expectations. Where those limits are not pushed but elevated is where you find the opportunity to grow your practice. For example, through added services that are appropriate to your specialty, training, and market you may grow revenue, and you fill a need within your market and enhance your traffic, retention or patient satisfaction. You may choose to add providers that complement your specialty, training, and market to provide added services, to improve personalized service or to keep pace with the demands on your practice. Additional facilities, whether complementary, enhanced, or improved, overcome space limitations or provide easier access for patients who may be geographically more distant, or may simply be served more conveniently.

Simply adding services, providers, or facilities may extend your physical abilities. But unless these are congruent to or enhance your current image, brand, and mission and fit within your strategic plans, and they succeed in your ability to fulfill the desires of those you treat, they are not contributing to your success; they are only extending your operations. The choice is yours, whether you take the opportunity to truly improve your model or grow your practice, or you simply extend your operations:

- Adding personnel who excel presents an opportunity for efficiency and improved services. Adding more staff to take on an overflow of tasks simply adds to overhead and adds more individuals in the chain of communication, increasing the potential for error.

- Services that improve treatment options, abilities, safety, or comfort present an opportunity to provide something better for your patients whether in overall experience or outcome. Adding another device or procedure to your service menu when you are not certain of the demand for it or what to expect of its performance, and have not performed a feasibility analysis to anticipate how to market it, will simply dilute your service menu.

- Adding providers who will expand the scope of services, and who have appropriate credentials and skill, with practice philosophies and values that are congruent to yours will expand your ability to treat more clients/patients. Adding service providers without defining the limitations, supervision, and their appropriate interface within your practice simply takes you out of the patient/provider relationship and thus alienates you from your patients.

- Expanding your facility to provide more room, greater flexibility for patients, and enhanced comfort, luxury, and safety for patients presents an opportunity to improve your image, privacy, services, and patients' overall experience. Growing, remodeling, changing, or adding facilities without taking into account your image, your market's needs and expectations, or the pace necessary to justify expansion will simply add to your debt load.

When you find you have reached your limit, if you expand without taking the time to excel, you will not add to your success; you will simply extend your operations.

Clearly, one of the greatest opportunities to contribute to your success is careful planning when you choose to expand staff, providers, services, or facilities. Your motivation for expansion should be to extend service, enhance your image, refine your brand, and elevate your mission. Maximize the opportunity that physical limits provide, not only by physical growth and improvement, but also by communicating the value this provides to those you serve. Communicate the strategies you undertake to your patients and your market; let them know you are improving. Internally, communicate to staff that as a result of opportunity and new strategies, thanks to the efforts of the team, you are also elevating your goals and expectations. You are the provider, but your practice requires a team effort. Changes may require new goals, new skills, or a new pace for your staff. Communicate this through messages that foster loyalty and empower others to help you meet these new goals.

How you manage your physical limitations, including those that hinder your ability to meet goals and have an impact on your bottom line, will undoubtedly present financial considerations. Money is the single variable to which any aspect of practice goals, growth, and development equate. Every action has a corollary monetary limit, just as any provider or practice has physical limits.

IN PRACTICE: Operation

A provider was in such high demand that he was performing multiple surgeries per day and was heavily booked in consultations and office visits before, between, and beyond time in the operating room.

When we met, he stated that he had a problem, and it was not a bad one to have. His physical limits to providing the quality care that patients had grown to expect and that had gained him ample referrals was clearly going to suffer if he continued to practice in this manner.

His first inclination was to cut back on services. That, however, would cut back his revenue without reducing his overhead expenses. His second impulse was to raise fees. This is not a very good move unless you truly expect that your market will bear this increase. He then thought he might eliminate certain services that took greater productivity but garnered less in fees. That too was not a perfect solution, because there was no one he felt comfortable referring certain services to, and moreover, most services he provided were interrelated in some way or at some time, and people had grown to trust him. He did not want to send someone outside his door.

Therein lay the answer to all of his physical limitations: he would need to not just extend, but to excel. Adding a like provider would not yield enough initially to keep them both busy. Bringing on a fellow was viewed as a temporary fix, because young providers seem to stay long enough to build a name and then move on. Bringing on a complementary provider, one who could take on certain services and then further build a practice extension of services, was my answer. However, the busy provider did not like the idea of having a "competitor" right in his own practice. He felt that this would diminish the strong image of his specialty.

- We started by looking at his service menu for a 2-year period. We evaluated:

- The number of surgeries by procedure

- The average time in surgery by procedure

- The net revenue by procedure (we deducted the cost of implants or special equipment for example, and adjusted for procedures that could be reimbursed or discounted)

- The average wait time to schedule surgery

- The procedures the doctor truly enjoyed performing

A clear trend emerged. The physician had his preferences, and it showed in procedures that were booked sooner, drew more revenue, and were among the procedures most frequently performed. We looked at the category of procedure that he didn't enjoy as much and that were performed less frequently and found that these procedures overlapped with a "competing" specialty. In a short time we were able to find a young physician in a complementary specialty (or competing specialty, depending on your point of view) who excelled at the procedures the practice owner didn't really enjoy, and this young physician performed other procedures that the practice owner did not. The two had like philosophies, a good rapport, and within a short time

Continued

🦋 IN PRACTICE: Operation—cont'd

they were practicing together. By carefully planning to overcome the limitations on his time, the physician not only had more time for his patients, was able to see and schedule patients for surgery sooner, but he also was able to improve his overall net revenue—he and the new doctor were now two revenue streams sharing one overhead expense. In addition, new services were added, a large patient population was created, and overall everyone was well served when the doctor chose to add a "competitor" to his practice.

This is an issue at the heart of the industry of aesthetic medicine. Each specialty claims ownership of certain procedures, but while some segments of aesthetic medical operations are appropriate to only one specialty, there are as many or more treatments or operational segments that cross over the boundaries of defined specialties. When you reach your physical limits, adding like services while enhancing service extends your ability to serve your audience. You reduce the need to refer outside your practice. You enhance the productivity of shared services and the opportunity for patients to engage these, and you may very well invite new target audience members to your door. These may be individuals who were not previously interested in your practice segment but are now interested in your complementary practice segment.

The value here is immense. In every sense it increases your ability to serve your existing clients and patients. Exposure and traffic opportunities for your practice as a whole will increase with a broader range of service. When your productivity is pushed to physical limits, it is a sign that you are doing something right and need to effectuate the proper support for your services so that quality of care is not compromised, and nothing goes wrong.

FINANCIAL LIMITS

Whether you have reached your physical limits or not, in any business there are always financial limits to consider. Even an "unlimited" cash flow has limits. Why spend something that will not result in a positive return for your practice? If your answer is merely because you want to, and you have not done the groundwork to ensure that this contemplated expenditure will yield a benefit to your practice, then that purchase is not for the benefit or success of your practice; it is for your own personal benefit or pleasure.

A financial limit is simple: it is the limit of what a provider is able to or willing to spend on any given item. It is not how one overcomes financial limits that contribute to the success of a practice; what contributes to or influences your ability to succeed is how you approach financial limits, including allocations or adjustments of expenditures, or the demands you place on productivity or operations to maximize your return on those expenditures, and the adjustment of goals and objectives. Quite simply, in business there are three options to addressing financial limits: borrow, decrease expenses, or increase revenue.

Will borrowing directly contribute to your success? Hardly. It will have an impact on your bottom line by requiring interest payments on debt. While that is straightforward, borrowing will contribute to your success only if it includes well-reasoned related approaches to either decreasing expenses or increasing revenue through enhanced services, operations, or image, or all of these things.

Decreasing expenses in aesthetic medicine can be done, but it must be done in such a way that it does not damage your practice, image, brand, and mission. For example, you may find a staff member or two who are paid higher than average for their positions. But isn't an individual's loyalty and the contributions he or she makes to serving the interests of patients and your practice worth that extra expense? You can trim little bits all around, such as finding a more economical supplier and rethinking utilities providers, insurance, or even your communications budget. The sum of a little can result in a lot of savings, but only if it does not diminish service, jeopardize the quality of care, or lead you to fall short of your goals. If you must take steps, consider what is nonessential or what is not fundamental to providing the services that drive your practice revenue. What you reduce or spend must all be equated in value. If there is real value in an expense to your practice, and trimming or cutting that expense will have a negative impact on your practice, you must make a value judgment. What is worth more—the possible savings by a reduction in expenses, or maintaining something of value that upholds your image, brand, and mission and is vital to your success? Financial limits are directly tied to your success. When you approach those limits with considerations of reallocating or adjusting expenditures, make certain you are doing so to maximize quality and value to your practice and those you serve.

The third option for addressing financial limits is increasing revenue. Will a slight increase in fees affect traffic? Can productivity be enhanced to make more time for billable services, and if so, how might this affect quality of care? Can conversion or retention be improved? Can traffic be increased? What will any of these things cost to accomplish?

Increasing revenue should reflect the success of your practice, but only when it is relative to the effort and expense necessary to do so, and when it does not have an impact on what those you serve expect of you. When you make any change in demands on productivity or operations, it must not only maintain quality and value, it must also maximize your return on the expenditures incurred to make that change.

Whether borrowing, decreasing expenses, or setting strategies to increase revenue, when you determine how you will approach your financial limitations, you need to adjust your goals and strategic, financial, and applied plans. Define what you will do to address and resolve your financial limitations in your strategic plan. Revise your budgets and projections accordingly. Track all that you do and its resulting impact on your practice. Unless you do this, you will not know (1) if your approach was correct, (2) where it may have faltered or failed you, and (3) what is most important, where to make adjustments and corrections.

A Little Leverage

At any time, whether building your practice, retooling, or simply keeping pace, you will probably need a little leverage to borrow money for your business/practice and to make enough money through your business efforts to repay existing loans, with reasonable return, or interest.

First, let's be clear that even though you may have the personal funds to resolve any financial limits you may have, you should not use those personal funds for business purposes, unless you as an individual formally lend the necessary funds to the practice. Why? Because when you start expending your own resources without attaching the same conditions any outside lender would attach to a loan or line of credit—leverage—you are digging a hole you may never be able to crawl out of. What does a lender expect of any business that intends to borrow money?

- A business plan that includes valid income and expense projections and a fiscal plan that demonstrates how the loan will be realistically and comfortably repaid

- Data that validate the business owner's personal and professional financial accountability (tax returns and financial statements)

Whether you go to a bank or any other outside financial resource for a loan or line of credit on your business, take out a personal loan or line of credit to use for your business, or use your own resources to fund your business's needs, you need to have a business plan and to demonstrate financial accountability. This can be a daunting task, but you need not go it alone. The assistance of qualified financial professionals, namely, your financial advisor or accountant, is essential not only in compiling the data and tax returns necessary but also in proffering their candid and experienced advice. If you and your professional resources have done your homework and have built solid and realistic strategic, financial, and applied plans, the task should be simple, and the loan should be easy to obtain, or the value of borrowing should be easy to validate.

Plan progressively from the core of your practice, defining it and the market demographics it serves as well as the potential that market holds for retaining your services. Apply reasonable and attainable productivity goals as well as realistic expenses. Include a return on investment that can easily repay any loan principal and interest. With such a plan, your ability to respond to financial limits by leveraging will be a very swift and validating process. When outsiders will not lend or extend a line of credit, it is likely the result of one of two things: either your plan lacks validity or realism, or your lender does not understand your business. Both can be overcome, but neither should occur if your plan is thorough and has a sound basis for leveraging.

RELATIVE WISDOM: Budget Yourself

A man was a true hard worker. He had a full-time job, and he did side jobs related to his skill to earn extra money. He seemed to have it all: a lovely home, cars, and took wonderful trips. Then one day, he put his home up for sale. He was desperate to find more side jobs, and did not hesitate to tell others he had to tape his credit cards to the ceiling so he could not use them. This man had been living beyond his means for several years, and suddenly it all caught up with him—the cost of his lifestyle had led him to max out his credit cards, and he was unable to pay his property taxes and mortgage. He was dazed, trying to figure out how it all happened.

How it happened was quite simple: he started with good credit. This made him a desirable customer for more credit. He had multiple cards with multiple limits, from general cards to one for every department store in town. He had separate financing for his furniture, home electronics, cars, and he had even charged the supplies he used for his side business. He was a good consumer, quickly taking advantage of every offer without thinking through how these short-term decisions would affect his long-term financial situation.

Relative wisdom: When you face a financial limit, don't just look at solutions in the short term; consider how these will impact your current finances, your short- and long-term obligations, and what that short-term solution will eventually cost you. Adding a piece of equipment that will enhance your service menu is an attractive opportunity, but before you lease or buy, consider how and what you will pay, and what your practice and your patients will receive in return. Smart financial moves are measured in short- or long-term value, depending on your realistic goals and plans, not in simply accepting every offer that comes along.

LEGAL LIMITS

What exactly are legal limits? How do they contribute to the success of your practice? Unlike physical or financial limits, there is no positive outcome in attempting to overcome legal limits. Rather, the positive, or influence on the success of your business, rests in accepting these limits and recognizing the value legal limits have in serving the public and upholding the respect and value of your specialty.

Legal limits on the practice of aesthetic medicine are numerous, and generally fall under the following:

- The fundamental governing principle of medicine—the Hippocratic oath every graduating medical student takes to preserve human life: "Above all, do no harm"

- The laws of national, state, and local governments, including regulation by health care agencies, such as the Food and Drug Administration (FDA), the Occupational Safety and Health Administration (OSHA), departments of professional regulation, and boards of health

- The "laws" of the medical boards by which you are certified and in whose specialty you practice

- The "laws" of your professional affiliations: medical societies, accreditation organizations, hospitals, or business resources such as your insurer

- The laws of ethics, as defined by all of the above and further elevated by your own personal standards

- The laws of privacy: actual statutes and regulations or standards set by your expectations and those you serve

All of these laws have context for the aesthetic medicine practitioner, and the everyday practice of medicine requires that you evaluate and understand these laws and regulations. Are there legitimate shades of gray? Is using a drug off-label violating FDA regulations? It is a violation only when that use is not for the basis of accredited research, is not recognized as an acceptable practice by your specialty, or is incongruent with the use for which the drug or treatment is approved. It is not legal if you fail to follow proper informed consent procedures. Beyond this, you are clearly flirting with legal limits. This includes physically leaving the country in which you practice and in which your patients reside to treat these patients with nonapproved drugs or devices. If you are licensed to practice in a country, you must respect the laws of that country. If you feel there is greater good in providing treatment by crossing borders and legal limits than there is participating in research or simply waiting, then share this with your liability insurer before your decide to give it a try.

The laws of medical boards exist for two reasons: (1) to maintain the integrity of your specialty and (2) to uphold excellence in patient care through your specialty. If you feel you must cross the legal limits as defined by your board certification, you are diminishing the value of the specialty; you should not use your credentials of board certification, nor should you practice in your specialty. Your medical board affiliation exists solely to verify your competence in practicing within a defined specialty. Your ability to continue practicing your specialty requires that you meet or exceed the requirements and review of the medical board by which you are certified.

The laws of your professional affiliations are much like those of your board certification, but to a greater degree. It is not your board that mounts public education campaigns. It is not your board that reviews and certifies the safety of your facilities. It is not your board that supports you in practice. It is your professional affiliations that support you in your specialty, practice, and community. But if you are not upholding the "legal" limits of your board, do not expect to maintain your professional affiliations. There is value to the self-policing of these organizations. These actions uphold the overall image of your profession and consumer confidence in that image. For example, there has been a trend toward medical providers naming procedures or techniques after themselves and seeking recognition or profit from these actions. This is far different from the recognition one may receive when others credit or name a procedure or device for the founder, such as Fredrick Mohs, who developed the micrographic procedure known as *Mohs surgery*. He did not name the procedure for himself; others in the medical profession named the technique after him. Clearly, it is against the policies of the American Medical Association to trademark a procedure, yet we know there are trademarked face lifts and other procedures with coined names aimed at marketing, with serious legal machines behind them, or named for a physician as though the procedure was his or her development alone. Clearly, these violate what is appropriate and "legal" in the sense of limitations in aesthetic medicine.

A SURGEON'S INTEGRITY AND NAVIGATING
PLASTIC SURGEON–CORPORATE RELATIONSHIPS

Bradley P. Bengtson, MD, FACS

One of the most important things I have, both personally and in my clinical plastic surgery practice, is my integrity. A good friend once told me that you can pay a marketing firm a lot of money to make you sound better than you actually are, but you cannot buy your reputation.

A challenging dichotomy exists in medicine today in which a surgeon with the most experience with a product or device is clearly the most desirable for a company as their spokesperson and champion, but he or she must also withstand increasing accusations of bias based on physician-industry collaboration. The physicians and surgeons with the most experience should be the ones on the podium teaching about their experiences with a product, device, or technique. Where it gets tricky is when they are asked to divert from the science to opinion or marketing messages or are asked to deliver scripted messages. I truly believe that surgeons, to remain credible, must stick to the data and the science and let the science drive the marketing. We may give an opinion based on experience or ensure that information is scientifically accurate, but I believe we should remain out of the major marketing message efforts.

We can't have it both ways. I have witnessed many physicians who "go into administration" in a hospital system, only to quickly become integrated into the corporate structure, and though they try to remain physician advocates, they cannot; they have lost credibility from the physicians' side.

One of my favorite movies is *The Fugitive.* In fact, I watched it again last weekend. I believe there is a common misconception among the public, and certainly among government officials and the FDA, that most physicians are easily biased by a company that provides them with perks, products, or services. Such was the case in the film, when Dr. Charles Nichols falsified his research with a drug, Provasic, that he was working on clinically. In his efforts to cover up his altered data about the side effects of the drug, he went so far as to kill the wife of Harrison Ford's character, Dr. Richard Kimball—and we all know you should never threaten or kill one of Harrison Ford's family members in any movie.

The perception that doctors will say or do anything for money is a disservice to our profession. Unfortunately, the public and lawmakers are all too quick to believe this. On the contrary, I believe that the vast majority of physicians have a very high degree of personal integrity and credibility.

Continued

A SURGEON'S INTEGRITY AND NAVIGATING PLASTIC SURGEON–CORPORATE RELATIONSHIPS—cont'd

There is one area that does need to be exposed and remedied, however. One of my professors used to say, "Be careful what you hear from the podium. If someone is speaking about his 'experience,' he may be speaking about just one case. His 'series' may actually be just two cases, and three or more cases may be what he finds 'time after time after time.' "

Although it is usually quite obvious when we are hearing bias from the podium, we have allowed an unspoken lack of transparency into our profession by permitting the presentation of limited procedures or "experiences" as the rule, when in fact they may be the exception. Or we allow data to be presented with very few actual numbers of patients who have had a certain procedure performed or device placed. I find myself asking, "What is the 'N' "? During my presentations I have begun following my corporate disclosure slides, which I do believe are important, with a "study disclosure slide." It lists the actual number of patients in the study who have undergone a specific procedure or technique, the complication rate, including operative and nonoperative complications, and revision rates.

I believe that this is the greatest potential for bias in our profession: not being completely transparent about our actual experience. We should simply present our data, let it speak for itself, and let the marketing message be derived from the data.

Because of the high profile and keen public interest in plastic surgery, we are often introduced to a new product through a marketing piece or on *Oprah,* rather than first seeing it presented at a scientific meeting or in a peer-reviewed journal. It is important, just as in every other surgical profession, to base our clinical decisions and what procedures we perform on the science. If the products or devices are equivalent, then we may base our decision on other factors. For instance, a large percentage of my practice is breast related. Although the studies on breast implants were certainly not designed to compare one manufacturer's devices to another, the spherical or round smooth implants are essentially equivalent among manufacturers. There are minor variations in the shells and patches, but the gel filler is essentially the same, and the reported premarket approval data are well within the standard deviation ranges. If we are choosing between two manufacturers of devices that are essentially the same, why do we choose one versus the other? It is then based on the relationship with the manufacturer, pricing, service, how congenial the sales reps are, and so on.

To circle back, we should make surgical decisions based on the science and data. If we do not have the science and the data, we need to be honest about that, describe what the trends are, and report the data as preliminary. If there is a brand new product or device about which little is known, we should be honest about that as well, and be clear about what is marketing driven. Further, we should not give opinions about products or procedures with which we have little or no experience.

Each profession should set the bar higher in its standards of what will be allowed to be promoted and presented. We must strive for a high level of honesty and transparency in our scientific meetings and personal presentations. If we actually track our own patient data and present the information for the benefit of our colleagues and patients, we must strive for an exceptionally high level of integrity and develop a "we can all learn from the mistakes of others" mentality. If we present data and patient information to try to make ourselves look good and to make it all about us, we will underreport complications and tend to overstate the actual numbers of patients and procedures. I would challenge each of us to begin rigorously tracking our patients, procedures, and true complication rates, and to strive to be part of the former group.

Corporate relationships are and will be getting more complex in the future, with a great deal of increased governmental and regulatory oversight. I encourage physicians and corporations to continue in the direction they appear to be moving—to engage doctors with the most integrity and experience with their products or devices to help them develop educational curricula, instructional videos for the benefit of all our patients and colleagues, and to help make the surgery safer, decrease the learning curve, and reduce complications. If one patient is saved a complication or suboptimal result, it will be worth it.

If we all stay focused on this approach and off the marketing or previous "consultant" ideology, it will give us a great deal more credibility and provide our best chance to stay above the fray when questions of bias and controversy arise.

The laws of ethics and your own personal standards are, most would say, clearly subjective. Do not overlook defining your own legal limits or standards, and make certain every individual who supports you in your practice or comes in contact with your practice fully understands and accepts these limits. The term *zero tolerance policy* is something everyone understands. Your staff, your professional resources, and your patients should understand where you draw the line, and where you absolutely will not make exceptions.

Privacy laws are so fundamental to the industry and practice of aesthetic medicine and to your success as a provider of aesthetic medicine that an entire chapter of this book has been devoted to this subject (see Chapter 15). Accept, embrace, uphold, and respect privacy. In addition, always share your standards and expectations with all those who work for you or with you, or seek out your work.

🌿 IN PRACTICE: A Legal Evolution

As the demand for aesthetic medical treatment and its various specialties continues to grow, and as the way in which all medicine is practiced evolves, including aesthetic medical treatment, the need for regulations to evolve is clear. But who takes the lead? The order of legal limits in the broadest sense begins with the laws of medicine and leads narrowly to your own ethics and personal standards. In the evolution of regulation, this order is the reverse: It begins with you. For example, as a provider, even though you may not be required to accredit your ambulatory surgical facility or office, you take the stand to do so voluntarily.

I have to commend the American Society of Plastic Surgeons and the American Society for Aesthetic Plastic Surgery, who as of July 1, 2002, required all members to use only surgical facilities that hold specific, recognized accreditation. The American Academy of Facial Plastic and Reconstructive Surgery has now embraced this doctrine. This was not some arbitrary move by a few outside the specialty to impose regulations on those inside. This was a move by two organizations of committed, board-certified specialists to further elevate their very strict laws of membership to uphold the integrity of the specialty and the laws of medicine by imposing the highest standards of patient safety.

Now that there are "laws" among the specialty for requiring accreditation of surgical fees, the specialties continue to promote self-regulation and self-policing efforts to improve the quality of care and the image of the specialties. Medical spas, physician extenders, supervision of nonphysician providers, the use of unapproved, illegal, or imported drugs and devices are all under scrutiny, by the professional societies, and in some cases by individual states and by regulatory agencies such as the FDA.

Physicians who are caught purchasing or administering counterfeit or unapproved drugs or devices are being investigated and prosecuted. From the time the first edition of this book was published in 2004 through July 2008, there were 68 arrests and 29 convictions reported by the FDA of physicians who injected patients with illegal or counterfeit Botox injections.

As the consumer demand for cosmetic medicine grows, and as the number of unqualified providers and poor safety incidents grows, the legal limits governing aesthetic medicine will continue to evolve to protect patient safety. Self-imposed regulation, through evolution, makes any specialty, this industry, and certainly any segment of medicine more visibly committed to upholding the highest standards of patient care. If you are one who imposes your own high standard of ethics and safety on your practice, you have nothing to do but applaud such evolution. If you are one who waits for this evolution, forget about success. You are missing the fundamental message of success in aesthetic medicine: practicing excellence.

SOCIAL LIMITS

Physical limits present opportunities in some cases. Financial limits are important to discovering the true value of strategies or goals. Legal limits are important to respect and to define for your practice. Social limits are those things that you simply have to have the intuition, common sense, or the good taste to understand.

Influence   You have influence over others, including your staff, your patients, perhaps your peers. Recognize the responsibility that comes with this: lead by example. Never pressure—educate and encourage. Likewise, there may be outside sources who have influence over you, your practice, your patients, or your peers. Genuine intentions are self-motivated, not driven by the actions of others. For example, if you have a staff member influencing you to offer cocktails at a "ladies' night out" because this is what your guests will expect, but you are uneasy with this, realize that your guests will hold you accountable for any repercussions. Stand your ground.

Acceptance   People want to feel as though they are accepted in their social groups. You want your market to accept you and your practice and the services you provide. But to use acceptance as a means to motivate others to your services is simply wrong. I once heard a physician tell his patient. "Well, you don't want to be the only mom at the pool who won't wear a swimsuit" in response to her request for a specific procedure. He was using peer acceptance to compel her to feel her desire was justified. If his intentions were genuinely to support her goals for surgery, he might have said, "You should feel confident wearing a swimsuit or anything else you feel is appropriate for you."

Rhetoric   Some of us may use language more skillfully or persuasively than others, but regardless of how well you communicate, you must distinguish between education and persuasion. There is nothing wrong with responding to objections—with education.

Flippancy or Humor   Making flip remarks or using questionable humor can backfire when discussing a person's sincere desires for enhancing their appearance. Everyone has a different threshold for attempts at banter, and using facetious remarks risks causing distaste or disgust among your audience. There are limits to poking fun or exploiting appearances. You don't want to be the provider whose tactics or taste is questionable.

I knew a physician whose favorite line to any patient who accepted treatment was, "Now you're one of my girls! I have them all over town, and I love every one of you." He of course thought he was cute; many of his patients thought he was boorish.

With social limits, there is no absolute, no one to define the rules but you. My advice is, if you have to think about it for a moment, if anyone calls your words or actions into question, you are pushing social limits. Accept the repercussions—that you may offend or lose patients, or bring your image into question—or decide that you must alter your behavior.

Limits exist for a reason, and that reason is a signal of change, evolution, or even caution. In practicing aesthetic medicine for success, once you have defined and embraced the final element of how to succeed—recognizing, respecting, setting, and elevating your limits— you will come full circle. You recognize the value of your resources and relationships, your professional standards, your staff, and your own personal influence in truly making success in aesthetic medicine possible.

CHAPTER 21

How Do You Optimize Resources and Relationships?

> *Oh, I get by with a little help from my friends*
> *Mm, gonna try with a little help from my friends*
> — JOHN LENNON AND PAUL MCCARTNEY,
> "WITH A LITTLE HELP FROM MY FRIENDS"

Individually people can accomplish great things, but without the acknowledgment, support, influence, and accolades of others, what value does accomplishment have? As a medical provider, you cannot do it alone. You need individuals to provide service to, to directly support and assist in the service you provide, and other individuals and resources to support your specialty. Those who do support you must be carefully chosen to meet and exceed your expectations and standards. These standards in turn must be founded on the standards of your board certification, specialty, and the professional groups and credentials by which you define yourself. They are enhanced and elevated by your professional and personal influence. The staff members you empower and entrust must accept and support these standards. Without consistent, congruent, and skilled efforts by those who support you in the operation of your business, even the best-laid plans of a clearly defined practice cannot succeed.

There is a delicate balance in managing your business and productively treating individuals to fulfill their personal desires for appearance enhancement. Finding that balance requires knowing all of the variables, responsibilities, and actions necessary to manage your business and serve your patients. You must empower others to support you. This requires that you:

- Function as the CEO—the director and decision-maker—while simultaneously realizing you are your business's chief product

- Provide aesthetic services, which is at the heart of satisfying your customer and creating value; these services are the means for generating revenue

- Select and train, encourage and evaluate, empower and entrust staff and professional resources

- Lead by example and demonstrate the professional standards of medicine and your specialty

- Define and display, with integrity and commitment, your personal influence

Although others will support you in your endeavors, the course of your success is charted by you alone. Your staff, the colleagues to whom you refer patients, and your patients must be chosen by you, guided by your profession's standards and by your image, brand, mission, and personal standards.

BRAND

Julius W. Few, MD, FACS

After 8 years of practice in a major metropolitan academic plastic surgery practice, I opened The Few Institute for Aesthetic Plastic Surgery. The day after our opening, I immediately realized the demand for our brand. Despite being in an academic practice, I strive for basic components that define my brand. I have always put the patient first, emphasizing the value of his or her time and effort to seek out plastic surgery.

The brand is simple: excellence in service, care, and custom attention. I put a great deal of time into the development of a system that would maximize efficiency for the patient and the staff. We relied more on word-of-mouth referrals than on direct marketing. In addition, the Few brand emphasizes patient selection over financial reward.

I have always believed that a patient must be a good fit for the given service to maximize positive outcomes and to reinforce the selective nature of the brand. Ultimately, if a patient is offered a service, he or she is part of a select 65% who are candidates for service at The Few Institute (TFI). This selective approach has been a vital part of our brand and emphasizes the integrity of the practice. The selectivity and emphasis on the patient experience have been refined in the opening of TFI. The Few Institute has no waiting room, allowing maximized privacy and special care. The brand emphasizes luxury without overindulgence. Patients are never made to feel they are paying for the experience; it is truly value-added, making the practice more resistant to economic fluctuations. The concepts we have enlisted are approaches other industries have been using for years. Furthermore, they embody the age-old precept, "Do unto others as you would have them do unto you."

STAFF

You rely on your staff members as your front line, your extra sets of hands; they provide the follow-through for all your practice goals. They provide the gentle, caring touches your patients value; they support your practice and business efforts. They support your patients' desires and help them achieve those desires. Without them, how could you practice? With them, how do you practice? Not only must you select, train, and communicate with staff and empower them to excel and grow, you must also continually monitor how they influence the success of your practice. Staff members must be more than mere functionaries; they must be integral to your plan. If they do not uphold your standards and values and do not project and practice your image, brand, and mission, they are a detriment to you. If they do not uphold the most stringent protocols of quality care, they are a detriment to your patients.

The staff you choose must be an extension of you. Mutual respect, trust, and understanding must be ever-present in your relationship with staff and in the relationship among staff. Staff members must work toward the goals you define for them. Make a daily effort to "catch people doing something right," remark on it with sincere praise, and you will reap enormous dividends in the loyalty and productivity this simple recognition engenders.

When planning your practice, you develop your staffing needs. As you grow and evolve, these needs change. Have you ever paused to consider the value that each staff member contributes to the success of your practice? They contribute to productivity and to your revenue base, or serve as an extension of you. If your staffing mix is not yet ideal, where can you improve? Where can you grow? Where are you consistent, or inconsistent? Where does conflict exist?

You must plan your staffing tactically (by tasks), financially (what each one contributes or generates to the revenue of the practice as well as the cost to the practice in salary, benefits, and potential liability), and as needed to meet the goals and expectations you have for them. Consider your office manager, reception staff (a position that may very well be held by the office manager), nursing staff, personal services providers, and retail support, as well as your partners or other providers whom you have hired to work in your practice. How exactly do team members contribute to your success, and is there anywhere they fail you?

- Job descriptions are fundamental to implementing training, goals, and cross-training.

- Documentation of salary schedules, scheduled performance, and financial reviews is important structurally to your business.

- Employment policies and guidelines are spelled out in a comprehensive manual that each staff member accepts, acknowledges by signature, and retains; this manual defines your practice rules, expectations, and benefits.

- Regular interface in one-to-one praise, teaching, or feedback helps keep staff on track.

- Regular team meetings and consistent team-building efforts are important to share information in a concerted setting with no distractions.

The key questions to ask yourself in evaluating staff members are simple and direct.

- Are staff properly trained and eager to learn in their practice roles? Are their roles defined in a job description, accepted by staff, and regularly reviewed and adjusted?

- Do staff understand and uphold my standards of quality care and patient comfort? Do they realize that the result of every action is to effectively serve a patient need or desire?

- Do staff uphold my practice image, brand, and mission? Do they practice together as a team that reflects me, and individually take responsibility for their own actions that inevitably reflect on me?

- Do staff practice my standards of communication with me, other staff members, resource people, and patients? Do they understand that protecting privacy is not an imposition, but a part of how we communicate and practice?

- Do staff respect and follow procedure? As individuals, are they limited in the functions they perform, or are they appropriately cross-trained to function daily as a team, and independently when necessary to fulfill the role of another team member?

- Do staff reach beyond my expectations of them? Do they exhibit pride in their efforts and in my work, and pride in being part of the team?

- Do staff take initiative with permission or act independently? Can I trust staff to act independently when necessary?

- When I am unavailable and something requires an immediate response, will staff members act intelligently and calmly to handle the situation? Can they be depended on to use their safety and emergency training, to act autonomously, and to report appropriately?

Unless you can confidently answer "Yes" to these questions about each member of your team, not only should you reconsider your staffing as it relates to your success, but also as it might be to your detriment.

You cannot succeed without staff. Staff development is an ongoing process, as is developing your practice. If you stop developing and growing, you are coasting—making minimal progress with little or no effort. In the rapidly changing and demanding world of aesthetic medicine, you and your staff cannot succeed by coasting.

IN PRACTICE: Higher Up

A well-established aesthetic provider chose to add a physician extender to his practice. He hired a physician assistant (PA) from across town who demonstrated high productivity and the ability to pull in a lot of revenue. She was fabled for persuading a patient who came in for something as simple as a wart removal to undergo a Botox injection on the spot. She was fast with the needle in every sense, and even faster with putting clinical skin care products in every patient's hands. She could talk anyone into a peel and accepted "No" from no one. In no time she was surpassing the established providers in volume of aesthetic services. The provider/proprietor was impressed at her quick start and never questioned how or why this was accomplished. He simply accepted this with glee.

Soon after that, however, the entire practice was falling hard. The practice, the provider/proprietor, and the new provider were slapped with a very public lawsuit involving negligence and incompetence by the new provider that left a woman hospitalized 1 week after a cosmetic injection for which there was no protocol for off-label use or otherwise. No informed consent process had been followed; the woman had originally visited the practice to have a suspicious lesion removed from her forearm. What began as this extender's flying high in this established and reputable practice wound up bringing risk and a damaged reputation to the practice. It became clear that she had been reckless. She was not identifying the best possible treatments for her patients, but persuading them to agree to various aesthetic services. Furthermore, she was not properly trained, and she prescribed treatment without the physician's direction or supervision. It also became clear that she had been careless, overlooking the fundamentals of practice, such as informed consent and patient education. Finally, her salesmanship was simply that—enticing patients to undergo a treatment they hadn't known they wanted by offering extremely attractive pricing. She was discounting everything, and making it up as she went along.

When the provider called me to work on his practice plan to try to undo the damage, he thought that he could just sweep her out and move forward. However, she was not so much the core of the problem as she was simply a manifestation of poor staff planning. The provider/proprietor had made several significant errors. He hadn't evaluated the hands-on ability and communication style of this new provider, nor had he communicated his standards to her. He had never defined procedures, nor had he encouraged staff members to speak up when things were amiss. Above all, he had failed to impress upon the new provider and staff members what he expected, other than to contribute to the growth of his practice.

The lesson here: Everyone and everything in your practice has the potential to contribute to your success or your downfall—most critically your staff. No plan, standards, image, brand, or mission will lead you to success if you do not communicate all of these to your staff and evaluate whether they are fulfilling the expectations you define.

PROFESSIONAL RESOURCES

Professional resources may be the outside services you hire to provide essential services that for reasons of economy, time constraints, or preference you choose not to have in-house. They are also your industry and professional support. So often physicians focus on the essential services and overlook the value of other professional resources.

Professional Specialty Groups   You pay dues and belong to specific groups that represent your specialty and interests. Belonging or being elected to an association or society represents more than simply a credential or affiliation: these groups represent you, so get involved. Read their newsletters and releases to stay abreast of what is happening, and what others are doing, thinking, and reacting to. Attend their meetings, join committees, and evaluate and consider the tools, products, and resources these groups have and use those that are right for you.

Pharmaceutical, Device, and Product Representatives or Consultants
There was a time when these individuals were all called "sales reps," and today, although they have several different titles, their primary function is to sell their product *and* provide service to you, their customer. If you have questions, service problems, or specific needs, these representatives should be ready to respond. If you have special plans, events, or needs for more education or support in public education, these individuals should connect you to or provide you with the resources you need. If you treat reps as simply suppliers, that is who they will be to your practice. If you develop a working relationship with them and communicate your expectations of them, those who truly are interested in your business will service first, then sell.

Advertising/Marketing Representatives   Whether from the local newspaper, your web design and hosting service, or other contacts, impose the same expectations of your advertising and external marketing resources that you do industry resources. Expect service first, then the sale, if valid for your needs and goals. Those who push the sale without providing information and answers are clearly not concerned about servicing your practice; they are solely there to make the sale.

Financial and Legal Services   Your banker, accountant, lawyer, insurance broker, and all others who provide financial services to your practice are invaluable resources who should not only respond when you need them, but also be proactive in determining how they can best serve you. For example, an insurance agent who doesn't provide you options for your annual renewals is simply making easy money. A banker who waits until you ask for direct deposit services is simply responding to your needs, not being responsible to you.

Never overlook anyone whose service to your practice contributes to your success. Can you do it without them? Yes, but you will likely be doing it alone or replacing them at some point. Make certain that any outside resource is the most beneficial for you and understands your expectations, just as any patient would select services from you because he or she trusts your skill and accepts your standards.

A professional resource must first know what your expectations are and how any plan or objective you present is intended to affect you and your practice. Although you hire consultants to support your practice in areas that you cannot and, in some cases, should not have in-house, the expertise they provide must be:

- Individualized to your needs, goals, and plans

- Focused on serving your needs

- Congruent with your standards as they relate to your practice

- Directed toward providing you with advice and manageable solutions

- Dedicated to working with you and for you to meet your expectations and achieve full satisfaction

If you cannot confidently affirm all of the above, keep looking for a resource that will understand, approach, and serve your interests on an individual basis to fulfill all of these criteria.

Where do you find such resources? How do most of your patients find you? The answer to both is through appropriate referral and through professional and certified directories.

CAVEAT: When you find resources that seem ideal for serving you and your practice, always confirm that the approach and the services you receive will be individualized to your needs. A successful practice is not modeled after anyone else's; rather, it is unique to its provider, market, and certainly bears a unique image, brand, and mission and distinctive objectives and goals. Therefore the practice must be serviced as the unique entity it is. Just as similar and successful outcomes for two different patients may be achieved through two very different approaches, there will not be a "one size fits all" approach that will suit your practice. Your professional resources must meet your unique needs and be individualized to your practice.

LEGAL WISDOM

Steven M. Harris, Esq.

Too often lawyers and physicians are pitted against each other because of the inherent conflict that exists in professional liability litigation. This is a shame, because each profession has so much to offer the other, especially when it comes to partnering in the business of medicine.

Unlike medical training, legal education provides a general curriculum of core courses designed to introduce law students to many areas of law, but because there are no residencies or fellowships in law, attorneys need to obtain specific training on the job. It is only there that areas of concentration or, in some cases, specialization are developed.

It is important to recognize this dynamic and to seek an attorney who understands the complicated legal and regulatory environment facing aesthetic surgeons. When selecting counsel, ask appropriate questions. None is more important than the attorney's experience in the particular transaction or matter in which you are about to engage. Please read the previous sentence again, especially the part that states, "the particular transaction or matter in which *you are about to engage.*"

If you plan to make a material commitment of time and capital, first protect your investment by retaining an attorney at the inception of the process. Attorney creativity and physician options are limited if contracts have been signed and understandings reached before experienced counsel can weigh in. There are always options in the design and approach to a deal. Keep them open as you assess the risk and profitability of your business plan.

An equally important caveat applies after you retain counsel. Remember, your attorney works for you. Although deferring to advice may be prudent, your attorney is rarely your business partner. (Note to attorneys reading this book: If you are business partners with a physician, decline to represent the transaction and see that independent counsel is hired.) That means the physician should make decisions after receiving the advice and counsel of trusted advisors such as consultants, accountants, insurance professionals, and bankers, in addition to lawyers. Do not let any one person or persons on your team dominate the decision-making process. Rather, gather appropriate advice and develop reasonable, calculated strategies.

Following these seminal yet simple rules will offer you the very best opportunity to develop effective partnerships with your attorney and professional team. The effort will pay off abundantly.

PROFESSIONAL STANDARDS

In addition to industry or business resources, you have great opportunities to support and be supported by other medical professionals. Connecting with your immediate peers in your community or your specialty can provide mutual support, understanding, and opportunity.

Peers Within Your Specialty   Whether you are a plastic surgeon, a dermatologist, or a facial plastic surgeon, there are individuals who share your specialty in your community or state, or through national organizations, and it is likely you will come to know these peers. You may be acquainted from the time of training to later phases in your practice. Stay connected to those you relate to and in time of need or doubt, for advice or just to exchange ideas, you have an ideal connected group of specialists who understand your practice and the nature of the challenges you face.

Other Physicians and Health Care Professionals   Whether part of your specialty community, your geographic region, your training, or simply through acquaintance, other physicians and health care professionals can be great resources to share information, experience, leads, or simply to problem-solve together.

COMPETITORS WORKING TOGETHER

Mark L. Jewell, MD

During my tenure as President of the American Society for Aesthetic Plastic Surgery in 2006, I was successful in developing a coalition of core-trained specialty societies to address the important topic of injectable safety. Since 1991, ASAPS has been very involved in patient safety in surgery. With the rapid increase in the use of cosmetic injectables (neurotoxins and tissue fillers), I thought that this was an area that similarly required patient safety.

There are many different specialties that use cosmetic injectables, including dermatology, plastic surgery, facial plastic surgery, and oculoplastic surgery. This group consists of practitioners who have received core training in the use of cosmetic injectables. Additionally, each group offers specific aesthetic surgical procedures, depending on training and scope of practice. Each of the core-trained groups' respective professional organizations offers

Continued

COMPETITORS WORKING TOGETHER—cont'd

CME-based education and instructional courses for cosmetic injectables. But training and CME was focused on the technical matters; there was minimal emphasis on patient safety and processes.

Formerly, there was limited interaction between professional societies in the area of aesthetic surgery and cosmetic medicine. I was fortunate to have developed personal friendships with leaders in other core-trained specialties. We had similar interests in the areas of patient safety and differentiation of those with core training in injectables from those with less training. The concept of a coalition of like-minded professional societies to promote patient safety with injectables suddenly had enormous support, even between groups that formerly had been adversaries. Our goal was not to conduct a defensive program that was designed to scare consumers regarding unsafe injectable practices, but to educate them about the benefits that cosmetic injectables have for patients when provided by a qualified, core-trained injector. Consumers have been historically poorly informed regarding the qualifications of injectors and understanding that injectables are medical treatments that may produce unexpected results, especially when provided by untrained injectors.

Cosmetic injectables have proved attractive to noncore physicians as a way to enhance practice revenue. Although any licensed physician can buy injectables, lasers, or implantable devices, most physicians lack substantive training in their safe use. Their use of cosmetic injectables may be unidimensional, since they lack surgical training to comprehensively address patient needs. There are other areas of concern related to unapproved injectors offering "Botox in the mall" or those who offer unapproved injectables from off-shore vendors.

A coalition of core-trained specialty professional organizations was developed by ASAPS that initially included the American Academy of Facial Plastic Surgery (AAFPS), the American Academy of Oculoplastic and Reconstructive Surgery (AORS), the American Society for Aesthetic Plastic Surgery, and the American Society of Dermatologic Surgeons (ASDS). This was the first time that competing professional societies were successful in putting differences aside and working together to address patient safety with cosmetic injectables. The message that was developed centered on "Doctor, Brand, Safety."

This was a significant event in which agreement was achieved on a vital topic: injector qualifications, legitimate products, and the safe use of injectables. The Coalition's website, *www.injectablesafety.org*, has been a great resource for patients about which injectables are approved and what questions they should be thinking about when considering cosmetic injectable treatments.

The Physician's Coalition for Injectable Safety has grown to become an international organization with the addition of the Canadian Society for Aesthetic Plastic Surgery (CSAPS) and the International Society for Aesthetic Plastic Surgery (ISAPS). As of July 2009, ASDS and the American Society of Plastic Surgeons (ASPS) have joined the Coalition. This comprises approximately 18,000 core-trained injectors, the largest organization of its kind in the world.

The Coalition has been successful in developing a training curriculum for subordinate injectors, working under the direct supervision of member physicians. Additionally, the latest offering of the Coalition is a comprehensive workbook, *Safety With Injectables,* that provides a framework for members to develop programs of injectable safety within their offices and clinics. The workbook addresses important topics of informed consent, staff training, infection control, and safety engineering to prevent mistakes and medication errors.

As the number of providers attempting to enter into the business of cosmetic medicine grows outside the core specialties, it is those groups once thought to be competitors—plastic surgeons, facial plastic surgeons, dermatologists, and oculoplastic surgeons—that will be the force that together can protect the image of cosmetic medicine as well as the safety of patients. Whether within your own community, your state, or on the national level, it is the spirit of competition that will drive physicians with similar goals to uphold and preserve fairness in a very dynamic market.

Personal Service Professionals   Physicians dislike being compared with hair stylists, personal trainers, or even personal therapists and counselors, and while you are clearly different in the services you provide and your level of personal preparation, you all do provide personal services that make individuals feel better about themselves. These relationships can be valuable in treating the whole person, in referrals, or simply in complementing each other or sharing market ideas.

Hospital Staff   Aesthetic physicians don't spend much time in the hospital. Even if you operate at the hospital, it is likely you only connect with the immediate individuals who serve your patients. Next time you are in the hospital, reach out—stroll through the emergency department and connect. Visit the doctors' lounge and take a few moments to share ideas or simply to make your presence known. Get involved, and others will be involved with you and your practice by referring patients, or simply by offering mutual support and validation.

Competitors   There is merit in the aphorism, "Keep your friends close and your enemies closer." The reality is that you should know your fair competitors. By name, by recognition, and certainly with mutual respect, even though you are all pursuing the same goal and potentially the same patients, you also share some commonalities—your specialty and the desire to excel. Be aware of who the staff are at your competitor's office; they may be "spies" calling or visiting your practice for information.

PERSONAL INFLUENCE

You cannot succeed alone. You need the identity and support of your profession to define your credibility and your role as a provider of aesthetic medicine. You need your professional resources to support your practice. You need your staff to operate your practice. Needing others is fundamental to your ability to succeed, but who those others are and how they will help you succeed can only be defined by you, based on your personal standards and influence. Your spouse or partner, parents or siblings, children, and close friends all have an influence on you and can be assets to your ability to practice or in simply supporting your goals and challenges.

Your personal influence is largely what will distinguish you, your practice, image, brand, mission, goals, communications, plans, and success in your specialty and in the world. Look around you: Where do you see your personal influence, your power to make things happen in your practice? Where do you not see it? Everywhere from patient care, to business operations, to communications, you must demonstrate, with integrity and commitment, your own personal influence. The center of your practice is you, the provider, and around you all other things must revolve. Again, you must define and display (preach and practice) with integrity and commitment (sincerely and consistently) the power and expectations you have as the provider and proprietor (the primary source of service and the business owner) of your practice.

- Who you are as a provider is meaningless unless you can define it from credentials through to personal influence and uphold it.

- What you practice in serving your clients and patients cannot exist without your personal influence, consistently applied.

- Communication with others would at best be generic and uninspired without your personal vision and influence as a provider in this highly personal field of aesthetic medicine.

- When you act, and the manner in which you act, requires individuality and character—your personal influence.

- Why you practice and treat others requires your personal influence primarily as basis, but what is most important, to achieve excellence.

- How this all coalesces is based on your personal influence—your ability to make things happen.

As a provider and proprietor, your personal influence is the catalyst that sets things in motion. Is that influence founded simply on your personal beliefs, or is it founded on how you blend and shape all the variables that contribute to the success of your practice based on your beliefs and expectations?

RELATIVE WISDOM: What to Expect

My grandmother taught me at an early age to never expect more from others than you are willing to commit to and carry out yourself. Never impose upon others standards that are higher than you would impose upon yourself and will consistently demonstrate. Never demand more from others than you know you can provide if demanded of you.

It is a logical lesson, yet so often our personal and professional standards and view of others can overlook how we in turn measure up ourselves.

How high have you set the bar? How do those who surround you in your practice see you? Do your staff, professional resources, colleagues, competitors, and patients define you in the same terms that you would define yourself? Does that definition exceed your expectations of yourself? Or are the terms by which others define you and your standards less than you might expect? Set the bar. Measure how others view you and see just where you fall, or if you stand tall.

PARTNERS IN LIFE

Victoria Hulett-Gross

I have experienced many different levels of involvement with my husband's practice. I was supportive of him through his residency, a full-time academic position, and then I worked full-time in his private practice, then not. The constant has always been that it is easy to support someone who truly loves what he is doing, but the practice is still a business.

A plastic surgery practice is always evolving, and I have come to realize that it is very much like parenting, with the practice being the "baby." As in parenting, each parent brings something different to the table, a different perspective. Each parent has weaknesses and strengths, but combined they form a powerful unit, with the best interests and intentions for the well-being of the baby.

It is very helpful to your practice as well as your relationship for a partner to have a solid peripheral view, plus a clear understanding of the inner workings of the office, finances, employees, and flow. Many times a partner can see what the other can't and can proactively protect the practitioner from the things that might not be evident. Working in a spouse's office can be a dubious role, and as a wife, sometimes it can be a no-win situation. If not handled carefully and intelligently, this can often change your relationship or result in the "good cop, bad cop" syndrome with employees. If the goal is truly looking after the best interests of the practice and maintaining a healthy relationship, then the best advice I can give is for both partners to approach this parenting by setting aside considerations of ego, accepting the contribution and assurance of another eye on the baby.

Ultimately, as a partner in life, I have found that there is a better function with limited day-to-day time in the office, and that I can better support the practice with my knowledge from a more global overview, though not as a complete outsider. In reality, no one is going to look after your practice as you would, and this provides a comfort level for both. It enables an exchange without becoming immersed in the daily frustrations of wondering if someone will ever change the toilet paper roll without you!

HOW? FULL CIRCLE

It is appropriate that this guide to growing in the practice of aesthetic medicine has now come full circle. It began to build your plan for success by defining who you are as a provider. It now comes back to who you are, not defined by credentials, but by your influence and standards as the finishing and most essential part of your plan for success. You are—not at both ends but throughout planning and practicing for success—the greatest variable in attaining success.

Success results when you take legitimate and appropriate variables and shape these to accomplish valid objectives and attain realistic goals:

1. Practice what you are qualified to do, and treat those who are appropriate candidates.

2. Recognize the principles of the practice of medicine and the business of personal services; you must uphold both.

3. Strive to provide value, not only in outcomes but in your patient's entire experience.

4. Define, work toward, and continuously measure your goals and the goals of those you serve.

5. Connect and communicate continuously with your market, patients, staff, resources, and peers.

6. Always keep an eye on your future and the future of those you serve and your industry.

7. Uphold your own standards and efforts and the standards of those who surround you.

8. You don't have to do it alone; empower a trusted team and connect yourself to trusted resources.

9. Recognize that safety is essential in aesthetic medicine.

10. Define whether you want to be at the core of your industry and practice, or whether you are just a slice of the pie. Empower your own success.

In February 2007, at the invitation of Dr. Renato Saltz, I spoke to the Rocky Mountain Society of Plastic Surgeons and presented a talk in which I defined the role of aesthetic physicians in the competitive marketplace as either the core of the industry or a slice of it. My metaphor has drawn some attention, and I hope that it helps you to put into perspective the many elements of growing, sustaining and succeeding in your practice:

> *Core:* You are the essential part, the center of all that exists in your practice.

> *Slice:* You are a portion of a piece of your practice, removed from the whole.

Consider this metaphor as you practice today, and plan for tomorrow.

❧ IN PRACTICE: Where Am I?

Throughout my career, I have had the honor and most deeply appreciated personal privilege of working for and knowing pioneers in aesthetic medicine and aesthetic medical services. The medical specialties that appropriately include aesthetic services have existed for decades; however, the segments devoted to enhancing function or appearance, not restoring it, have really only begun to evolve in their own subspecialty identities since the latter decades of the twentieth century.

You cannot write a guide to succeeding in the practice of aesthetic medicine without a nod to those who are models of success. History and experience, as we know, can be a great lesson. I have had the opportunity to know many gifted physicians. But to have the privilege to learn from a practitioner who in himself is history is a remarkable experience. He is my mentor, although he is a surgeon, and I am not. His career as a surgeon was brilliant, and although he no longer practices aesthetic medicine, he remains active in his profession, in educating future physicians, and in educating the public. As I came to the conclusion of this book, I thought about this extraordinary man and what was the true force behind his success and passion, and here is what I learned.

The lesson here: Never become complacent. Never stop asking questions, and always offer sincere and direct answers. Remain focused and skilled, and communicate candidly and with compassion. Never lose sight of the fact that your actions and your influence can touch or change the lives of others, and never overlook your obligation to serve those who cannot reach out to you. Practice with integrity and passion and don't plan for success. Plan for excellence, and success will always be in sight.

AFTERWORD

By Nicholas Kuechel and Andy Kuechel
With an introduction by Marie Czenko Kuechel

There is no time for cut-and-dried monotony.
There is time for work. And time for love.
That leaves no other time!
— GABRIELLE BONHEUR "COCO" CHANEL

As I was working on this second edition of my book, the economy was teetering. The largest stimulus package in U.S. history was enacted by Congress to stabilize the economy, with criticisms and claims of success daily. Doctors worried about whether patients would continue to seek aesthetic medicine at a time when thousands of people were losing their jobs, hundreds of thousands of mortgages were in foreclosure, the stockmarket was in decline, and banks were closing. Economic experts predicted a slow, tortuous recovery.

At such a time in our history, you may question the relevance of this book, filled with concepts, definitions, guidelines, and anecdotes intended to help you establish or enhance an aesthetic practice that will meet your professional and personal goals. You may be expecting clearcut solutions, a template you can use to make your practice an immediate and guaranteed success.

But success doesn't happen that way; there is no one-size-fits-all pattern for success. It requires a process of self-examination, goal-setting, establishing an intelligent, individualized business model, hiring the right professionals, and maintaining a clear vision of why you wanted to practice aesthetic medicine.

Only two things in life remain constant for those of us who want to succeed: the love of work, and the need for love in our lives. I love my work because of my desire to see people happy and fulfilled and because of the truly amazing people I meet and interact with daily.

I've been advised to employ apprentices, to train others to my vision. But I don't want to manage people; I don't want to build an empire. I'd rather write a book that I hope will help you. I don't see or measure my success in growing a business by numbers. For me, success lies in challenging myself, using my skills and new ideas to achieve my ultimate goal: helping patients have safe and positive experiences in aesthetic medicine. Moreover, success for me is being able to work in such a way that my family, the loves in my life, can be near to my heart and my hands at every possible moment. To remain successful, I make time for my work. But like you, I often feel there simply isn't enough time to accomplish all that needs doing; sometimes the time for love is what is left after the work is done.

Whether you are contemplating starting, growing, changing, or improving your practice or are simply reflecting on how you can be a more successful practitioner of aesthetic medicine, I advise you to take a moment to contemplate not just your time at work, but your time for love. What follows was written by my sons, Nicholas, age 11, and Andrew, age 9, expressing their earnest desire to understand what makes adults work so hard.

❦

When you're a kid, you wonder why adults work so much. We know that working makes the money that gives us our house, food, and pays for the things we have, but working takes a lot of time, and sometimes adults don't seem to have time for anything else.

Our mom spent a lot of time writing her book to help doctors be better doctors, she says. She asked if we wanted to write something for her book. She said that sometimes kids have important things to say. We thought about it and decided that we would. Our message is about what kids see and feel when their parents work, and why people who work sometimes need to think like kids.

We see you when you're busy. We see you talking on the phone, and staring at the computer. We don't see you in your office very much, but we wonder what happens when you're there. You do a lot of work at home, and you work when you're with us. Sometimes it feels like you forget that we need you as much as your work does.

We hope your work is fun, because you spend so much time on it. But we need time with you too just to laugh and have fun. We want you to enjoy time with us as much as you like your work. You always tell us that we have work too because we go to school and learn. But we also spend time playing with our friends or in sports, and sometimes we do nothing much at all—just hang out.

Kids do what we want first; we always put off what we don't want to do, which is why sometimes we feel like you want to do your work and not do the fun things. Play is work. Play is learning. Play is exercise. No matter how bad you feel, playing a sport, a game, some music, even playing with each other can make you feel better. It can make you smile. Sometimes just hanging out with nothing to do is a good thing.

Andrew: I'm a kid; I need to explore, not just to grow bigger, not just older, but to grow experience. You need to try new things, new experiences. Like when I wanted to go bungee jumping—my dad said no; my mom said as long as it was safe, that she would go with me. If you are going to try new things, make sure you are safe.

Nicholas: One more thing: When your family needs you, stop working for a while and pay attention, because family should come first. It doesn't matter if you will get a lot of money or if you have a big, important meeting. You might miss out on the most important thing in your life.

Everyone has someone in life who loves them, and who they love. And even though you need to work, you need love more. You need people more than work and you need to find the time to be with the people you love. Work will always be there, it doesn't go away, it seems to find you. Love and fun and learning, spending time together are always there, they won't go away either. But you need to come to them, they won't find you.

We hope you find something in our mom's book that helps you in your work. We just want to tell you that you are more than someone who works. You are someone in a world of other people, of friends, of family, a world we hope is always one where kids can learn about work, have fun at work and learning, and feel loved. No matter if you are a president or king, doctor or rock star, you have work and play. And whether you are working or playing, no matter how much fun, how hard, or how stressful things can be, making other people happy and being happy with what you do makes you a success.

INDEX